Statistics for Biology and Health

Series Editors:
M. Gail
K. Krickeberg
J. Samet
A. Tsiatis
W. Wong

For further volumes:
http://www.springer.com/series/2848

Jianguo Sun · Xingqiu Zhao

Statistical Analysis of Panel Count Data

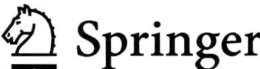

Jianguo Sun
Department of Statistics
University of Missouri
Columbia, MO, USA

Xingqiu Zhao
Department of Applied Mathematics
The Hong Kong Polytechnic University
Hong Kong, Hong Kong SAR

ISSN 1431-8776
ISBN 978-1-4614-8714-2   ISBN 978-1-4614-8715-9 (eBook)
DOI 10.1007/978-1-4614-8715-9
Springer New York Heidelberg Dordrecht London

Library of Congress Control Number: 2013947164

© Springer Science+Business Media New York 2013
This work is subject to copyright. All rights are reserved by the Publisher, whether the whole or part of the material is concerned, specifically the rights of translation, reprinting, reuse of illustrations, recitation, broadcasting, reproduction on microfilms or in any other physical way, and transmission or information storage and retrieval, electronic adaptation, computer software, or by similar or dissimilar methodology now known or hereafter developed. Exempted from this legal reservation are brief excerpts in connection with reviews or scholarly analysis or material supplied specifically for the purpose of being entered and executed on a computer system, for exclusive use by the purchaser of the work. Duplication of this publication or parts thereof is permitted only under the provisions of the Copyright Law of the Publisher's location, in its current version, and permission for use must always be obtained from Springer. Permissions for use may be obtained through RightsLink at the Copyright Clearance Center. Violations are liable to prosecution under the respective Copyright Law.
The use of general descriptive names, registered names, trademarks, service marks, etc. in this publication does not imply, even in the absence of a specific statement, that such names are exempt from the relevant protective laws and regulations and therefore free for general use.
While the advice and information in this book are believed to be true and accurate at the date of publication, neither the authors nor the editors nor the publisher can accept any legal responsibility for any errors or omissions that may be made. The publisher makes no warranty, express or implied, with respect to the material contained herein.

Printed on acid-free paper

Springer is part of Springer Science+Business Media (www.springer.com)

To Xianghuan, Ryan, and Nicholas
To Feng and Jenna

Preface

Panel count data occur in studies that concern recurrent events, or event history studies, when study subjects are observed only at discrete time points. By recurrent events, we mean the event that can occur or happen multiple times or repeatedly. In other words, study subjects could experience recurrences of the same event and the resulting data are usually referred to as event history data. Examples of recurrent events include disease infections, hospitalizations or tumor occurrences in medical studies and warranty claims of automobiles or system break-downs in reliability studies. There also exist many other fields that often yield event history data such as demographic studies, economic studies and social sciences.

The event history study can be generally classified into two types. One is the studies that monitor study subjects continuously and the resulting data are usually referred to as recurrent event data (Cook and Lawless, 2007). In this case, the times of all occurrences of the event of interest are recorded. That is, one has complete data or sample paths on the underlying point or recurrent event process that characterizes the occurrence of the recurrent event of interest. The other is the studies in which study subjects are observed only at discrete time points and thus they produce panel count data. In this situation, one knows only the numbers of occurrences of the event between observation times and thus has incomplete data or sample paths on the underlying recurrent event process. The occurrence of panel count data could be due to many different reasons. For example, it may be too expensive, impossible, or not realistic to conduct continuous follow-ups.

For the analysis of recurrent event data, there exists a great deal of literature, especially a couple of excellent books. For example, Andersen et al. (1993) provide a comprehensive coverage of counting process approaches for the analysis of recurrent event data. Cook and Lawless (2007) give a relatively complete and thorough review of the recent literature on recurrent event data. Comparatively, only sparse literature exists on the analysis of panel count data. It is of interest and helpful to mention that in addition to the amount of relevant information available being different between recurrent event data and panel count data, yet another key difference is the observation process. In the case of the former, the observation process means the length of the whole follow-up, while in the case of the latter, it also includes a sequence of consecutive observation times. Also to analyze recurrent event data, it is common and convenient to characterize the occurrences of recurrent events by point processes and to model the intensity process of the point process. On the other hand, for the analysis of panel count data, it is usually more convenient to work directly on the mean function of the point processes due to the incomplete nature of the observed information.

This book is intended to provide an up-to-date reference for those who are conducting research on the analysis of panel count data as well as those who need to analyze panel count data to answer practical questions. It can also be used as a text for a graduate course in statistics or biostatistics that has basic knowledge of probability and statistics as a prerequisite. The main focus of the book is on methodology, but some applications of the methods to real data are also provided.

Chapter 1 contains introductory material and surveys basic concepts and point process models commonly used for the analysis of panel count data. Examples of panel count data as well as recurrent event data are discussed, and some key features of panel count data are described. Chapter 2 discusses some Poisson assumption-based models and inference procedures with the focus on parametric approaches. To be complete, regression analysis of simple count data is first briefly considered.

Chapters 3–6 concern nonparametric and semiparametric approaches for panel count data. Specifically, Chap. 3 deals with one-sample analysis of panel count data with the focus on nonparametric estimation of the mean function of the underlying recurrent event process of interest. In Chap. 4, the two-sample comparison problem for panel count data and some nonparametric procedures are discussed. Regression analysis of panel count data is the topic of Chaps. 5 and 6. In Chap. 5, we discuss the situation where the observation process is independent of the underlying recurrent event process given covariate processes. In this case, the inference can be made conditional on the observation process. Chapter 6 considers the situation where the observation process may be related to the underlying recurrent event process, and some joint modeling inference procedures are described.

Through Chaps. 2–6, it is assumed that there exists only one recurrent event process of interest. Sometimes there may exist several related recurrent event processes of interest and in this case, we have multivariate panel count data. Chapter 7 considers the analysis of multivariate panel count data with the focus on nonparametric treatment comparison and semiparametric regression analysis. To keep the book at a reasonable length, many important topics about panel count data cannot be investigated in details. Chapter 8 provides some brief investigation on several such topics. They include variable selection with panel count data, the analysis of mixed recurrent event and panel count data, and the analysis of panel count data arising from multi-state models. In addition, some discussions are given on Bayesian approaches for the analysis of panel count data and the analysis of panel count data arising from mixture models or with measurement errors.

In all chapters except Chap. 8, we have used references sparsely except in the last section of each chapter, which provides bibliographical notes including related references. Also we have chosen not to provide in-depth coverage of the asymptotic results related to the approaches described in the book as well as counting process and martingale theory needed for the derivation of the asymptotic results.

We owe thanks to many persons who have contributed directly and indirectly to this book. First we are indebted to Xin He, Yang Li, Do-Hwan Park, Hui Zhao and Qingning Zhou, who either read parts of the draft and gave their important comments or provided great computational help. We want to thank many of our collaborators on the subject over the years including Narayanaswamy Balakrishnan, Richard Cook, Joan Hu, Jack Kalbfleisch, Ni Li, Liuquan Sun, Xingwei Tong, LJ Wei, and Liang Zhu, whose collaborations and contributions to the field made this book possible. Also, we would like to express our thanks to Howard Bailey and KyungMann Kim for kindly providing the skin cancer panel count data.

Finally, we thank our family and especially Xianghuan (Jianguo's wife) and Feng (Xingqiu's husband) for their patience and support during this project.

Columbia, MO, USA Jianguo Sun
Hong Kong, China Xingqiu Zhao

Contents

1 **Introduction** 1
   1.1 Event History Studies 1
       1.1.1 Failure Time Data on Remission Times of Acute Leukemia Patients 3
       1.1.2 Recurrent Event Data on Times to Mammary Tumors 4
   1.2 Panel Count Data 5
       1.2.1 Reliability Study of Nuclear Plants 5
       1.2.2 National Cooperative Gallstone Study 6
       1.2.3 Bladder Cancer Study 7
       1.2.4 Skin Cancer Chemoprevention Trial 9
   1.3 Some Notation and Basic Concepts About Counting Processes 10
       1.3.1 Counting Processes and Martingales 10
       1.3.2 Some Commonly Used Models and Counting Processes .. 12
   1.4 Analysis of Recurrent Event Data 14
       1.4.1 Nonparametric Estimation 15
       1.4.2 Nonparametric Treatment Comparison 16
       1.4.3 Regression Analysis Under the Cox Intensity Model ... 17
   1.5 Analysis of Panel Count Data 18
       1.5.1 Some Features of Panel Count Data 19
       1.5.2 Outline 20

2 **Poisson Models and Parametric Inference** 23
   2.1 Introduction 23
   2.2 Regression Analysis of Count Data 24
       2.2.1 Likelihood-Based Procedures 24
       2.2.2 Estimating Equation-Based Procedures 26
       2.2.3 Discussion 27
   2.3 Parametric Maximum Likelihood Estimation of Panel Count Data 29
       2.3.1 Analysis Under Poisson Models 29

		2.3.2	Analysis Under Mixed Poisson Models	30
		2.3.3	An Illustration	32
		2.3.4	Discussion	33
	2.4	Regression Analysis with Piecewise Models		34
		2.4.1	Likelihood-Based Approach	35
		2.4.2	Estimating Equation-Based Approach	39
		2.4.3	An Illustration	42
		2.4.4	Discussion	43
	2.5	Bibliography, Discussion, and Remarks		44

3 Nonparametric Estimation 47
- 3.1 Introduction 47
- 3.2 Likelihood-Based Estimation of the Mean Function 48
  - 3.2.1 Non-homogeneous Poisson Process-Based Estimator .. 49
  - 3.2.2 Other Likelihood-Based Estimators 50
- 3.3 Isotonic Regression-Based Estimation of the Mean Function . 52
  - 3.3.1 Isotonic Regression Estimator 52
  - 3.3.2 Illustrations 53
  - 3.3.3 Discussion 56
- 3.4 Generalized Isotonic Regression-Based Estimation of the Mean Function 57
  - 3.4.1 Generalized Isotonic Regression Estimators 57
  - 3.4.2 Determination of the GIRE 59
  - 3.4.3 An Illustration 61
- 3.5 Estimation of the Rate Function 62
  - 3.5.1 Raw Estimators of the Rate Function 62
  - 3.5.2 Smooth Estimators of the Rate Function 64
  - 3.5.3 Illustrations 65
  - 3.5.4 Discussion 67
- 3.6 Bibliography, Discussion, and Remarks 69

4 Nonparametric Comparison of Point Processes 71
- 4.1 Introduction 71
- 4.2 Two-Sample Comparison of Cumulative Mean Functions 72
  - 4.2.1 Nonparametric Test Procedure I 72
  - 4.2.2 Nonparametric Test Procedure II 74
  - 4.2.3 Discussion 75
- 4.3 General p-Sample Comparison of Cumulative Mean Functions 77
  - 4.3.1 NPMPLE-Based Nonparametric Procedures 77
  - 4.3.2 NPMLE-Based Nonparametric Procedures 78
  - 4.3.3 Discussion 80
- 4.4 Numerical Comparison and Illustration 81
  - 4.4.1 Analysis of National Cooperative Gallstone Study 82
  - 4.4.2 Numerical Comparison of the Test Procedures 82

	4.5		Comparison of Cumulative Mean Functions with Different Observation Processes	84
		4.5.1	Test Statistics	84
		4.5.2	An Application	86
		4.5.3	Discussion	87
	4.6		Bibliography, Discussion, and Remarks	89
5	**Regression Analysis of Panel Count Data I**			91
	5.1		Introduction	91
	5.2		Analysis by the Likelihood-Based Approach	92
		5.2.1	A Semiparametric Maximum Pseudo-likelihood Estimation Procedure	93
		5.2.2	A Semiparametric Spline-Based Maximum Likelihood Estimation Procedure	95
		5.2.3	Discussion	96
	5.3		Analysis by the Estimating Equation Approach I	97
		5.3.1	Assumptions and Models	98
		5.3.2	Estimation of All Regression Parameters	99
		5.3.3	Estimation with Same Follow-Up Times	102
	5.4		Analysis by the Estimating Equation Approach II	103
		5.4.1	A Conditional Estimating Equation Procedure	103
		5.4.2	An Unconditional Estimating Equation Procedure	106
		5.4.3	Discussion	108
	5.5		Analysis with Semiparametric Transformation Models	109
		5.5.1	Assumptions and Models	109
		5.5.2	Estimation Procedure	110
		5.5.3	Determination of Estimators	113
		5.5.4	A Goodness-of-Fit Test	115
	5.6		Analysis of National Cooperative Gallstone Study	116
	5.7		Bibliography, Discussion, and Remarks	119
6	**Regression Analysis of Panel Count Data II**			121
	6.1		Introduction	121
	6.2		Analysis by a Joint Modeling Procedure	122
		6.2.1	Assumptions and Models	122
		6.2.2	Estimation of Parameters	124
		6.2.3	Discussion	128
	6.3		Analysis by a Robust Estimation Procedure	129
		6.3.1	Assumptions and Models	130
		6.3.2	Inference Procedure	130
		6.3.3	Analysis of Bladder Cancer Study	133
		6.3.4	Discussion	135
	6.4		Analysis with Semiparametric Transformation Models	136
		6.4.1	Assumptions and Models	136
		6.4.2	Inference Procedure	138

		6.4.3 An Illustration 139

        6.4.3 An Illustration 139
        6.4.4 Discussion 141
  6.5 Analysis with Dependent Terminal Events 142
        6.5.1 Assumptions and Models 143
        6.5.2 Estimation of Regression Parameters................ 145
        6.5.3 Reanalysis of Bladder Cancer Study 149
        6.5.4 Discussion 151
  6.6 Bibliography, Discussion, and Remarks 152

7 Analysis of Multivariate Panel Count Data 155
  7.1 Introduction 155
  7.2 Nonparametric Comparison of Cumulative Mean Functions .. 156
        7.2.1 Two-Sample Nonparametric Test Procedures......... 157
        7.2.2 An Application 158
        7.2.3 Discussion 159
  7.3 Regression Analysis with Independent Observation Processes. 161
        7.3.1 Assumptions and Models 161
        7.3.2 Estimation Procedure............................. 163
        7.3.3 Analysis of Psoriatic Arthritis Data................. 166
        7.3.4 Discussion 169
  7.4 Joint Regression Analysis with Dependent Observation
      Processes 170
        7.4.1 Assumptions and Models 171
        7.4.2 Inference Procedure 172
        7.4.3 Analysis of Skin Cancer Chemoprevention Trial 175
        7.4.4 Discussion 177
  7.5 Conditional Regression Analysis with Dependent
      Observation Processes................................... 178
        7.5.1 Assumptions and Models 178
        7.5.2 Estimation Procedure............................. 179
        7.5.3 Determination of Estimators 181
        7.5.4 Reanalysis of Skin Cancer Chemoprevention Trial 183
        7.5.5 Discussion 185
  7.6 Bibliography, Discussion, and Remarks 186

8 Other Topics 189
  8.1 Introduction 189
  8.2 Variable Selection with Panel Count Data 190
        8.2.1 Assumptions and Penalty Functions 191
        8.2.2 Variable Section Procedure 192
        8.2.3 An Illustration 195
        8.2.4 Discussion 197
  8.3 Analysis of Mixed Recurrent Event and Panel Count Data ... 199
        8.3.1 Introduction 199
        8.3.2 Regression Analysis of Mixed Data 200

		8.3.3	Analysis of the Childhood Cancer Survivor Study 202
		8.3.4	Discussion 204
	8.4	Analysis of Panel Count Data from Multi-state Models 205	
		8.4.1	Introduction 205
		8.4.2	Maximum Likelihood Estimation with Homogeneous Finite State Markov Models 207
		8.4.3	Discussion 210
	8.5	Bayesian Analysis and Analysis of Nonstandard Panel Count Data 212	
		8.5.1	Bayesian Analysis of Panel Count Data 212
		8.5.2	Analysis of Panel Count Data with Measurement Errors 214
		8.5.3	Analysis of Panel Count Data from Mixture Models .. 217
	8.6	Concluding Remarks 220	

9 Some Sets of Data 223

References 253

Index 267

1
Introduction

1.1 Event History Studies

The event history study refers to the study concerning the patterns of the occurrences of certain events and is often seen in many fields. Among them, two that have seen or used such studies most are probably medical research and social sciences (Allison, 1984; Kalbfleisch and Prentice, 2002; Klein and Moeschberger, 2003; Nelson, 2003; Vermunt, 1997; Yamaguchi, 1991). In medical research, the event under study can be the occurrence of a disease or death, the hospitalization of certain patient, or the occurrence of some infection. In social sciences, examples of the subjects for event history studies include occurrence rates of births, deaths, marriages and divorces in demographic studies, and the employment or unemployment history of certain populations in social studies. In addition to these two, other fields that often see event history studies include reliability studies and tumorigenicity experiments.

The events concerned in event history studies can be generally classified into two types. One is the type of events that can occur only once and the other is the type of events that can occur repeatedly, which are usually referred to as recurrent events. For the first type of events, it can be the case that the event itself can indeed occur only once such as death. It can also happen that the event itself may occur repeatedly but the focus or objective is the first occurrence of the event such as the first marriage. There exists a great deal of literature on statistical methods for dealing with the first type of events, in particular in medical context (Kalbfleisch and Prentice, 2002; Klein and Moeschberger, 2003). A typical example of this is described below. Examples of recurrent events include occurrences of the hospitalizations of intravenous drug users (Wang et al., 2001), occurrences of the same infection such as recurrent pyogenic infections among inherited disorder patients (Lin et al., 2000), repeated occurrences of certain tumors, and warranty claims for an automobile (Kalbfleisch et al., 1991). A specific example of such data on tumor occurrences is given below.

With respect to the event history data on recurrent events, they can also be generally classified into two types. One is from the event history studies that monitor study subjects continuously and consequently provide information on the times of all occurrences of the events. These data are usually referred to as recurrent event data (Cook and Lawless, 2007). The other type is the so-called panel count data, the focus of this book, and they arise when study subjects are examined or observed only at discrete time points (Kalbfleisch and Lawless, 1985; Sun, 2009; Zhao et al., 2011a). In this case, only the numbers of occurrences of the events between subsequent observation times are available, and the exact occurrence times of the events are unknown. The panel count data could occur for various reasons. For example, they may arise because continuous observation is too expensive or impossible, or when it is not practical to conduct continuous follow-ups of the subjects under study.

A special case of panel count data that often occurs in practice is that each subject is observed only once and such data are commonly referred to as current status data (Diamond and McDonald, 1991; Sun and Kalbfleisch, 1993). In this situation, only available information about the recurrent event of interest is the total number of the occurrences of the event up to the observation time. A common example of current status data arises in tumorigenicity experiments that concern the occurrence rate of certain tumors. In these experiments, it is often the case that only the number of tumors that have occurred before the death or sacrifice of the animal is known. Another area that frequently produces current status data is demographic studies (Diamond and McDonald, 1991). Note that in the statistical literature, current status data are sometimes also used to refer to the data from the event history study concerning an event that can occur only once and in which study subjects are observed only once (Sun, 2006). A more complete terminology for this latter type of data that is often used is current status failure time data.

Extensive literature has been developed for the analysis of both the event history study in which the event can occur only once and the study that gives rise to recurrent event data. This is especially the case for the former case and the resulting data are usually referred to as failure time or survival data. For example, among many others, Kalbfleisch and Prentice (2002) and Klein and Moeschberger (2003) give two excellent books on the topic. Among the existing literature for the latter (Cook and Lawless, 1996; Lawless and Nadeau, 1995; Lin et al., 2000; Pepe and Cai, 1993; Wang and Chen, 2000), there also exist two great books. One is Andersen et al. (1993), which provides a comprehensive coverage of counting process approaches for the analysis of recurrent event data. The other is Cook and Lawless (2007), which gives a relatively complete and thorough review of the recent literature. Comparatively, only sparse literature exists on the analysis of panel count data.

A key and distinguishing feature of failure time data is censoring and truncation, which may or may not exist in event history studies on recurrent events. One main difference between recurrent event data and panel count data is the amount of relevant information available and another key difference is the observation process. In the case of the former, the observation process means the length of the whole follow-up, while in the case of

1.1 Event History Studies

the latter, it also includes a sequence of consecutive observation times. This observation process may or may not be independent of the underlying point process generating the observed data. To analyze recurrent event data, it is common and convenient to characterize the occurrences of recurrent events by counting processes and to model the intensity process of the counting process (Andersen et al., 1993). On the other hand, for the analysis of panel count data, it is usually more convenient to work directly on the mean function of the counting processes due to the incomplete nature of the observed information. More discussion on this is given below.

Note that in practice, one could regard panel count data as a special type of longitudinal data and apply the methodology developed for general longitudinal data. However, a major drawback in this approach is that one would miss the special structure of panel count data. Moreover, some questions of interest in panel count data cannot be answered from the longitudinal data point of view.

To give a better idea about the types of the event history data described above, we describe two examples below. The first one is about failure time data and the second one is on recurrent event data. Examples of panel count data are provided in the next section.

1.1.1 Failure Time Data on Remission Times of Acute Leukemia Patients

Freireich et al. (1963) and Gehan (1965) discussed a set of data arising from a clinical trial on acute leukemia patients. The data, presented in Table 1.1, give the remission times in weeks for 42 patients in 2 treatment groups. One treatment is the drug 6-mercaptopurine (6-MP) and the other is the placebo treatment. The study was performed over a 1-year period and the patients were enrolled into the study at different times. The main goal of the study is to compare the two treatments with respect to their ability to maintain remission. In other words, it is of interest to know if the patients with drug 6-MP had significantly longer remission times than those given the placebo treatment.

Table 1.1. Remission times in weeks for acute leukemia patients

Treatment	Survival times in weeks
6-MP	6, 6, 6, 6*, 7, 9*, 10, 10*, 11*, 13, 16, 17*, 19*, 20*, 22, 23, 25* 32*, 32*, 34*, 35*
Placebo	1, 1, 2, 2, 3, 4, 4, 5, 5, 8, 8, 8, 8, 11, 11, 12, 12, 15, 17, 22, 23

This is a typical set of failure time data. For the observed information given in the table, the starred numbers represent censoring times or censored remission times. That is, such an observation is the amount of time from when the patient entered the study to the end of the study. These remission times were censored because these patients were still in the state of remission at the end of the trial. Thus their actual remission times were known only to be greater than the censoring times. For the other patients, their remission times were observed exactly. This situation commonly occurs in failure time studies, and the resulting data are usually referred to as right-censored failure time data. In addition to Freireich et al. (1963) and Gehan (1965), many other authors discussed this set of right-censored failure time data such as Kalbfleisch and Prentice (2002).

Table 1.2. Times to tumor for 48 female rats (# in parentheses are # of tumors)

Treatment group		Control group
ID	Times to tumor	ID Times to tumor (in days)
1	182	1 63, 102, 119, 161(2), 172, 179
2		2 88, 91, 95, 105, 112, 119(2), 137, 145, 167, 172
3	63, 68	3 91, 98, 108, 112, 134, 137, 161(2), 179
4	152	4 71, 174
5	130, 134, 145, 152	5 95, 105, 134(2), 137, 140, 145, 150(2)
6	98, 152, 182	6 68(2), 130, 137
7	88, 95, 105, 130, 137, 167	7 77, 95, 112, 137, 161, 174
8	152	8 81, 84, 126, 134, 161(2), 174
9	81	9 68, 77, 98, 102(3)
10	71, 84, 126, 134, 152	10 112
11	116, 130	11 88(2), 91, 98, 112, 134(2), 137(2), 140(2), 152(2)
12	91	12 77, 179
13	63, 68, 84, 95, 152	13 112
14	105, 152	14 71(2), 74, 77, 112, 116(2), 140(2), 167
15	63, 102, 152	15 77, 95, 126, 150
16	63, 77, 112, 140	16 88, 126, 130(2), 134
17	77, 119, 152, 161, 167	17 63, 74, 84(2), 88, 91, 95, 108, 134, 137, 179
18	105, 112, 145, 161, 182	18 81, 88, 105, 116, 123, 140, 145, 152, 161(2), 179
19	152	19 88, 95, 112, 119, 126(2), 150, 157, 179
20	81, 95	20 68(2), 84, 102, 105, 119, 123(2), 137, 161, 179, 182
21	84, 91, 102, 108, 130, 134	21 140
22		22 152, 182(2)
23	91	23 81
		24 63, 88, 134
		25 84, 134, 182

1.1.2 Recurrent Event Data on Times to Mammary Tumors

Table 1.2 presents a set of data on the times to mammary tumors in days for 48 female rats, reproduced from Gail et al. (1980). The data arose from a carcinogenicity experiment on the times to the development of mammary tumors in two treatment groups. At the beginning of the experiment, the rats were exposed to a carcinogen for 60 days and then randomized to receive either retinoid treatment or control. The total follow-up period is 122 days after randomization and during the period, the rats were examined every few days for the development of new tumors. A given animal may experience any number of tumors and one of the main objectives is to compare the tumor growth rates between the two treatment groups.

As mentioned above, for the recurrent event data such as these given in Table 1.2, the observed information includes the time of each occurrence of the event of interest during the follow-up period. As can be seen, the number of the occurrences of the event and the occurrence times differ from subject to subject, and there are two rats who never developed tumors during the follow-up. Note that sometimes one may be interested only in the occurrence time of the first tumor, and in this case, the data become right-censored failure time data on the time to the first tumor as these given in Table 1.1. For more discussion on this data set, readers are referred to as Cook and Lawless (2007) among others.

1.2 Panel Count Data

As described above, panel count data arise from event history studies in which study subjects are examined or observed only at discrete time points. Thus they give only the numbers of occurrences of the recurrent events of interest between subsequent observation times. In particular, the exact occurrence times of the events are unknown. In the following, we discuss four examples of panel count data. The first three examples concern univariate panel count data, while the last one discusses a set of panel count data that involves two types of related recurrent events, that is, bivariate panel count data.

1.2.1 Reliability Study of Nuclear Plants

Table 1.3 presents a set of panel count data arising from a reliability study of 30 nuclear plants on the loss of feedwater flow. The data are reproduced from Gaver and O'Muircheartaigh (1987) and Sun and Kalbfleisch (1995). They give the observation time (one per plant) and the corresponding observed number of losses of feedwater flow for each nuclear plant. In other words, only one observation was taken for each study subject and we actually have current status data.

Among others, one objective of this reliability study is to estimate the mean or average number of losses of feedwater flow based on the observed data. For this, one simple approach is to assume that the number of loss of feedwater flow follows a parametric model such as the Poisson distribution, and one can then carry out the maximum likelihood estimation. More generally, one may want to apply some nonparametric procedures. Among others,

Gaver and O'Muircheartaigh (1987) and Sun and Kalbfleisch (1995) analyzed this set of data.

Table 1.3. Observed numbers of loss of feedwater flow from 30 nuclear plants

\multicolumn{8}{c}{Observation time t_i (in years) and observed number n_i}
Plant	t_i n_i	Plant	t_i n_i	Plant	t_i n_i	Plant	t_i n_i
1	15 4	9	4 13	17	2 11	25	1 1
2	12 40	10	3 4	18	2 1	26	3 10
3	8 0	11	4 27	19	2 0	27	2 5
4	8 10	12	4 14	20	1 3	28	4 16
5	6 14	13	4 10	21	1 5	29	3 14
6	5 31	14	2 7	22	1 6	30	11 58
7	5 2	15	3 4	23	5 35		
8	4 4	16	3 3	24	3 12		

1.2.2 National Cooperative Gallstone Study

The National Cooperative Gallstone Study is a 10-year, multicenter, double-blinded, placebo-controlled clinical trial on the use of the natural bile acid chenodeoxycholic acid, cheno, for the dissolution of cholesterol gallstones. The original study consists of a total of 916 patients randomized into each of three treatments, placebo, low dose, and high dose, and they were treated for up to 2 years. One of the primary objectives of the study is to assess the impact of the treatments on the incidence of digestive symptoms commonly associated with the gallstone disease. The symptoms range from milder episodes of nausea/vomiting, dyspepsia, and diarrhea to more severe episodes of digestive colic, i.e., severe pain, and cholecystitis, i.e., digestive obstruction.

The data set I of Chap. 9, reproduced from Thall and Lachin (1988) and Sun (2006), gives the observed information on the incidence of nausea over the first 52 weeks follow-up on 113 patients with floating gallstones in high-dose (65) and placebo (48) groups. Nausea is an unpleasant sensation vaguely referred to the epigastrium and abdomen, often culminating in vomiting. It is very commonly associated with the gallstone disease and it is important for the investigators to determine whether there exists a significant difference between the incidence of nausea for the patients in the two groups. It was hypothesized that any treatment effect should be observed shortly after patients achieved maximal dose (usually by 3 months). The effect might later begin to dissipate.

During the study, the patients were scheduled to return for clinic observations at 1, 2, 3, 6, 9, and 12 months during the first year follow-up. However, actual visit or observation times differ from patient to patient. For example, the first observation times range from 3 to 9 weeks, and some patients

1.2 Panel Count Data

dropped out of the study early. At each visit, they were asked to report the total number of each type of symptom that had occurred between successive visits such as the number of the incidences of nausea. That is, the observed data include actual visit times and the numbers of the incidences or occurrences of nausea between the visits, and we have panel count data on the occurrence of nausea. For the analysis of the data here, several questions can be of interest. One is to estimate the pattern or average rate of the incidences of nausea and then to compare the patterns or average rates between the treatment groups. Also one may want to conduct regression analysis of these panel count data for treatment comparison and estimation of some covariate effects.

Table 1.4. Current status data for the placebo group of bladder cancer study

ID	Initial size	# of initial tumors	Follow-up time	# of tumors	ID	Initial size	# of initial tumors	Follow-up time	# of tumors
1	3	1	1	0	25	6	1	30	3
2	1	2	4	0	26	3	1	31	6
3	1	1	7	0	27	2	1	32	0
4	1	5	10	0	28	1	2	34	0
5	1	4	10	1	29	1	2	36	0
6	1	1	14	0	30	1	3	36	8
7	1	1	18	5	31	2	1	37	0
8	1	1	18	0	32	1	4	40	16
9	3	1	18	2	33	1	5	40	16
10	3	1	23	9	34	2	1	41	0
11	1	1	23	24	35	1	1	43	3
12	1	3	23	10	36	6	2	43	1
13	3	3	23	0	37	1	2	44	12
14	3	2	24	27	38	1	1	45	12
15	1	1	25	5	39	1	1	48	1
16	1	8	26	8	40	3	1	49	0
17	4	1	26	12	41	1	3	51	1
18	2	1	26	0	42	7	1	53	1
19	2	1	28	3	43	1	3	53	15
20	4	1	29	0	44	1	1	47	0
21	2	1	29	0	45	2	3	52	19
22	1	4	29	0	46	3	1	53	23
23	5	1	30	10	47	3	2	52	17
24	1	2	30	13					

1.2.3 Bladder Cancer Study

Table 1.4 gives a set of panel count data on the patients in the placebo group of the bladder cancer study conducted by the Veterans Administration Cooperative Urological Research Group (Byar, 1980; Byar et al., 1977). The study consists of the patients who had superficial bladder tumors when they entered the study, and they were randomly assigned to each of the three treatment groups, placebo, thiotepa and pyridoxine. For all patients, their initial tumors were removed transurethrally, and they had multiple recurrences of tumors during the study. To give a quick idea about panel count data and another example of current status data, the data in Table 1.4 are actually the summary data from the patients in the placebo group. Specifically, they only give the follow-up time and the total number of bladder tumors that occurred during the follow-up for each study subject. In other words, we have a set of current status data on the occurrence of bladder tumors, and this would be the case if each subject was examined only once. In addition, for each patient, the observed data also provide information on two potentially important baseline covariates. They are the size of the largest initial tumor and the number of initial tumors.

For each patient in the bladder cancer study, the observed data actually include a sequence of clinical visit times and the numbers of recurrent tumors that occurred between the visits. As the initial tumors, the recurrent tumors were also removed transurethrally at the patient's clinic visits. The data set II of Chap. 9, reproduced from Andrews and Herzberg (1985) and Sun and Wei (2000), gives the observed data on 85 patients in the placebo (47) and thiotepa (38) groups. Note that the data on the third treatment pyridoxine are not included here as many authors have showed that it did not have significant effect. The unit for observation times is a month with the largest observation time being 53 months.

For the analysis of this set of panel count data, several issues may be of interest as those for the data arising from the National Cooperative Gallstone Study discussed in the previous subsection. These include treatment comparison and regression analysis, and many authors have discussed these and others (He et al., 2009; Hu et al., 2003; Huang et al., 2006; Sun et al., 2007b; Sun and Wei, 2000; Wellner and Zhang, 2007; Zhang, 2006). In addition, among others, Sun and Wei (2000) noted that the observation process seems to depend on the treatment and covariates. Furthermore, He et al. (2009) and Sun et al. (2007b) pointed out that the underlying counting process representing the occurrence of bladder tumors may be related to the observation times. More discussion on this is given below.

1.2.4 Skin Cancer Chemoprevention Trial

Lee (2008) and Li (2011) discussed a set of panel count data arising from a skin cancer chemoprevention trial, funded by a NCI R01 grant and conducted by the University of Wisconsin Comprehensive Cancer Center in Madison, Wisconsin. It is a double-blinded and placebo-controlled randomized phase III clinical trial. The primary objective of this trial is to evaluate the effectiveness of $0.5\,\text{g/m}^2/\text{day}$ PO difluoromethylornithine (DFMO) in reducing new skin cancers in a population of the patients with a history of non-melanoma skin cancers: basal cell carcinoma and squamous cell carcinoma. The study consists of 291 patients randomized to either the placebo group (147) or the DFMO group (144). During the study, the patients were scheduled to be assessed or observed every 6 months for the development of new skin cancers of the two types.

The observed information is presented in data set III of Chap. 9, kindly provided by Dr. Howard Bailey, the PI of the study. For each patient, it gives a sequence of observation times and the numbers of occurrences of both basal cell carcinoma and squamous cell carcinoma between the observation times. As expected, these real observation times differ from patient to patient and so as the follow-up times. One difference between this set of panel count data and the data discussed in the previous examples is that here there exist two types of recurrent events defined by the two types of skin cancers. It is obvious that the incidences or occurrences of these two types of skin cancers, basal cell carcinoma and squamous cell carcinoma, are correlated. In other words, we have a set of bivariate panel count data.

The data set III of Chap. 9 actually includes only 290 skin cancer patients as one patient who did not give any observation was removed. It can be seen that among these patients, the number of observations ranges from 1 to 17. With respect to the number of the recurrent events, the number of new basal cell carcinoma ranges from 0 to 16, while the number of new squamous cell carcinoma ranges from 0 to 23. For each patient, in addition to the treatment indicator, information is also available on three baseline covariates. They are patient's gender, age at the diagnosis and the number of prior skin cancers from the first diagnosis to randomization. For the analysis, a simple and naive approach is to assess the treatment effects on each of the two types of skin cancers by conducting two separate analyses of univariate panel count data. It is clear that this would not be efficient and one may prefer some joint analysis of the two types of skin cancers together.

More examples of panel count data and their analyses are given throughout the book. In the next section, we introduce some notation and basic concepts about counting processes that are commonly used in practice and throughout the book.

1.3 Some Notation and Basic Concepts About Counting Processes

In this section, we introduce some notation and review some basic concepts and models about counting processes. They are the foundation of many approaches developed for the analysis of panel count data and also used throughout the book.

1.3.1 Counting Processes and Martingales

Counting processes have been playing an essential role in the development of statistical models and inferential procedures for event history analysis. Some of the early and significant contributions to this were given by Aalen (1975, 1978) and Andersen and Borgan (1985). They and others established the connection between counting process and event history analysis and showed how the theory of multivariate counting processes can provide a general framework and a useful tool for event history analysis. In particular, Andersen and Gill (1982) proposed the Cox type intensity model for counting processes, developed the partial likelihood estimation procedure for regression parameters, and established the large sample theory for the resulting estimators. For detailed description and discussion on these and general stochastic processes, readers are referred to Andersen et al. (1993) and Cox and Miller (1965) in addition to the references mentioned above.

Let $(\Omega, \mathcal{F}, \mathcal{P})$ be a probability space and $\mathcal{T} = [0, \tau)$ a continuous time interval, where τ is a given terminal time, $0 < \tau \leq \infty$. A stochastic process X is a family of random variables $\{X(t) : t \in \mathcal{T}\}$. A filtration or history $(\mathcal{F}_t : t \in \mathcal{T})$ is an increasing right-continuous family of sub-σ-algebras of $\mathcal{F}$ such that $\mathcal{F}_t$ contains all the information generated by the stochastic process X on $[0, t]$. The process X is said to be adapted to the filtration if $X(t)$ is $\mathcal{F}_t$-measurable for every $t \in \mathcal{T}$. A process X is predictable with respect to $\mathcal{F}_t$ if $X(t)$ is known given the history $\mathcal{F}_{t-}$ generated by $\{X(s) : 0 \leq s < t\}$.

A counting process is a stochastic process $\{N(t); t \geq 0\}$ with $N(0) = 0$ and $N(t) < \infty$ almost surely such that the path is right-continuous with probability one, piecewise constant, and has only jump discontinuities with jumps of size $+1$. To model a counting process, one usually employs its intensity process defined as

$$\lambda(t) = \lim_{\Delta t \downarrow 0} \frac{P\{N(t + \Delta t-) - N(t-) = 1 | \mathcal{F}_{t-}\}}{\Delta t}$$

and imposes some assumptions on its format. Given $\lambda(t)$, one can obtain the so-called cumulative intensity process $\Lambda(t) = \int_0^t \lambda(s) ds$ and could directly model $\Lambda(t)$ too. Suppose that there exists a vector of covariate process

1.3 Some Notation and Basic Concepts About Counting Processes

denoted by $\boldsymbol{Z}(t)$. Let $\mathcal{F}_t$ denote the history generated by $\{N(s), \boldsymbol{Z}(s): 0 \leq s < t\}$ and $\lambda_Z(t)$ the intensity process of $N(t)$ associated with $\mathcal{F}_t$. That is,

$$E\{dN(t)|\mathcal{F}_t\} = \lambda_Z(t)\, dt,$$

where $dN(t)$ denotes the increment $N((t+dt)-) - N(t-)$ of $N(t)$ over the small interval $[t, t+dt)$.

Of course, in practice, one usually faces more than one counting process. A K-dimensional multivariate counting process is a stochastic process $\{N_1(t), \ldots, N_K(t); t \geq 0\}$ with K components such that each component $N_k(t)$ is a counting process having jumps of size $+1$, no two components can jump simultaneously, and each $N_k(\infty)$ is almost surely finite. That is, multiple events cannot occur. The process defined above can be thought of as counting the occurrences of K different types of recurrent events. As the single counting process, the multivariate counting process is governed by its intensity process $\{\lambda_1(t), \ldots, \lambda_K(t); t \geq 0\}$, where $\lambda_k(t)$ corresponds to $N_k(t)$. For this, Aalen (1978) introduced the multiplicative intensity model defined as

$$\lambda_k(t) = \alpha_k(t)\, Y_k(t). \tag{1.1}$$

Here $\alpha_k(t)$ is a non-negative deterministic function and $Y_k(t)$ a non-negative predictable stochastic process, $k = 1, \ldots, K$. Usually one can regard $\alpha_k(t)$ as an individual intensity for the occurrence of the kth type of recurrent events and $Y_k(t)$ the risk indicator or the number of subjects at risk of experiencing the kth type of recurrent events at $t-$. If $\alpha_1(t) = \ldots = \alpha_K(t) = \alpha_0(t)$ in model (1.1), then it is easy to see that $N(t) = \sum_{k=1}^{K} N_k(t)$ is a counting process with the intensity process $\alpha_0(t)\, Y(t)$, where $Y(t) = \sum_{k=1}^{K} Y_k(t)$.

One major reason that counting processes have played fundamental and important roles for the analysis of event history studies is their link with martingales. The use of martingale methods makes it possible for the development and derivation of various statistical procedures. Let $M(t)$ denote an integrable stochastic process, that is, $E\{|M(t)|\} < \infty$ for all t, and $\mathcal{F}_t$ the associated history up to time t. We say that $M(t)$ is a martingale if

$$E\{M(t)|\mathcal{F}_s\} = M(s)$$

for all $s \leq t$. Let the $N_k(t)$'s and $\lambda_k(t)$'s be defined as above and define

$$dM_k(t) = dN_k(t) - \lambda_k(t)\, dt,$$

$k = 1, \ldots, K$. Then the processes

$$M_k(t) = N_k(t) - \int_0^t \lambda_k(s)\, ds, \ k = 1, \ldots, K$$

are martingales. In particular, we have $E\{M_k(t)\} = 0$.

For a martingale $M(t)$, its variance process is usually defined through

$$d<M>(t) = Var\{dM(t)|\mathcal{F}_{t-}\}.$$

For the martingales $M_k(t)$'s defined above, one can show that

$$d<M_k>(t) = Var\{dN_k(t)|\mathcal{F}_{t-}\} \approx \lambda_k(t)\,dt$$

and thus

$$<M_k>(t) = \int_0^t \lambda_k(s)\,ds,$$

$k = 1,\ldots,K$. Let $M_1(t)$ and $M_2(t)$ denote two martingales. Their covariance process $<M_1, M_2>$ is defined by the increments

$$d<M_1,M_2>(t) = Cov\{dM_1(t), dM_2(t)|\mathcal{F}_{t-}\}$$

and we say that they are orthogonal if $<M_1, M_2> = 0$. One can show that the martingales $M_k(t)$'s defined above are orthogonal. For more discussion on martingales and in particular on the martingale central limit theorems commonly used in event history studies, the readers are referred to the book Andersen et al. (1993).

1.3.2 Some Commonly Used Models and Counting Processes

For the analysis of recurrent event data, one of the most commonly used models on $\lambda_Z(t)$, the intensity process given the covariate process $\boldsymbol{Z}(t)$, is the Cox type intensity model

$$\lambda_Z(t) = \lambda_0(t)\,\exp\{\boldsymbol{\beta}^T \boldsymbol{Z}(t)\}, \qquad (1.2)$$

proposed by Andersen and Gill (1982). In the above, $\lambda_0(t)$ denotes an unspecified continuous function and $\boldsymbol{\beta}$ is a vector of regression parameters. In practice, the Cox intensity model (1.2) may be too restrictive (Lin et al., 2000) and corresponding to this, one may want to model the mean or rate function $r(t)$ of $N(t)$ defined by

$$E\{dN(t)\} = r(t)\,dt.$$

Given $r(t)$, the mean function $\mu(t)$ can be calculated as $\mu(t) = \int_0^t r(s)ds$. Note that it is easy to see that the mean or rate function cannot completely specify the counting process $N(t)$ and they are sometimes referred to as the marginal cumulative intensity or intensity function. One major advantage of dealing with the mean or rate function is that less assumptions are usually needed in modeling them compared to modeling the intensity process. As a consequence, one can expect more robust inferential procedures. Also it

1.3 Some Notation and Basic Concepts About Counting Processes

is apparent that they can be more intuitive than the intensity function in practice.

Given $\boldsymbol{Z}(t)$, a commonly used model for the rate function is the so-called proportional rate model

$$r_Z(t)\, dt \;=\; E\{\, dN(t)|\boldsymbol{Z}(t)\} \;=\; r_0(t)\,\exp\{\boldsymbol{\beta}^T \boldsymbol{Z}(t)\}\, dt\,, \qquad (1.3)$$

where $r_0(t)$ denotes an unknown baseline rate function and $\boldsymbol{\beta}$ regression parameters as above. Assume that $\boldsymbol{Z}$ is time-independent. Then from model (1.3), one can derive

$$\mu_Z(t) \;=\; E\{\, N(t)|\boldsymbol{Z}\,\} \;=\; \mu_0(t)\,\exp(\boldsymbol{\beta}^T \boldsymbol{Z})\,, \qquad (1.4)$$

where $\mu_0(t) = \int_0^t r_0(s)\, ds$. This is often referred to as the proportional mean model (Cook and Lawless, 2007; Lawless and Nadeau, 1995; Lin et al., 2000). One advantage of model (1.4) is that it is applicable to any counting process or can be used to model point processes with positive jumps of arbitrary sizes. In contrast, model (1.2) requires the Poisson structure (Lin et al., 2000). Of course, one could apply model (1.4) to time-dependent covariates too.

For an event history study concerning transitions among finite states, a commonly used model is the finite state Markov Chain model. Suppose that $\{X(t): t \ge 0\,\}$ is a continuous stochastic process with right continuous sample paths and state space $S = \{1, \ldots, m\}$. Let $\{q_{ij}(t): i \ne j = 1, \ldots, m\,\}$ be nonnegative left continuous functions satisfying $\int_0^t q_{ij}(s)\, ds < \infty$ for all $t > 0$. The process $\{X(t)\}$ is said to be a continuous time Markov Chain with intensities $q_{ij}(t)$ if

$$P\{X(t) = j | X(t-h) = i, X(s), 0 \le s < t-h\}$$
$$= P\{X(t) = j | X(t-h) = i\} \;=\; q_{ij}(t)h + o(h)$$

for small $h > 0$ and all $i \ne j$. Define $q_{ii}(t) = -\sum_{j \ne i} q_{ij}(t)$. Then $Q(t) = (\,q_{ii}(t)\,)_{m \times m}$ is usually referred to as the transition intensity matrix and often the target for inference. Given $Q(t)$, it is easy to see that one can determine the transition probability matrix $P(s,t) = (\,p_{ij}(s,t)\,)$ for $t > s$, where $p_{ij}(s,t) = P(X(t) = j | X(s) = i)$. If $q_{ij}(t) = q_{ij}$, independent of time t, for all (i,j), we usually say that the Markov Chain $X(t)$ is time homogeneous. In this case, we usually write $Q(t) = Q$ and $P(s,t)$ depends only on the difference $t - s$.

Let $X(t)$ be a continuous Markov Chain with the state space $S = \{1, \ldots, m\}$ as defined above. For each pair (i,j), define $N_{ij}(t)$ to be the cumulative number of transitions from state i to state j up to time t, $i \ne j = 1, \ldots, m$. Then $\{N_{ij}(t)\}$ is a $m(m-1)$-dimensional multivariate counting process. That is, one can transfer Markov Chain problems to counting process problems. Among the continuous Markov Chains, a simple and commonly used one is the three-state model. In this case, the three states could represent, for example, a health status, a disease status and death. Of course, in practice, one could also simply use a finite state model or the three-state model without imposing the Markov assumption. More discussion on Markov Chains and the three-state model is given in Sect. 8.4.

Among counting processes, the most commonly used one is perhaps the Poisson process $\{N(t); t \geq 0\}$ defined by

$$P\{N(t+dt) - N(t) = 1|\mathcal{F}_{t-}\} = \lambda(t)dt + o(dt)$$

and

$$P\{N(t+dt) - N(t) \geq 2|\mathcal{F}_{t-}\} = o(dt)$$

with $\lambda(t)$ being a left-continuous function. The definition above says that the Poisson process $N(t)$ has at most one jump over a small time interval and does not depend on its history. The process defined above is commonly referred to as a non-homogeneous Poisson process. If $\lambda(t)$ is a constant, the process is usually called a homogeneous Poisson process. For a Poisson process $\{N(t) : t \geq 0\}$, we have that at each t, $N(t)$ follows the Poisson distribution with $E\{N(t)\} = \Lambda(t) = \int_0^t \lambda(s)ds$. That is, $\Lambda(t)$ is also the mean function of the process and in this situation, we have that $r(t) = \lambda(t) = d\Lambda(t)/dt$.

Suppose that $N(t)$ is the non-homogeneous Poisson process defined above and let T_k denote the time to the occurrence of the kth event. Then it can be shown that T_1 has the density function

$$f_1(t) = \lambda(t) \exp\{-\Lambda(t)\}$$

and given $T_{k-1} = t_{k-1}$, T_k has the density function

$$f_k(t_k) = \lambda(t_k) \exp[-\{\Lambda(t_k) - \Lambda(t_{k-1})\}]$$

for $t_k > t_{k-1}$, $k \geq 2$. Also given $N(\tau) = n$, the joint density function of $T_1, \ldots, T_n$ has the form

$$f(t_1, \ldots, t_n) = \frac{n! \prod_{i=1}^n \lambda(t_i)}{\{\Lambda(\tau)\}^n}, \ 0 < t_1 < \ldots < t_n < \tau.$$

If $N(t)$ is homogeneous, that is, $\lambda(t) = \lambda$, then $T_1, T_2 - T_1, T_3 - T_2, \ldots$ are independent exponential variables with mean λ^{-1}.

1.4 Analysis of Recurrent Event Data

To help the discussion on the analysis of panel count data, we first in this section give a brief review of some of the commonly asked questions and the corresponding available approaches in the literature for the analysis of recurrent event data. This is because many of these questions are often of interest in the case of panel count data too. In addition, the ideas behind

1.4 Analysis of Recurrent Event Data

some of these approaches have been or can be easily generalized to the latter situation. Of course, as discussed above, there exist several differences between the two types of event history data, and as a consequence, there also exist some questions that are unique to panel count data.

Consider a study concerning a single type of recurrent events and consisting of n independent subjects. Define $N_i(t)$ to be the counting process representing the number of occurrences of the event over the interval $[0, t]$ for subject i, $i = 1, \ldots, n$. Assume that each subject is observed continuously up to time $\min(C_i, \tau)$, where C_i denotes the observation period or follow-up time for subject i and τ the study length. That is, we have recurrent event data on the $N_i(t)$'s. Define the left-continuous function $Y_i(t) = I(t \leq \min(C_i, \tau))$, indicating whether subject i is under observation at time t, $i = 1, \ldots, n$. Here we assume that the follow-up time C_i is independent of the counting process $N_i(t)$ completely or given covariates. In the following, we confine our discussion on three topics or questions, nonparametric estimation, nonparametric treatment comparison and regression analysis under the Cox intensity model.

1.4.1 Nonparametric Estimation

For the analysis of recurrent event data, one of the basic questions is to evaluate or estimate the occurrence rate of the recurrent event of interest. To address this, assume that all study subjects come from a homogeneous population and the intensity process $\lambda_i(t)$ for $N_i(t)$ has the form $\lambda_i(t) = \alpha(t) Y_i(t)$, where $\alpha(t)$ is a nonnegative deterministic function. Then the estimation of the occurrence rate becomes estimating the function $\alpha(t)$ or more conveniently the corresponding cumulative function $\Lambda(t) = \int_0^t \alpha(s) ds$. For this, motivated by the fact that $N_i(t) - \int_0^t \alpha(s) Y_i(s) ds$ is a martingale, a commonly used estimator is given by the so-called Nelson-Aalen estimator

$$\hat{\Lambda}(t) = \int_0^t \frac{J.(s) \, dN.(s)}{Y.(s)} \tag{1.5}$$

(Andersen et al., 1993). In the above, $N.(t) = \sum_{i=1}^n N_i(t)$, $Y.(t) = \sum_{i=1}^n Y_i(t)$ and $J.(t) = I(Y.(t) > 0)$. It is easy to see that $N.(t)$ and $Y.(t)$ denote the total number of occurrences of the event up to time t and the number of subjects still under observation at time t, respectively.

Let $t_1 < t_2 < \cdots$ denote the sequence of all distinct occurrence times of the recurrent events of interest. Then the Nelson-Aalen estimator can be rewritten as

$$\hat{\Lambda}(t) = \sum_{j:t_j \leq t} \frac{\Delta N.(t_j)}{Y.(t_j)},$$

where $\Delta N.(t_j) = N.(t_j) - N.(t_{j-1})$. Given $\hat{\Lambda}(t)$, it is obvious that one can estimate $\alpha(t)$ by

$$\hat{\alpha}(t) = \frac{\Delta N.(t)}{Y.(t)}, \qquad (1.6)$$

or more generally by a kernel estimator

$$\hat{\alpha}_K(t) = \frac{1}{h} \int_{t-h}^{t+h} K\left(\frac{t-s}{h}\right) d\hat{\Lambda}(s), \qquad (1.7)$$

where $K(t)$ is a kernel function and h is a positive constant called the bandwidth (Wand and Jones, 1995). It is easy to see that the estimator $\hat{\alpha}_K(t)$ is the average or smooth version of the raw estimator $\hat{\alpha}(t)$, and one can control the degree of the smoothness by choosing appropriate K and h.

In the case that the $N_i(t)$'s are non-homogeneous Poisson processes, one can easily show that the estimator $\hat{\Lambda}(t)$ is actually the nonparametric maximum likelihood estimator of the mean function of the processes (Cook and Lawless, 2007). Also some robust variance estimation for the Nelson-Aalen estimator can be developed (Cook and Lawless, 2007).

1.4.2 Nonparametric Treatment Comparison

To describe the treatment comparison problem, assume that one has a multivariate counting process $\{N_1(t), \ldots, N_K(t); t \geq 0\}$ satisfying the multiplicative intensity model (1.1). Also assume that one is interested in testing the hypothesis

$$H_0 : \alpha_1(t) = \ldots = \alpha_K(t).$$

Define $A_k(t) = \int_0^t \alpha_k(s) \, ds$ and $A(t) = \int_0^t \alpha(s) \, ds$, where $\alpha(t)$ denotes the common function of the $\alpha_k(t)$'s under H_0, $k = 1, \ldots, K$. Let $\hat{A}_k(t)$ denote the Nelson-Aalen estimator defined in (1.5) with replacing $N.(s)$, $Y.(s)$ and $J.(s)$ by $N_k(s)$, $Y_k(s)$ and $J_k(s) = I(Y_k(s) > 0)$, respectively, $k = 1, \ldots, K$. Also define

$$\hat{A}(t) = \int_0^t \frac{J(s)}{Y(s)} \, dN(s)$$

and

$$\tilde{A}_k(t) = \int_0^t J_k(s) \, d\hat{A}(s) = \int_0^t \frac{J_k(s)}{Y(s)} \, dN(s),$$

where $Y(t) = \sum_{k=1}^K Y_k(t)$, $N(t) = \sum_{k=1}^K N_k(t)$ and $J(t) = I(Y(t) > 0)$.

To test the hypothesis H_0, Andersen and Gill (1982) proposed to use the statistic $\{U_1(\tau), \ldots, U_K(\tau)\}$, where

$$U_k(t) = \int_0^t W_k(s) \, d(\hat{A}_k - \tilde{A}_k)(s)$$

1.4 Analysis of Recurrent Event Data

with the $W_k(t)$'s being some locally bounded predictable weight processes. Furthermore, they showed that the $U_k(t)$'s converge weakly to a K-variate Gaussian martingale under H_0 and $\{U_1(\tau), \ldots, U_K(\tau)\}$ is asymptotically multinormally distributed with mean zero. Hence one can perform a chi-squared test on the hypothesis H_0. It is easy to see that the basic idea behind the test statistics above is to compare the two estimators of $A_k(t)$. One is the estimator $\tilde{A}_k(t)$ obtained under the hypothesis H_0 and the other is the estimator $\hat{A}_k(t)$ independent of the hypothesis H_0. In the case of two-sample situations ($K = 2$), instead of the test statistic above, one could equivalently apply the statistic

$$\int_0^\tau W(t)\, d(\hat{A}_1 - \hat{A}_2)(t),$$

where $W(t)$ is a bounded predictable weight process as $W_k(t)$.

In practice, in addition to the hypothesis H_0, one may be interested in some other hypotheses about the $\alpha_k(t)$'s too. For example, again for the two-sample situation, a model of practical interest is the proportional intensity model

$$\alpha_1(t) = \theta\, \alpha_2(t),$$

and sometimes one may be interested in testing $\theta = 1$. Also as discussed above, instead of the intensity function, sometimes one may want to focus on the rate or mean functions of the underlying counting processes. Thus the hypothesis could be about the rate or mean functions. In these situations, one approach for the construction of test statistics is to directly apply the idea above to compare two sets of estimators of the rate or mean functions obtained with and without the hypothesis.

1.4.3 Regression Analysis Under the Cox Intensity Model

Let the $N_i(t)$'s and $Y_i(t)$'s be defined as before. Suppose that in addition, there exists a vector of covariate processes denoted by $\mathbf{Z}_i(t)$ for subject i, $i = 1, \ldots, n$, and the goal is to make inference about covariate effects. For this, assume that the intensity process of $N_i(t)$ has the form

$$\lambda_i(t) = Y_i(t)\, \lambda_0(t)\, \exp\{\boldsymbol{\beta}^T \mathbf{Z}_i(t)\}, \tag{1.8}$$

where $\lambda_0(t)$ and $\boldsymbol{\beta}$ are defined as in model (1.2). To estimate $\boldsymbol{\beta}$, Andersen and Borgan (1985) suggested to use the solution to the equation $\partial C(\tau; \boldsymbol{\beta})/\partial \boldsymbol{\beta} = 0$, where

$$C(t; \boldsymbol{\beta}) = \sum_{i=1}^n \int_0^t \boldsymbol{\beta}^T \mathbf{Z}_i(s)\, dN_i(s) - \int_0^t \log\left\{\sum_{i=1}^n Y_i(s)\, \exp\{\boldsymbol{\beta}^T \mathbf{Z}_i(s)\}\right\} d\bar{N}(s)$$

with $\bar{N}(t) = \sum_{i=1}^n N_i(t)$.

Let $U(t;\boldsymbol{\beta}) = \partial C(t;\boldsymbol{\beta})/\partial \boldsymbol{\beta}$ and

$$S^{(j)}(t;\boldsymbol{\beta}) = \frac{1}{n} \sum_{i=1}^{n} Y_i(t) \, \exp\{\boldsymbol{\beta}^T \boldsymbol{Z}_i(t)\} \, \boldsymbol{Z}_i^j(t) \, ,$$

$j = 0, 1$. Then we have

$$U(t;\boldsymbol{\beta}) = \sum_{i=1}^{n} \int_0^t \boldsymbol{Z}_i(s) \, dN_i(s) - \int_0^t \frac{S^{(1)}(s;\boldsymbol{\beta})}{S^{(0)}(s;\boldsymbol{\beta})} \, d\bar{N}(s)$$

$$= \sum_{i=1}^{n} \int_0^t \left\{ \boldsymbol{Z}_i(s) - \bar{\boldsymbol{Z}}(s;\boldsymbol{\beta}) \right\} Y_i(s) \, dN_i(s) \, , \qquad (1.9)$$

where $\bar{\boldsymbol{Z}}(t;\boldsymbol{\beta}) = S^{(1)}(t;\boldsymbol{\beta})/S^{(0)}(t;\boldsymbol{\beta})$. Let $\hat{\boldsymbol{\beta}}$ denote the estimator of $\boldsymbol{\beta}$ defined above. Given $\hat{\boldsymbol{\beta}}$, one can estimate $\Lambda_0(t) = \int_0^t \lambda_0(s) \, ds$ by

$$\hat{\Lambda}_0(t;\hat{\boldsymbol{\beta}}) = \sum_{i=1}^{n} \int_0^t \frac{Y_i(s) \, dN_i(s)}{n \, S^{(0)}(s;\hat{\boldsymbol{\beta}})} \, . \qquad (1.10)$$

Note that in the discussion above, it was assumed that there exists only one type of recurrent events. Sometimes there may exist K types of recurrent events and in this case, we could have a $n \times K$-dimensional multivariate counting process $\{ N_{ki}(t), k = 1, \ldots, K, i = 1, \ldots, n, \, t \geq 0 \}$. Here $N_{ki}(t)$ represents the cumulative numbers of the occurrences of the kth type of recurrent events from subject i up to time t. To model covariate effects, it is straightforward to generalize model (1.8) to

$$\lambda_{ki}(t) = Y_i(t) \, \lambda_{k0}(t) \, \exp\{\boldsymbol{\beta}^T \boldsymbol{Z}_i(t)\} \, ,$$

where the $\lambda_{k0}(t)$'s are unspecified type-specific underlying intensities as $\lambda_0(t)$. In the model above, one could also allow $Y_i(t)$ and $\boldsymbol{Z}_i(t)$ to depend on the type of the recurrent event. Andersen and Borgan (1985) considered this generalized intensity model and developed an estimation procedure for $\boldsymbol{\beta}$, which includes the estimation procedure described above for model (1.8) as a special case. Furthermore, they also discussed the situation where the $\lambda_{k0}(t)$'s can be described by some parametric models.

1.5 Analysis of Panel Count Data

As discussed above, in event history studies, the event of interest may occur only once or can occur multiple times. For the latter case, the event is usually referred to as a recurrent event. In the case that the event can occur only once or one is only interested in the first occurrence of a recurrent event, the resulting data are usually referred to as failure time data. Failure time data

1.5 Analysis of Panel Count Data

can occur in several formats and the two formats commonly seen in practice are right-censored data and interval-censored data (Kalbfleisch and Prentice, 2002; Sun, 2006). The latter type of data arises when study subjects are observed only at discrete time points instead of continuously. One can see that the structure difference between recurrent event data and panel count data is actually similar to that between the two types of failure time data.

1.5.1 Some Features of Panel Count Data

Compared to failure time data and recurrent event data, panel count data have some similarities as well as some unique features. In terms of the data structure or sampling scheme, panel count data are similar to interval-censored data as in both case, study subjects are observed only at discrete time points. As a consequence, one only knows the numbers of the occurrences of the event between observation times (Kalbfleisch and Lawless, 1985; Sun and Wei, 2000). Thus panel count data are also sometimes referred to as interval count data or interval-censored recurrent event data (Lawless and Zhan, 1998; Thall, 1988). One major difference between failure time data and the data on recurrent events is that with the former, the random variable of interest is always the time to an event and the event is treated as an absorbing event. This is clearly not the case in the latter situation. As a consequence, censoring plays a much more important role in the analysis of failure time data than that in the analysis of the data on recurrent events.

Let $N(t)$ be defined as in the previous section, a counting process denoting the number of occurrences of a recurrent event up to and including time t. In the case of recurrent event data, the whole sample path of $N(t)$ is known, while for panel count data, only the values of $N(t)$ at observation time points are known. In particular, we do not know the time points at which $N(t)$ jumps. It is easy to see that compared to recurrent event data, panel count data contain much less relevant information about the underlying recurrent event process. Some of the resulting consequences are that the inference for the latter is much harder than for the former, and also the models and inference goals for the latter often differ from these for the former. To give an example, consider an extreme and also simple case where all study subjects are observed only at one single time point t_0. In this case, it is clear that the only inference that one could make about the underlying recurrent event process is its behavior at t_0. On the other hand, if one has recurrent event data over the interval $[0, t_0]$, it is apparent that one would know or can say much more about the recurrent event process of interest.

Let $\lambda(t)$ and $\mu(t)$ denote the intensity process and mean function of $N(t)$ as before, respectively. It is obvious that if possible, one would prefer to know or make inference about $\lambda(t)$ as the intensity process completely determines the process $N(t)$. In general, this is possible if one has recurrent event data as discussed in the previous section. On the other hand, this would be difficult or impossible with panel count data. To see this, again consider the simple case discussed above where all study subjects are observed only at one single time point t_0. In this case, one can definitely estimate $\mu(t)$ at $t = t_0$, but it is clear that the data provide no definite information at all about $\lambda(t)$. Due to the same reason, for the analysis of panel count data, one usually focuses only on the mean function of the underlying recurrent event process. On the other hand, for the analysis of recurrent event data, one could choose to directly model either the intensity process or the mean function.

Assume that one observes panel count data and let $T_1 < \ldots < T_m$ denote the potential observation time points on $N(t)$. Define $\tilde{H}(t) = \sum_{j=1}^{m} I(t \geq T_j)$, which is often referred to as the observation process on $N(t)$. In practice, there usually also exists a follow-up time denoted by C, meaning that the subject is followed up to time C. As the result, the real observation process is $H(t) = \tilde{H}(\min(t, C))$, and with panel count data, one faces both the process of interest $N(t)$ and the observation process $H(t)$ in addition to the variable C or the count process $I(t \leq C)$. In other words, panel count data involve three processes and in contrast, recurrent event data involve only two processes $N(t)$ and $I(t \leq C)$. Of course, if all three processes are independent of each other, one only needs to focus on the recurrent event process $N(t)$ and can conduct the analysis conditional on the other two processes. In practice, however, it can happen that the recurrent event process of interest $N(t)$ and the observation process $\tilde{H}(t)$ are related. In this case, the analysis is much more difficult and the resulting panel count data are often referred to as panel count data with informative or dependent observation processes. More discussion on this is given below, particularly in Chap. 6. Also some discussion is given below for the case where the follow-up process $I(t \leq C)$ may be related with them as well.

1.5.2 Outline

As can be seen from the contents, this book discusses six different topics on the analysis of panel count data in details. In Chap. 2, we first consider the situation where the data can be described by non-homogeneous Poisson processes with the focus on parametric inference procedures. In other words, $N(t)$ or the $N_i(t)$'s defined above are Poisson processes, and it is reasonable to make some parametric assumptions about the intensity process $\lambda(t)$, the rate function $r(t)$ or the mean function $\mu(t)$. A key advantage of this assumption is that one can derive or write out the resulting likelihood function and thus can apply the maximum likelihood approach for inference. Note that this is also the major difference between Chap. 2 and most other parts of the book where it is difficult or impossible to employ the maximum likelihood approach. Also in this chapter, to make the book relatively complete, some discussion is provided on regression analysis of simple count data.

Chapters 3 and 4 are on nonparametric analysis of panel count data with the focus on the mean function of the underlying recurrent event process

1.5 Analysis of Panel Count Data

of interest. Specifically, Chap. 3 considers nonparametric estimation of the mean function $\mu(t)$ and several commonly used approaches are discussed and compared. Some simple estimators of the rate function $r(t)$ including kernel estimators are also described. In Chap. 4, we investigate the treatment comparison problem or the testing of the hypothesis formulated by the mean functions. Here it is assumed that study subjects are given several different treatments or there exist several different recurrent event processes, and the goal is to compare them in terms of their mean functions. For the problem, we discuss several procedures. The key idea behind all the procedures is to compare the estimated mean functions obtained under the null hypothesis and without the hypothesis, respectively.

Regression analysis of panel count data is the focus of Chaps. 5 and 6. In Chap. 5, we first consider the situation where the underlying recurrent event process and the observation process are independent completely or conditionally given covariate processes. Chapter 6 discusses the case where the two processes may be related or the observation process may contain relevant information about the recurrent event process of interest. For both cases, the focus is on estimation of the effects of covariates on the mean function of the recurrent event process. In other words, unlike in the analysis of recurrent event data, we model covariate effects through the mean function rather than the intensity process. To describe the relationship between the recurrent event process of interest and the observation process in Chap. 6, we consider both the joint modeling approach and the conditional modeling approach. For inference about or estimation of covariate effects, we mainly employ the estimating equation approach. Note that it is not hard to see that the maximum likelihood approach is not available here in general.

In all of the previous chapters, it has been assumed that there exists only one type of recurrent events of interest. Chapter 7 considers the situation where there exist two or more related types of recurrent events of interest, that is, the analysis of multivariate panel count data. As discussed before, in this case, one important issue that does not exist with univariate panel count data but needs to be taken into account is the relationship among different types of events. For the analysis of multivariate panel count data, the discussion mainly focuses on two problems, nonparametric treatment comparison and regression analysis. In both cases, as with univariate panel count data, we formulate the problems by using the mean functions of the underlying recurrent event processes. For inference, we focus on the robust methods that leave the relationship among different types of recurrent events arbitrary as it is usually difficult or unrealistic to model such relationship in general.

Chapter 8 briefly discusses several topics on the analysis of panel count data that are not touched in other chapters. These include variable selection, the analysis of mixed recurrent event and panel count data, and the analysis of panel count data arising from multi-state models. In addition, some discussions are also given on Bayesian approaches for the analysis of panel count data and the analysis of panel count data arising from mixture models or with measurement errors. For each of these topics, we mainly review the existing literature and discuss possible directions for future research. Note that most of these topics have been extensively discussed in some other fields but are relatively new in the area of panel count data. For example, there exists a great deal of literature on variable selection in the field of generalized linear model or on Bayesian approaches for the analysis of failure time data. Also note that for all these topics except the panel count data from multi-state models, the focus of the investigation is the same as with other chapters in terms of inference goals, the occurrence pattern of the recurrent events of interest. But for latter, one is usually interested in how long a subject stays at certain states or how often a subject transfers from one state to another state. In other words, a major target in this case is to estimate or make inference about the transition intensity or probability matrix. The chapter concludes with some final remarks for the book, including possible directions for future research and available software packages for the analysis of panel count data.

2
Poisson Models and Parametric Inference

2.1 Introduction

It is well-known that for the analysis of count data, Poisson model is perhaps the most commonly used model or assumption (Breslow, 1984, 1990; Cameron and Trivedi, 1998). Thus for the analysis of panel count data, it is helpful to first consider Poisson-based approaches for the motivation of more general inference procedures and their comparison. As mentioned before, the focus of this chapter is on parametric approaches, which also can be seen as a motivation to many semiparametric inference procedures discussed later.

To be complete, we start with the discussion on regression analysis of simple count data in Sect. 2.2. Count data can be seen as a special case of panel count data in which all study subjects are observed only once at the same time point. They occur in many fields including actuarial studies, demography, economics, political and social sciences, and reliability studies. Examples of count data include the occurrences of certain tumors and the frequency of recurrent events such as auto accidents and visits to doctor's offices or clinics. For inference about regression parameters, both the likelihood-based method and the estimating equation-based method are described. The former is developed under the Poisson assumption and the latter can be regarded as a generalization of the former. Section 2.3 considers regression analysis of panel count data with the focus on the maximum likelihood approach. For this, two situations are discussed. One is that the underlying recurrent event processes of interest are non-homogeneous Poisson processes and the other is that the recurrent event processes are mixed Poisson processes (Dean, 1991; Lawless, 1987a,b).

As mentioned above, the focus of this book is on nonparametric and semiparametric inference procedures. One reason for the discussion of parametric methods is that the development of the former is often motivated by the latter. Of course, the latter itself could be useful too when the parametric assumption used is reasonable. Sometimes one may prefer some approaches or compromises between the two types of procedures. One such type of approaches is piecewise procedures that are essentially parametric methods but can be made to be close to nonparametric or semi-parametric inference methods. Section 2.4 describes two piecewise approaches for regression analysis of panel count data. Similar to the two methods discussed in Sect. 2.2 for count data, one is a likelihood-based method and the other is an estimating equation-based method. In Sect. 2.5, some bibliographical notes and remarks are given. Throughout the chapter, it is assumed that the observation process is independent of the underlying recurrent event process of interest.

2.2 Regression Analysis of Count Data

Consider a recurrent event study that consists of n independent subjects and in which the observed information from each subject is only the number of the events that have occurred over some time interval. For subject i, let N_i denote the observed count and suppose that there exists a vector of covariates $\boldsymbol{Z}_i$, $i = 1, \ldots, n$. Then the observed data are $\{(N_i, \boldsymbol{Z}_i); i = 1, \ldots, n\}$. It is assumed that the main goal is to make inference about the effects of covariates on the occurrence rate of the event of interest.

To describe the covariate effects, we assume that given $\boldsymbol{Z}_i$, the conditional mean of N_i has the form

$$E(N_i|\boldsymbol{Z}_i) = \exp(\boldsymbol{\beta}^T \boldsymbol{Z}_i), \quad (2.1)$$

where $\boldsymbol{\beta}$ denotes the vector of regression parameters. Note that an alternative or a more natural choice is to assume $E(N_i|\boldsymbol{Z}_i) = \alpha \exp(\boldsymbol{\beta}^T \boldsymbol{Z}_i)$, a special case of the proportional mean model (1.4), where α is an unknown parameter. It is easy to see that model (2.1) includes this latter choice as a special case by setting the first component of $\boldsymbol{Z}_i$ as one. For inference about $\boldsymbol{\beta}$, in the following, we first discuss some likelihood-based procedures developed for the situation where the N_i's follow the Poisson distribution. Some estimating equation-based procedures are then presented that do not require the Poisson assumption and followed by some discussions.

2.2.1 Likelihood-Based Procedures

In this subsection, we suppose that the N_i's follow Poisson distributions with the mean given by model (2.1). Then it is easy to see that the log-likelihood function of $\boldsymbol{\beta}$ is proportional to

$$l(\boldsymbol{\beta}) = \sum_{i=1}^{n} \left\{ N_i \boldsymbol{\beta}^T \boldsymbol{Z}_i - \exp(\boldsymbol{\beta}^T \boldsymbol{Z}_i) \right\}.$$

It follows that the maximum likelihood estimator, denoted by $\hat{\boldsymbol{\beta}}_P$, of $\boldsymbol{\beta}$ is given by the solution to the score estimating equation

2.2 Regression Analysis of Count Data

$$\sum_{i=1}^{n} \mathbf{Z}_i \left\{ N_i - \exp(\boldsymbol{\beta}^T \mathbf{Z}_i) \right\} = 0. \quad (2.2)$$

It is easy to show that $\hat{\boldsymbol{\beta}}_P$ is consistent and its distribution can be approximated by the normal distribution with mean $\boldsymbol{\beta}_0$, the true value of $\boldsymbol{\beta}$, and the covariance matrix

$$V_{ML}(\boldsymbol{\beta}) = n^{-1} \left\{ \sum_{i=1}^{n} \mathbf{Z}_i \mathbf{Z}_i^T \exp(\boldsymbol{\beta}^T \mathbf{Z}_i) \right\}^{-1}$$

with $\boldsymbol{\beta}$ replaced by $\hat{\boldsymbol{\beta}}_P$.

Under the Poisson assumption, we have that $Var(N_i|\mathbf{Z}_i) = E(N_i|\mathbf{Z}_i)$ and it is well-known that this often does not hold in practice. To relax this restriction, one common approach is to assume that there exists a latent variable ν_i and given ν_i, N_i follows the Poisson distribution with the mean

$$E(N_i|\mathbf{Z}_i, \nu_i) = \nu_i \exp(\boldsymbol{\beta}^T \mathbf{Z}_i), \quad (2.3)$$

$i = 1, \ldots, n$. That is, the N_i's follow the mixed Poisson distribution. Here it is assumed that the ν_i's are i.i.d. with $E(\nu_i) = 1$ and $Var(\nu_i) = \sigma_\nu^2$. Under the model above, it is easy to show that

$$E(N_i|\mathbf{Z}_i) = \mu_i = \exp(\boldsymbol{\beta}^T \mathbf{Z}_i), \ Var(N_i|\mathbf{Z}_i) = \mu_i (1 + \sigma_\nu^2 \mu_i).$$

That is, the variance of N_i can be equal to or larger than its mean.

Now we assume that the ν_i's follow the Gamma distribution with the density function

$$g(\nu; \gamma) = \frac{\gamma^{-1/\gamma}}{\Gamma(\gamma^{-1})} \nu^{\gamma^{-1}-1} e^{-\nu/\gamma},$$

where $\Gamma(a) = \int_0^\infty t^{a-1} \exp(-t) \, dt$, the Gamma function. In this case, we have $\sigma_\nu^2 = \gamma$. Then the marginal density function of N_i is given by

$$f(N_i|\boldsymbol{\beta}, \gamma) = \frac{\Gamma(\gamma^{-1} + N_i)}{\Gamma(\gamma^{-1}) \Gamma(N_i + 1)} \left(\frac{\gamma^{-1}}{\gamma^{-1} + \mu_i} \right)^{\gamma^{-1}} \left(\frac{\mu_i}{\mu_i + \gamma^{-1}} \right)^{N_i}.$$

That is, N_i follows the negative binomial distribution. It follows that the log likelihood function of $\boldsymbol{\beta}$ and γ is proportional to

$$l(\boldsymbol{\beta}, \gamma) = \sum_{i=1}^{n} \left\{ \sum_{j=0}^{N_i - 1} \log(j + \gamma^{-1}) - (N_i + \gamma^{-1}) \log(1 + \gamma \mu_i) \right. \\ \left. + N_i \log \gamma + N_i \boldsymbol{\beta}^T \mathbf{Z}_i \right\}.$$

Let $\hat{\boldsymbol{\beta}}_{NB}$ and $\hat{\gamma}_{NB}$ denote the resulting maximum likelihood estimators of $\boldsymbol{\beta}$ and γ, respectively. Then they can be obtained by solving the score equations

$$\sum_{i=1}^{n} \frac{N_i - \mu_i}{1 + \gamma \mu_i} \, \boldsymbol{Z}_i = 0$$

and

$$\sum_{i=1}^{n} \left\{ \frac{1}{\gamma^2} \left(\log(1 + \gamma \mu_i) - \sum_{j=0}^{N_i - 1} \frac{1}{j + \gamma^{-1}} \right) + \frac{N_i - \mu_i}{\gamma(1 + \gamma \mu_i)} \right\} = 0$$

together. One can easily show that $\hat{\boldsymbol{\beta}}_{NB}$ and $\hat{\gamma}_{NB}$ are consistent. Furthermore, their joint distribution can be asymptotically approximated by the multivariate normal distribution with mean $(\boldsymbol{\beta}_0^T, \gamma_0)^T$ and the covariance matrix determined by

$$Var(\hat{\boldsymbol{\beta}}_{NB}) = n^{-1} \left(\sum_{i=1}^{n} \frac{\hat{\mu}_i}{1 + \tilde{\mu}_i} \, \boldsymbol{Z}_i \boldsymbol{Z}_i^T \right)^{-1},$$

$$Var(\hat{\gamma}_{NB}) = n^{-1} \left\{ \sum_{i=1}^{n} \left(\log(1 + \tilde{\mu}_i) - \sum_{j=0}^{N_i - 1} \frac{1}{j + \hat{\gamma}_{NB}^{-1}} \right)^2 + \frac{\hat{\mu}_i}{\hat{\gamma}_{NB}^2 (1 + \tilde{\mu}_i)} \right\}^{-1}$$

and $Cov(\hat{\boldsymbol{\beta}}_{NB}, \hat{\gamma}_{NB}) = 0$. That is, $\hat{\boldsymbol{\beta}}_{NB}$ and $\hat{\gamma}_{NB}$ are asymptotically independent. In the above, again $\boldsymbol{\beta}_0$ and γ_0 denote the true values of $\boldsymbol{\beta}$ and γ, respectively, $\hat{\mu}_i = \exp(\hat{\boldsymbol{\beta}}_{NB}^T \boldsymbol{Z}_i)$ and $\tilde{\mu}_i = \hat{\gamma}_{NB} \hat{\mu}_i$.

2.2.2 Estimating Equation-Based Procedures

As mentioned above, under the negative binomial model, the variance of N_i does not have to be equal to its mean as under the Poisson model, but cannot be smaller than its mean. It is obvious that this may still be too restrictive in reality. In this subsection, we assume that the N_i's still satisfy model (2.1) but do not make any assumption about the distribution of the N_i's. By following the estimating equation theory, it is clear that one can still employ the estimating Eq. (2.2) and to use its solution, denoted by $\hat{\boldsymbol{\beta}}_{PP}$, to estimate $\boldsymbol{\beta}$. Again by using the estimating equation theory (White, 1982), one can show that $\hat{\boldsymbol{\beta}}_{PP}$ is consistent and its distribution can be asymptotically approximated by the normal distribution with mean $\boldsymbol{\beta}_0$ and the covariance matrix

$$Var(\hat{\boldsymbol{\beta}}_{PP}) = n^{-1} \left(\sum_{i=1}^{n} \hat{\mu}_i \, \boldsymbol{Z}_i \boldsymbol{Z}_i^T \right)^{-1} \left(\sum_{i=1}^{n} w_i \, \boldsymbol{Z}_i \boldsymbol{Z}_i^T \right) \left(\sum_{i=1}^{n} \hat{\mu}_i \, \boldsymbol{Z}_i \boldsymbol{Z}_i^T \right)^{-1}, \quad (2.4)$$

2.2 Regression Analysis of Count Data

where $\hat{\mu}_i = \exp(\hat{\boldsymbol{\beta}}_{PP}^T \boldsymbol{Z}_i)$ and $w_i = Var(N_i|\boldsymbol{Z}_i)$, $i = 1, \ldots, n$. The estimator $\hat{\boldsymbol{\beta}}_{PP}$ is often referred to as the Poisson pseudo- or quasi-maximum likelihood estimator.

To use the formula (2.4), one usually needs to specify the variance function w_i's. For this, one common choice is to let

$$w_i = \phi \mu_i, \qquad (2.5)$$

where ϕ is an unknown parameter. In this case, the formula reduces to

$$Var(\hat{\boldsymbol{\beta}}_{PP}) = \frac{\phi}{n} \left(\sum_{i=1}^n \hat{\mu}_i \boldsymbol{Z}_i \boldsymbol{Z}_i^T \right)^{-1}$$

and one can estimate ϕ empirically by

$$\hat{\phi} = \frac{1}{n-p} \sum_{i=1}^n \frac{(N_i - \hat{\mu}_i)^2}{\hat{\mu}_i},$$

where p denotes the dimension of $\boldsymbol{\beta}$. Another common choice for the w_i's is to assume that

$$w_i = \mu_i + \alpha \mu_i^2 \qquad (2.6)$$

with α being an unknown parameter as ϕ. Under the model above, we have

$$Var(\hat{\boldsymbol{\beta}}_{PP}) = n^{-1} \left(\sum_{i=1}^n \hat{\mu}_i \boldsymbol{Z}_i \boldsymbol{Z}_i^T \right)^{-1} \left(\sum_{i=1}^n (\hat{\mu}_i + \alpha \hat{\mu}_i^2) \boldsymbol{Z}_i \boldsymbol{Z}_i^T \right) \left(\sum_{i=1}^n \hat{\mu}_i \boldsymbol{Z}_i \boldsymbol{Z}_i^T \right)^{-1}$$

and one can also estimate α empirically by

$$\hat{\alpha} = \frac{1}{n-p} \sum_{i=1}^n \frac{\{(N_i - \hat{\mu}_i)^2 - \hat{\mu}_i\}}{\hat{\mu}_i^2}.$$

Of course, sometimes one may not want to impose any form on the w_i's. In this case, assuming that we can treat $\{(N_i, \boldsymbol{Z}_i)\}_{i=1}^n$ as i.i.d., one can estimate $Var(\hat{\boldsymbol{\beta}}_{PP})$ by the robust estimator

$$n^{-1} \left(\sum_{i=1}^n \hat{\mu}_i \boldsymbol{Z}_i \boldsymbol{Z}_i^T \right)^{-1} \left(\sum_{i=1}^n (N_i - \hat{\mu}_i)^2 \boldsymbol{Z}_i \boldsymbol{Z}_i^T \right) \left(\sum_{i=1}^n \hat{\mu}_i \boldsymbol{Z}_i \boldsymbol{Z}_i^T \right)^{-1}. \qquad (2.7)$$

2.2.3 Discussion

There exists extensive literature on the analysis of count data (Cameron and Trivedi, 1998; Vermunt, 1997). For example, Cameron and Trivedi (1998) discussed the count data arising from natural and social sciences. Also they gave a relatively complete review of the analysis approaches commonly used in the field. In particular, in these books, one can find some real count data and the applications of the methods discussed above to real count data. As mentioned before, the main purpose of this section is to give some introduction of the existing literature as the count data can be regarded as a special case of panel count data. More importantly, the methods described above serve as a motivation to many inference procedures discussed below for the analysis of panel count data.

To relax the Poisson assumption used in Sect. 2.2.1, instead of using the mixed Poisson model, an alternative is to develop a latent class-based Poisson model as follows (Wedel et al., 1993). Suppose that study subjects are from K unknown classes and each subject belongs to one and only one class. Let α_k denote the unknown probability that a subject belongs to class k with $\sum_{k=1}^{K} \alpha_k = 1$. It is assumed that conditional on subject i belonging to class k, N_i follows the Poisson distribution with mean

$$\lambda_{i|k} = \exp(\boldsymbol{\beta}_k^T \boldsymbol{Z}_i),$$

where $\boldsymbol{\beta}_k$ is a vector of unknown regression parameters as $\boldsymbol{\beta}$, $i = 1, \ldots, n$, $k = 1, \ldots, K$. Then the likelihood function of the $\boldsymbol{\beta}_k$'s and α_k's has the form

$$L(\boldsymbol{\beta}_k's, \alpha_k's) = \prod_{i=1}^{n} \sum_{k=1}^{K} \alpha_k \exp\left\{-\exp(\boldsymbol{\beta}_k^T \boldsymbol{Z}_i)\right\} \frac{\exp(N_i \boldsymbol{\beta}_k^T \boldsymbol{Z}_i)}{N_i!}.$$

It follows that one can naturally estimate the $\boldsymbol{\beta}_k$'s and α_k's by their maximum likelihood estimators.

For estimation of $\boldsymbol{\beta}$ in model (2.1) without making a distribution assumption, instead of the estimating Eq. (2.2), one can use its weighted version given by

$$\sum_{i=1}^{n} w_i \boldsymbol{Z}_i \left\{ N_i - \exp(\boldsymbol{\beta}^T \boldsymbol{Z}_i) \right\} = 0,$$

where the w_i's are some weights. One can easily show that the estimator of $\boldsymbol{\beta}$ given by the solution to the equation above is consistent. Furthermore, one can asymptotically approximate its distribution by the normal distribution with mean $\boldsymbol{\beta}_0$ and the covariance matrix

$$n^{-1} \left(\sum_{i=1}^{n} w_i \hat{\mu}_i \boldsymbol{Z}_i \boldsymbol{Z}_i^T \right)^{-1} \left(\sum_{i=1}^{n} w_i^2 (N_i - \hat{\mu}_i)^2 \boldsymbol{Z}_i \boldsymbol{Z}_i^T \right) \left(\sum_{i=1}^{n} w_i \hat{\mu}_i \boldsymbol{Z}_i \boldsymbol{Z}_i^T \right)^{-1}$$

with $\boldsymbol{\beta}$ replaced by its estimator. It is easy to see that the estimator above reduces to (2.7) if one takes $w_i = 1$ for all i.

2.3 Parametric Maximum Likelihood Estimation of Panel Count Data

Consider an event history study concerning certain recurrent events that involves n independent subjects and in which each subject gives rise to a counting process $N_i(t)$. Here $N_i(t)$ represents the total number of the occurrences of the recurrent event of interest from subject i up to time t, $i = 1, \ldots, n$. For each subject, as before, suppose that there is a p-dimensional vector $\boldsymbol{Z}_i$ of covariates whose effects on $N_i(t)$ are of main interest. Also suppose that $N_i(t)$ is observed only at finite time points $t_{i,1} < \cdots < t_{i,m_i}$, where m_i denotes the number of observation times, $i = 1, \ldots, n$. That is, we only observe panel count data given by

$$\{ (t_{i,j}, n_{i,j} = N_i(t_{i,j}), \boldsymbol{Z}_i) \, ; \, j = 1, \ldots, m_i, i = 1, \ldots, n \} \, .$$

For estimation of the effects of covariates on the $N_i(t)$'s, in the following, we first consider the situation where it is reasonable to assume that the $N_i(t)$'s are non-homogeneous Poisson processes. A more general situation where the $N_i(t)$'s are mixed Poisson processes is then discussed and followed by an illustrative example and some discussions.

2.3.1 Analysis Under Poisson Models

In this subsection, we assume that the N_i's are non-homogeneous Poisson processes with the rate function

$$E\{ dN_i(t) | \boldsymbol{Z}_i \} = r(t; \boldsymbol{\beta}, \boldsymbol{Z}_i) \, dt = r_0(t; \boldsymbol{\beta}_1) \exp(\boldsymbol{\beta}_2^T \boldsymbol{Z}_i) \, dt \, , \qquad (2.8)$$

$i = 1, \ldots, n$. In the above, $\boldsymbol{\beta} = (\boldsymbol{\beta}_1^T, \boldsymbol{\beta}_2^T)^T$ denotes the unknown parameters and $r_0(t; \boldsymbol{\beta}_1)$ is a function of t known up to $\boldsymbol{\beta}_1$. Some simple and commonly used choices for $r_0(t; \boldsymbol{\beta}_1)$ include $r_0(t; \boldsymbol{\beta}_1) = \boldsymbol{\beta}_1^T \boldsymbol{\phi}(t)$ and

$$r_0(t; \boldsymbol{\beta}_1) = \exp\left\{ \boldsymbol{\beta}_1^T \boldsymbol{\phi}(t) \right\} . \qquad (2.9)$$

In the above, $\boldsymbol{\phi}(t)$ is a vector of known functions of t such as $\boldsymbol{\phi}(t) = (1, t, \log(t))^T$ or

$$\boldsymbol{\phi}(t) = (1, t, \ldots, t^q)^T \qquad (2.10)$$

with q being a known integer.

It is apparent that under the formulation (2.9), the rate function $r(t; \boldsymbol{\beta}, \boldsymbol{Z}_i)$ can be rewritten as

$$r(t; \boldsymbol{\beta}, \boldsymbol{Z}_i) = \exp\left\{ \boldsymbol{\beta}^T \boldsymbol{Z}_i^*(t) \right\} ,$$

where $Z_i^*(t) = (\phi^T(t), Z_i^T)^T$. Also the likelihood function of β is proportional to

$$L(\beta) = \prod_{i=1}^{n} L_i(\beta)$$

$$= \prod_{i=1}^{n} \prod_{j=1}^{m_i} \exp\{-\Delta\mu_{i,j}(\beta)\} \{\Delta\mu_{i,j}(\beta)\}^{\Delta n_{i,j}}$$

$$= \prod_{i=1}^{n} \exp\{-\mu_i(\beta)\} \prod_{j=1}^{m_i} \{\Delta\mu_{i,j}(\beta)\}^{\Delta n_{i,j}},$$

where $\Delta\mu_{i,j}(\beta) = \int_{t_{i,j-1}}^{t_{i,j}} r(t; \beta, Z_i)\, dt$, $\mu_i(\beta) = \int_0^{t_{i,m_i}} r(t; \beta, Z_i)\, dt$ and $\Delta n_{i,j} = n_{i,j} - n_{i,j-1}$ with $t_{i,0} = 0$ and $n_{i,0} = 0$. It follows that one can obtain the maximum likelihood estimator of β, which is consistent and asymptotically has a normal distribution. The determination of the estimator is discussed in more details in the next subsection for a more general situation.

Suppose that $t_{1,m_1} = \cdots = t_{n,m_n}$. That is, all subjects have the same last observation time point. In this case, for inference about β_2, a conditional likelihood can actually be derived as

$$L_c(\beta) = \exp\left(\sum_{i=1}^{n} n_{i,m_i} \beta_2^T Z_i\right) \left\{\sum_{i=1}^{n} \exp(\beta_2^T Z_i)\right\}^{-\sum_{i=1}^{n} n_{i,m_i}}.$$

It is easy to see that for this simple situation, the inference about β_2 depends only on the observed numbers of the events at the last observation time or the total numbers of occurrences of the events during the whole follow-up period. In other words, the number of observations and observation times before the last observation time do not contain relevant information about β_2.

2.3.2 Analysis Under Mixed Poisson Models

Similar to the situation considered in Sect. 2.2, the Poisson process assumption used in the previous subsection may be questionable in practice, and one way to relax it is to consider mixed Poisson processes (Thall, 1988). More specifically, assume that there exists a latent variable ν_i and given ν_i and Z_i, $N_i(t)$ is a non-homogeneous Poisson process with the rate function

$$E\{dN_i(t)|Z_i, \nu_i\} = \nu_i\, r(t; \beta, Z_i)\, dt = \nu_i\, r_0(t; \beta_1) \exp(\beta_2^T Z_i)\, dt. \quad (2.11)$$

Here β and $r_0(t; \beta_1)$ are defined as in model (2.8). Furthermore, it is assumed that the ν_i's are i.i.d. with the density function $g(\nu; \alpha)$ known up to the unknown vector of parameters α. Then it is easy to see that the likelihood function of $\theta = (\beta^T, \alpha^T)^T$ is proportional to

2.3 Parametric Maximum Likelihood Estimation of Panel Count Data

$$L(\boldsymbol{\theta}) = \prod_{i=1}^{n} L_i(\boldsymbol{\theta})$$

$$= \prod_{i=1}^{n} \int_0^\infty \prod_{j=1}^{m_i} \exp\{-\nu\,\Delta\mu_{i,j}(\boldsymbol{\beta})\}\,\{\nu\,\Delta\mu_{i,j}(\boldsymbol{\beta})\}^{\Delta n_{i,j}}\,g(\nu;\boldsymbol{\alpha})\,d\nu$$

$$= \prod_{i=1}^{n} \int_0^\infty \exp\{-\nu\,\mu_i(\boldsymbol{\beta})\} \prod_{j=1}^{m_i} \{\nu\,\Delta\mu_{i,j}(\boldsymbol{\beta})\}^{\Delta n_{i,j}}\,g(\nu;\boldsymbol{\alpha})\,d\nu\,.$$

It follows that one can estimate both $\boldsymbol{\beta}$ and $\boldsymbol{\alpha}$ by maximizing the likelihood function above.

Suppose that the baseline rate function $r_0(t;\boldsymbol{\beta}_1)$ has the form (2.9) and the latent variables ν_i's follow the gamma distribution with the density function

$$g(\nu;\alpha_1,\alpha_2) = \frac{\nu^{\alpha_1-1}}{\alpha_2^{\alpha_1}\,\Gamma(\alpha_1)}\,\exp(-\nu/\alpha_2)\,,\,\nu > 0\,.$$

That is, the $N_i(t)$'s are negative binomial processes (Lawless, 1987b). Then one can show that $L_i(\boldsymbol{\theta})$ is equivalent to

$$L_i(\boldsymbol{\theta}) = \frac{\Gamma(\alpha_1+n_{i,m_i})}{\Gamma(\alpha_1)}\,\alpha_2^{-\alpha_1}\,(\mu_i(\boldsymbol{\beta})+\alpha_2^{-1})^{-(n_{i,m_i}+\alpha_1)}\,\prod_{j=1}^{m_i}(\Delta\mu_{i,j}(\boldsymbol{\beta}))^{\Delta n_{i,j}}\,.$$

Define $\mathbf{a}_i^T = (\Delta\mu_{i,1},\ldots,\Delta\mu_{i,m_i})$, $\mathbf{a}^T = (\mathbf{a}_1^T,\ldots,\mathbf{a}_n^T)$,

$$W = \frac{\partial \log L(\boldsymbol{\theta})}{\partial \mathbf{a}} = (W_1^T,\ldots,W_n^T)^T$$

with $W_i = \partial \log L(\boldsymbol{\theta})/\partial \mathbf{a}_i$, and

$$D = \frac{\partial \mathbf{a}}{\partial \boldsymbol{\beta}} = \begin{bmatrix} D_1 \\ \vdots \\ D_n \end{bmatrix} = \begin{bmatrix} \partial \mathbf{a}_1/\partial \boldsymbol{\beta} \\ \vdots \\ \partial \mathbf{a}_n/\partial \boldsymbol{\beta} \end{bmatrix} = \begin{bmatrix} \mathrm{diag}(\mathbf{a}_1)\,\mathbf{X}_1 \\ \vdots \\ \mathrm{diag}(\mathbf{a}_n)\,\mathbf{X}_n \end{bmatrix},$$

where $\mathbf{X}_i = (\mathbf{Z}_i^{*T}(t_{i,1}),\ldots,\mathbf{Z}_i^{*T}(t_{i,m_i}))$. Then we have

$$\log L_i(\boldsymbol{\theta}) \propto I(n_{i,m_i} > 0)\sum_{k=0}^{n_{i,m_i}-1}\log(\alpha_1+k) - \alpha_1\log(\alpha_2)$$

$$- (n_{i,m_i}+\alpha_1)\log\left(\mu_{i,m_i}+\alpha_2^{-1}\right) + \sum_{j=1}^{m_i}\Delta n_{i,j}\log(\Delta\mu_{i,j})\,,$$

$i = 1,\ldots,n$. It follows that the score function $U(\boldsymbol{\beta}) = \partial \log L(\boldsymbol{\theta})/\partial\boldsymbol{\beta}$ has the form

$$U(\boldsymbol{\beta}) = D^T W = \sum_{i=1}^{n} D_i^T W_i$$

$$= \sum_{i=1}^{n} \mathbf{X}_i^T \left(\Delta \mathbf{n}_i - \frac{n_{i,m_i} + \alpha_1}{\mu_{i,m_i} + \alpha_2^{-1}} \mathbf{a}_i \right)$$

since

$$W_{i,j} = \frac{\Delta n_{i,j}}{\Delta \mu_{i,j}} - \frac{n_{i,m_i} + \alpha_1}{\mu_{i,m_i} + \alpha_2^{-1}},$$

where $\Delta \mathbf{n}_i = (\Delta n_{i,1}, \ldots, \Delta n_{i,m_i})^T$. The computation of the score function $U(\boldsymbol{\alpha}) = \partial \log L(\boldsymbol{\theta})/\partial \boldsymbol{\alpha}$ is straightforward.

It follows that one can obtain the maximum likelihood estimators, denoted by $\hat{\boldsymbol{\beta}}_{MPL}$ and $\hat{\boldsymbol{\alpha}}_{MPL}$, of $\boldsymbol{\beta}$ and $\boldsymbol{\alpha}$ by solving the score equations $U(\boldsymbol{\beta}) = 0$ and $U(\boldsymbol{\alpha}) = 0$ together. By the standard maximum likelihood theory, $\hat{\boldsymbol{\beta}}_{MPL}$ and $\hat{\boldsymbol{\alpha}}_{MPL}$ are consistent and have joint asymptotic normal distribution with their covariance matrix consistently estimated by the observed Fisher information matrix. Note that in general, there is no closed form for the integration involved in the likelihood function $L(\boldsymbol{\theta})$ and thus some numerical algorithms have to be used. Some discussions on this can be found in Thall (1988) among others.

2.3.3 An Illustration

To illustrate the maximum likelihood estimation procedures described above, we apply them to a set of current status data arising from a tumorigenicity experiment on multiple incidental tumors. The experiment consists of 99 female and 100 male rats. The observed data, presented in Table 2.1 and reproduced from Ii et al. (1987) and Sun and Kalbfleisch (1993), give the total numbers of the tumors that each rat had developed up to the 10-week interval within which they died. In other words, each animal is observed only once at the death and the death times are given by 10-week intervals. For the convenience, it is assumed below that the observation is at the endpoint of each 10-week interval. The number in the table denotes the number of rats which died in the ith interval and in which k tumors were found. Note that the term incidental means that the presence of such tumors has no effect on the death rate. In other words, the death or observation time is independent of the occurrences of the tumors.

To compare the tumor occurrence rates between female and male rats, let $N_i(t)$ denote the number of tumors that have occurred up to time t for the ith animal and define $Z_i = 1$ if animal i is male and 0 otherwise, $i = 1, \ldots, 199$. Suppose that the $N_i(t)$'s are mixed Poisson processes with the rate function

$$E\{dN_i(t)|Z_i, \nu_i\} = \nu_i \exp(\beta_1 + \beta_2 Z_i) \, dt.$$

2.3 Parametric Maximum Likelihood Estimation of Panel Count Data

Table 2.1. Observed number of k-tumored animals at interval i

		(a) Males k	(b) Females k
Week	Interval i	0 1 2 3 4 5 6 7	0 1 2 3 4 5 6 7
1–10	1		
11–20	2		
21–30	3		
31–40	4	3	
41–50	5	11	9 1
51–60	6		2 1
61–70	7	17 1	12 2
71–80	8	2	
81–90	9	3 1	2
91–100	10	5 3 1	1 1 2 2
101–110	11	5 7 1 2	5 4 1 2
111–120	12	8 5 2 1	9 5 3 1
121–130	13	6 1	1 4 3 3
131–140	14	1 4 1 1	2 5 4 3 1 1
141–150	15	3 2 2 1	1 2 1 3

In the above, the ν_i's are defined as in model (2.11) with the density function $g(\nu; \alpha_1, \alpha_2)$ given in the previous subsection. The application of the maximum likelihood estimation procedure given above yields $\hat{\beta}^*_{MPL,1} = \exp(\hat{\beta}_{MPL,1}) = 0.421$ and $\hat{\beta}_{MPL,2} = -0.601$ with the estimated standard errors of 0.066 and 0.165, respectively. This indicates that the male rats seem to have a significantly lower tumor occurrence rate than the female rates. By assuming $E(\nu_i) = 1$ for all i, we obtain $\hat{\beta}^*_{MPL,1} = 0.120$ and $\hat{\beta}_{MPL,2} = -0.601$ with the estimated standard errors being 0.011 and 0.155, which give the same conclusion.

2.3.4 Discussion

The focus of this section has been on the Poisson process and parametric analysis. It is apparent that it is straightforward to generalize the inference procedures described above to or develop similar parametric inference procedures under different parametric models. Some references on this include Albert (1991), Lawless (1987a), Thall (1988) and Thall and Lachin (1988).

It is well-known that in general, parametric models and analyses should be preferred than nonparametric and semiparametric models and analyses if there is some evidence indicating or suggesting that the parametric models are reasonable or appropriate. In addition to being more efficient, parametric analyses are usually more straightforward than nonparametric and semi-parametric analyses. On the other hand, in many situations, there may not exist such evidence or appropriate parametric models, or there do not exist data or information that can be used to assess the appropriateness of an assumed parametric model. In consequence, one may want to employ or rely on nonparametric and semiparametric models and the corresponding inference procedures. One advantage is that they could avoid making assumptions on parametric models and give more reasonable and/or robust analysis results. It is apparent that these general arguments apply to the analysis of panel count data considered here.

In addition to the two types of procedures mentioned above, sometimes one may prefer a third type of models or procedures or a compromise between the two. One such procedure is described in the next section, which models the baseline rate function $r_0(t)$ in model (1.3) or $r_0(t; \boldsymbol{\beta}_1)$ in model (2.8) by using a piecewise constant function (Lawless and Zhan, 1998). It is obvious that by controlling the number of steps, one can push the resulting analysis procedure more similar to either a parametric procedure or a semiparametric procedure. As another compromise between parametric and semiparametric procedures, instead of using the piecewise step function, one can employ some smooth functions such as monotone splines (Lu et al., 2009). More discussions on this are given below. Of course, as mentioned above, nonparametric and semiparametric procedures for the analysis of panel count data are discussed in later chapters.

2.4 Regression Analysis with Piecewise Models

In this section, we consider the same problem and also the same type of inference procedures in nature as those discussed in the previous section. On the other hand, as mentioned above, the inference procedures to be described can also be regarded as compromises between parametric and semiparametric procedures. Specifically, consider a recurrent event study for which we only observe panel count data. Let the $N_i(t)$'s, $\boldsymbol{Z}_i$'s, $t_{i,j}$'s, m_i's, $n_{i,j}$'s and $\Delta n_{i,j}$'s be defined as in the previous section and suppose that one is mainly interested in estimating the effects of the covariates $\boldsymbol{Z}_i$'s on the $N_i(t)$'s as before.

To describe the effects of the covariates, we assume that there exist i.i.d. latent variables $\{\nu_i\}_{i=1}^n$ with $E(\nu_i) = 1$ and given ν_i and $\boldsymbol{Z}_i$, the rate function of $N_i(t)$ has the form

$$E\{dN_i(t)|\boldsymbol{Z}_i, \nu_i\} = \nu_i\, r_0(t)\, \exp(\boldsymbol{\beta}^T \boldsymbol{Z}_i)\, dt, \tag{2.12}$$

2.4 Regression Analysis with Piecewise Models

$i = 1, \ldots, n$. In the above, $r_0(t)$ denotes an unknown baseline rate function and β is a vector of regression parameters. Furthermore, it is assumed that there exists a prespecified partition $0 = s_0 < \cdots < s_k < \infty$ such that $r_0(t) = \alpha_l$ for $t \in S_l = (s_{l-1}, s_l]$, where the α_l's are unknown constants. That is, the baseline rate function $r_0(t)$ is a step function. It is apparent that the model above can be seen a special case of model (2.11) and implies the proportional rate model (1.3).

For estimation of the regression parameter β in model (2.12), in the following, we consider two inference procedures. First we assume that the $N_i(t)$'s are non-homogeneous Poisson processes and develop the maximum likelihood estimation procedure. A generalized estimating equation procedure is then discussed and followed by an illustration and some discussions.

2.4.1 Likelihood-Based Approach

In this subsection, we assume that the $N_i(t)$'s are non-homogeneous Poisson processes with the rate function given by model (2.12). It follows that we have

$$E\{ N_i(t) | Z_i, \nu_i \} = \nu_i \mu_0(t) \exp(\beta^T Z_i), \qquad (2.13)$$

where $\mu_0(t) = \sum_{l=1}^{k} \alpha_l u_l(t)$ with $u_l(t) = \max\{0, \min(s_l, t) - s_{l-1}\}$, representing the length of the intersection of the two intervals $(0, t]$ and S_l. For each (i, j), define $\mu_{i,j} = \mu_0(t_{i,j}) \exp(\beta^T Z_i)$ and

$$\Delta \mu_{i,j} = \mu_{i,j} - \mu_{i,j-1} = \mu_{0,i,j} \exp(\beta^T Z_i),$$

$j = 1, \ldots, m_i$, $i = 1, \ldots, n$. Here $\mu_{0,i,j} = \sum_{l=1}^{k} \alpha_l u_l(i, j)$ and

$$u_l(i, j) = \max\{ 0, \min(s_l, t_{i,j}) - \max(s_{l-1}, t_{i,j-1}) \},$$

denoting the length of the intersection of the two intervals $(t_{i,j-1}, t_{i,j}]$ and S_l, $l = 1, \ldots, k$. Then under the assumption above, one can easily show that

$$E\{ N_i(t_{i,j}) - N_i(t_{i,j-1}) | Z_i, \nu_i \} = \nu_i \Delta \mu_{i,j}.$$

For the simplicity, we assume that the ν_i's follow the gamma distribution with the density function $g(\nu; \gamma)$ given in Sect. 2.2.1. That is, the ν_i's have the mean one and variance γ. It follows that the likelihood function of β, $\alpha = (\alpha_1, \ldots, \alpha_k)^T$ and γ is proportional to

$$L(\beta, \alpha, \gamma) = \prod_{i=1}^{n} \int_0^{\infty} \prod_{j=1}^{m_i} \exp(-\nu_i \Delta \mu_{i,j}) (\nu_i \Delta \mu_{i,j})^{\Delta n_{i,j}} g(\nu_i; \gamma) \, d\nu_i$$

or

$$L(\boldsymbol{\beta},\boldsymbol{\alpha},\gamma) = \prod_{i=1}^{n} \left(\prod_{j=1}^{m_i} \Delta\mu_{i,j}^{\Delta n_{i,j}} \right) \frac{\Gamma(n_{i,m_i} + 1/\gamma)\,\gamma^{n_{i,m_i}}}{\Gamma(1/\gamma)\,(1 + \gamma\mu_{i,m_i})^{n_{i,m_i}+1/\gamma}}.$$

The resulting log likelihood function has the form

$$l(\boldsymbol{\beta},\boldsymbol{\alpha},\gamma) = \sum_{i=1}^{n} \left\{ \sum_{j=1}^{m_i} (\Delta n_{i,j} \log \Delta\mu_{i,j}) + n_{i,m_i} \log \gamma + \log \Gamma \left(n_{i,m_i} + \frac{1}{\gamma} \right) \right.$$
$$\left. - \log \Gamma \left(\frac{1}{\gamma} \right) - \left(n_{i,m_i} + \frac{1}{\gamma} \right) \log(1 + \gamma\mu_{i,m_i}) \right\}.$$

For the determination of the maximum likelihood estimators of $\boldsymbol{\beta}$, $\boldsymbol{\alpha}$ and γ, we need their score functions, which have the form

$$\frac{\partial l(\boldsymbol{\beta},\boldsymbol{\alpha},\gamma)}{\partial \boldsymbol{\beta}} = \sum_{i=1}^{n} \frac{n_{i,m_i} - \mu_{i,m_i}}{1 + \gamma\mu_{i,m_i}} \boldsymbol{Z}_i, \qquad (2.14)$$

$$\frac{\partial l(\boldsymbol{\beta},\boldsymbol{\alpha},\gamma)}{\partial \alpha_l} = \sum_{i=1}^{n} \sum_{j=1}^{m_i} \frac{(\Delta n_{i,j} - \Delta\mu_{i,j}) u_l(i,j) \exp(\boldsymbol{\beta}^T \boldsymbol{Z}_i)}{\Delta\mu_{i,j}}$$
$$- \sum_{i=1}^{n} \frac{\gamma(n_{i,m_i} - \mu_{i,m_i}) u_l(i,+) \exp(\boldsymbol{\beta}^T \boldsymbol{Z}_i)}{1 + \gamma\mu_{i,m_i}}, \qquad (2.15)$$

and

$$\frac{\partial l(\boldsymbol{\beta},\boldsymbol{\alpha},\gamma)}{\partial \gamma} = \sum_{i=1}^{n} \left\{ \frac{n_{i,m_i} - \mu_{i,m_i}}{\gamma(1 + \gamma\mu_{i,m_i})} + \gamma^{-2} \log(1 + \gamma\mu_{i,m_i}) \right\}$$
$$- \gamma^{-1} \sum_{i=1}^{n} \sum_{s=1}^{n_{i,m_i}} \{1 + \gamma(s-1)\}^{-1},$$

respectively, where $u_l(i,+) = \sum_{j=1}^{m_i} u_j(i,j)$, $l = 1,\ldots,k$. Thus it is natural to solve the score equations

$$\frac{\partial l(\boldsymbol{\beta},\boldsymbol{\alpha},\gamma)}{\partial \boldsymbol{\beta}} = 0,\ \frac{\partial l(\boldsymbol{\beta},\boldsymbol{\alpha},\gamma)}{\partial \alpha_l} = 0,\ \frac{\partial l(\boldsymbol{\beta},\boldsymbol{\alpha},\gamma)}{\partial \gamma} = 0,\ l = 1,\ldots,k$$

together by using, for example, the Newton-Raphson algorithm. As an alternative, one could apply the EM algorithm (Dempster et al., 1977) given below and developed by Lawless and Zhan (1998).

To define the pseudo-complete data, assume that one observes the ν_i's and c_{ijl}, the number of the occurrences of the recurrent event of interest within the intersection of S_l and $(t_{i,j-1}, t_{i,j}]$, $j = 1,\ldots,m_i$, $i = 1,\ldots,n$,

2.4 Regression Analysis with Piecewise Models

$l = 1, \ldots, k$. Define $u_{ijl} = \alpha_l\, u_l(i,j)\, \exp(\boldsymbol{\beta}^T \boldsymbol{Z}_i)$. Then the log likelihood function based on the pseudo-complete data ν_i's and c_{ijl}'s can be written as

$$l_{pl}(\boldsymbol{\beta}, \boldsymbol{\alpha}, \gamma) = l_{pl,1}(\gamma) + l_{pl,2}(\boldsymbol{\beta}, \boldsymbol{\alpha}),$$

where

$$l_{pl,1}(\gamma) = -n\left\{\log \Gamma\left(\frac{1}{\gamma}\right) + \frac{\log \gamma}{\gamma}\right\} + \gamma^{-1} \sum_i (\log \nu_i - \nu_i)$$

and

$$l_{pl,2}(\boldsymbol{\beta}, \boldsymbol{\alpha}) = \sum_{i=1}^n \sum_{j=1}^{m_i} \sum_{l=1}^k c_{ijl} \log u_{ijl} - \sum_{i=1}^n \nu_i\, \mu_{i,m_i}.$$

Denote $\boldsymbol{\theta} = (\boldsymbol{\beta}^T, \boldsymbol{\alpha}^T, \gamma)^T$. The EM algorithm can be carried out as follows.

Step 1. Choose an initial estimator $\boldsymbol{\theta}^{(0)}$.

Step 2. E-step. At the mth iteration, compute

$$l_{pl,1}^{(m)}(\gamma \mid \boldsymbol{\theta}^{(m-1)}) = E\left\{l_{pl,1}(\gamma \mid n'_{i,j}s, \boldsymbol{\theta}^{(m-1)})\right\}$$
$$= -n\left\{\log \Gamma\left(\frac{1}{\gamma}\right) + \frac{\log \gamma}{\gamma}\right\} + \gamma^{-1} \sum_i \left(\widetilde{\log \nu_i}^{(m)} - \widetilde{\nu}_i^{(m)}\right)$$

and

$$l_{pl,2}^{(m)}(\boldsymbol{\beta}, \boldsymbol{\alpha} \mid \boldsymbol{\theta}^{(m-1)}) = E\left\{l_{p,2}(\boldsymbol{\beta}, \boldsymbol{\alpha} \mid n'_{i,j}s, \boldsymbol{\theta}^{(m-1)})\right\}$$
$$= \sum_{i=1}^n \sum_{j=1}^{m_i} \sum_{l=1}^k \widetilde{c}_{ijl}^{(m)} \log u_{ijl} - \sum_{i=1}^n \widetilde{\nu}_i^{(m)} \mu_{i,m_i}.$$

In the above,

$$\widetilde{\log \nu_i}^{(m)} = \Phi(C_{i1}^{(m)}) - \log(C_{i2}^{(m)}),$$

$$\widetilde{\nu}_i^{(m)} = \frac{C_{i1}^{(m)}}{C_{i2}^{(m)}},$$

and

$$\widetilde{c}_{ijl}^{(m)} = \frac{\Delta n_{i,j}\, \alpha_l^{(m-1)}\, u_l(i,j)}{\sum_{b=1}^k \alpha_b^{(m-1)}\, u_b(i,j)},$$

where

$$C_{i1}^{(m)} = n_{i,m_i} + \frac{1}{\gamma^{(m-1)}}, \quad C_{i2}^{(m)} = \mu_{i,m_i}^{(m-1)} + \frac{1}{\gamma^{(m-1)}}$$

and $\Phi(t) = d \log \Gamma(t)/dt$.

Step 3. M-step. Maximize $l_{pl,1}^{(m)}(\gamma \mid \boldsymbol{\theta}^{(m-1)})$ and $l_{pl,2}^{(m)}(\boldsymbol{\beta}, \boldsymbol{\alpha} \mid \boldsymbol{\theta}^{(m-1)})$ with respect to $\boldsymbol{\theta}$ to obtain the estimator $\boldsymbol{\theta}^{(m)}$.

Step 4. Repeat Steps 2 and 3 until the convergence.

To implement the EM algorithm above, one needs to choose an initial estimator $\boldsymbol{\theta}^{(0)}$ and a convergence criterion. For the former, a simple and natural approach is to set $\nu_i = 1$ for all i and the α_l's to be identical in (2.13) and then to employ the resulting estimators as the initial estimators of $\boldsymbol{\beta}$ and $\boldsymbol{\alpha}$. For the parameter γ, one can use the moment estimator given by

$$\frac{1}{n} \sum_{i=1}^n \left\{ \frac{n_{i,m_i}}{\mu_0(t) \exp(\boldsymbol{\beta}^T \boldsymbol{Z}_i)} - 1 \right\}^2$$

with replacing $\mu_0(t)$ and $\boldsymbol{\beta}$ by their initial estimators. In practice, of course, one may want to employ several different initial estimators to hope that they all result in the same final estimators. For the convergence criterion, a common one is to compare the consecutive values of the estimators $\boldsymbol{\theta}^{(m-1)}$ and $\boldsymbol{\theta}^{(m)}$ or the values of the log likelihood function $l_{pl}(\boldsymbol{\beta}, \boldsymbol{\alpha}, \gamma)$ at $\boldsymbol{\theta}^{(m-1)}$ and $\boldsymbol{\theta}^{(m)}$. More specifically, for given positive numbers ϵ_1 and ϵ_2, one can stop the iteration if

$$\max_l |\theta_l^{(m)} - \theta_l^{(m-1)}| \leq \epsilon_1$$

or

$$|l_{pl}(\boldsymbol{\theta}^{(m)}) - l_{pl}(\boldsymbol{\theta}^{(m-1)})| \leq \epsilon_2,$$

where the maximum above is over all components of $\boldsymbol{\theta}$. An alternative, suggested by Lawless and Zhan (1998), is to use

$$\max_l \frac{|\theta_l^{(m)} - \theta_l^{(m-1)}|}{|\theta_l^{(m-1)}| + 10^{-5}} \leq \epsilon_1$$

and

$$\frac{|l_{pl}(\boldsymbol{\theta}^{(m)}) - l_{pl}(\boldsymbol{\theta}^{(m-1)})|}{|l_{pl}(\boldsymbol{\theta}^{(m-1)})| + 10^{-5}} \leq \epsilon_2$$

together.

Let $\hat{\boldsymbol{\theta}}_L = (\hat{\boldsymbol{\beta}}_L^T, \hat{\boldsymbol{\alpha}}_L^T, \hat{\gamma}_L)^T$ denote the maximum likelihood estimator of $\boldsymbol{\theta}$ obtained above. Then it follows from the standard maximum likelihood theory that $\hat{\boldsymbol{\theta}}_L$ is consistent and asymptotically follows a multivariate normal distribution. Furthermore, its covariance matrix can be consistently estimated by the observed Fisher information matrix or the negative second derivative of the log likelihood function $l(\boldsymbol{\beta}, \boldsymbol{\alpha}, \gamma)$ calculated at the maximum likelihood estimator. For this, one can directly find the second derivative or use the EM algorithm (Louis, 1982).

2.4.2 Estimating Equation-Based Approach

As discussed in Sect. 2.2, the Poisson process or mixed Poisson process assumption may not hold in practice, and one way to address it is to employ the estimating equation or generalized estimating equation approach (McCulluagh and Nelder, 1989). The general idea behind the latter approach is to only model the mean function and the covariance matrix of the underlying response process or the recurrent event process, and the resulting estimation procedure is usually robust. Also to follow the idea discussed in Sect. 2.2, for estimation of $\boldsymbol{\beta}$ and $\boldsymbol{\alpha}$, one could directly employ the score functions given in (2.14) and (2.15) and solve the estimating equations

$$\frac{\partial l(\boldsymbol{\beta},\boldsymbol{\alpha},\gamma)}{\partial \boldsymbol{\beta}} = 0 \, , \quad \frac{\partial l(\boldsymbol{\beta},\boldsymbol{\alpha},\gamma)}{\partial \alpha_l} = 0 \, , \, l = 1,\ldots,k$$

while ignoring the mixed Poisson process assumption. In the following, we describe this using the generalized estimating equation theory (McCulluagh and Nelder, 1989).

In this subsection, we use the same notation defined in the previous subsection. Also define $\boldsymbol{Y}_i = (\Delta n_{i,1}, \cdots, \Delta n_{i,m_i})^T$, $\boldsymbol{a}_i = (\Delta \mu_{i,1}, \cdots, \Delta \mu_{i,m_i})^T$ as in Sect. 2.3.2, and $\boldsymbol{b}_i = \text{diag}(\boldsymbol{a}_i)$, $i = 1, \ldots, n$. Then it is easy to see that the covariance matrix of $\boldsymbol{Y}_i$ under the mixed Poisson model specified in the previous subsection has the form

$$\boldsymbol{V}_i = \boldsymbol{b}_i + \gamma\, \boldsymbol{a}_i\, \boldsymbol{a}_i^T \, . \tag{2.16}$$

Now assume that the recurrent event processes $N_i(t)$'s only satisfy (2.13) and (2.16), and let $\boldsymbol{D}_i = \partial \boldsymbol{a}_i/\partial(\boldsymbol{\beta}^T, \boldsymbol{\alpha}^T)$ and $\boldsymbol{S}_i = \boldsymbol{Y}_i - \boldsymbol{a}_i$. Then by following the generalized estimating equation theory, for estimation of $\boldsymbol{\beta}$ and $\boldsymbol{\alpha}$, we have the generalized estimating equations

$$\boldsymbol{U}_1(\boldsymbol{\beta},\boldsymbol{\alpha},\gamma) = \sum_{i=1}^{n} \boldsymbol{D}_i^T \boldsymbol{V}_i^{-1} \boldsymbol{S}_i = 0 \, . \tag{2.17}$$

One can easily show that

$$\boldsymbol{U}_1(\boldsymbol{\beta},\boldsymbol{\alpha},\gamma) = \begin{pmatrix} \frac{\partial l(\boldsymbol{\beta},\boldsymbol{\alpha},\gamma)}{\partial \boldsymbol{\beta}} \\ \frac{\partial l(\boldsymbol{\beta},\boldsymbol{\alpha},\gamma)}{\partial \alpha_1} \\ \cdots \\ \frac{\partial l(\boldsymbol{\beta},\boldsymbol{\alpha},\gamma)}{\partial \alpha_k} \end{pmatrix} \, .$$

That is, the equations defined in (2.17) are the same as those used in the previous subsection for estimation of $\boldsymbol{\beta}$ and $\boldsymbol{\alpha}$. Note that $\boldsymbol{V}_i$ given in (2.16) is a working covariance matrix, which may be correct or may not, and also one may use other forms. For the estimation of $\boldsymbol{\beta}$ and $\boldsymbol{\alpha}$, a simple approach is to adopt (2.16) and solve the Eqs. (2.17) based on a given value of γ such as $\gamma = 0$. Alternatively and more generally, one may want to develop an additional estimating equation for γ and estimate all parameters together.

One such estimating equation for γ is the simple moment equation

$$U_2(\boldsymbol{\beta}, \boldsymbol{\alpha}, \gamma) = \sum_{i=1}^{n} w_i \left\{ (n_{i,m_i} - \mu_{i,m_i})^2 - \sigma_i^2 \right\} = 0, \tag{2.18}$$

suggested by Lawless and Zhan (1998), where

$$\sigma_i^2 = \text{Var}(n_{i,m_i}) = \mu_{i,m_i} + \gamma \mu_{i,m_i}^2$$

and the w_i's are some weights. Some simple choices for the weights include $w_i = 1$, $w_i = 1/\sigma_i^2$ and $w_i = \mu_{i,m_i}^2/\sigma_i^4$. Now one can estimate $\boldsymbol{\beta}$, $\boldsymbol{\alpha}$ and γ by iteratively solving the Eqs. (2.17) and (2.18) as follows.

Step 1. Choose an initial estimator $\boldsymbol{\theta}^{(0)}$.

Step 2. At the mth iteration, obtain the updated estimators of $\boldsymbol{\beta}$ and $\boldsymbol{\alpha}$ as

$$\begin{pmatrix} \boldsymbol{\beta}^{(m)} \\ \boldsymbol{\alpha}^{(m)} \end{pmatrix} = \left\{ \begin{pmatrix} \boldsymbol{\beta} \\ \boldsymbol{\alpha} \end{pmatrix} + \left(\sum_{i=1}^{n} \mathbf{D}_i^T \mathbf{V}_i^{-1} \mathbf{D}_i \right)^{-1} \right.$$
$$\left. \times \left(\sum_{i=1}^{n} \mathbf{D}_i^T \mathbf{V}_i^{-1} \mathbf{S}_i \right) \right\} \bigg|_{\boldsymbol{\beta}=\boldsymbol{\beta}^{(m-1)}, \boldsymbol{\alpha}=\boldsymbol{\alpha}^{(m-1)}, \gamma=\gamma^{(m-1)}}.$$

Step 3. Also at the mth iteration, obtain the updated estimator of γ as

$$\gamma^{(m)} = \gamma^{(m-1)} - \left\{ \left(\frac{\partial U_2}{\partial \gamma} \right)^{-1} U_2 \right\} \bigg|_{\boldsymbol{\beta}=\boldsymbol{\beta}^{(m)}, \boldsymbol{\alpha}=\boldsymbol{\alpha}^{(m)}, \gamma=\gamma^{(m-1)}}.$$

Step 4. Repeat Steps 2 and 3 until the convergence.

It is apparent that the discussion on the selection of initial estimators and the convergence criterion given in the previous subsection applies here. Let $\hat{\boldsymbol{\theta}}_E = (\hat{\boldsymbol{\beta}}_E^T, \hat{\boldsymbol{\alpha}}_E^T, \hat{\gamma}_E)^T$ denote the estimator of $\boldsymbol{\theta}$ defined above. Then it can be shown by using the estimating equation theory that under some mild conditions, $\hat{\boldsymbol{\beta}}_E$ and $\hat{\boldsymbol{\alpha}}_E$ are consistent and their joint distribution can be asymptotically approximated by a multivariate normal distribution (Lawless and Zhan, 1998; Liang and Zeger, 1986; White, 1982). These results hold no matter whether the covariance matrices V_i's specified by (2.16) are correct or not.

For estimation of the covariance matrix of $\hat{\boldsymbol{\beta}}_E$ and $\hat{\boldsymbol{\alpha}}_E$, define

$$\boldsymbol{\Sigma}_n(\boldsymbol{\beta}, \boldsymbol{\alpha}, \gamma) = \begin{pmatrix} \boldsymbol{\Sigma}_{n,11} & \boldsymbol{\Sigma}_{n,12} \\ \boldsymbol{\Sigma}_{n,21} & \boldsymbol{\Sigma}_{n,22} \end{pmatrix}$$

2.4 Regression Analysis with Piecewise Models

and
$$\Gamma_n(\boldsymbol{\beta}, \boldsymbol{\alpha}, \gamma) = \begin{pmatrix} \Gamma_{n,11} & \Gamma_{n,12} \\ \Gamma_{n,21} & \Gamma_{n,22} \end{pmatrix}.$$

In the above,
$$\Sigma_{n,11} = \frac{1}{n} E\left\{-\frac{\partial \mathbf{U}_1}{\partial(\boldsymbol{\beta}^T, \boldsymbol{\alpha}^T)}\right\} = \frac{1}{n} \sum_{i=1}^{n} \mathbf{D}_i^T \mathbf{V}_i^{-1} \mathbf{D}_i$$

$$\Sigma_{n,12} = \frac{1}{n} E\left(-\frac{\partial \mathbf{U}_1}{\partial \gamma}\right) = 0,$$

$$\Sigma_{n,21} = \frac{1}{n} E\left\{-\frac{\partial U_2}{\partial(\boldsymbol{\beta}^T, \boldsymbol{\alpha}^T)}\right\} = \frac{1}{n} \sum_{i=1}^{n} w_i \left(1 + 2\gamma \mu_{i,m_i}\right) \frac{\partial \mu_{i,m_i}}{\partial(\boldsymbol{\beta}^T, \boldsymbol{\alpha}^T)},$$

$$\Sigma_{n,22} = \frac{1}{n} E\left(-\frac{\partial U_2}{\partial \gamma}\right) = \frac{1}{n} \sum_{i=1}^{n} w_i \mu_{i,m_i}^2,$$

$$\Gamma_{n,11} = \frac{1}{n} \sum_{i=1}^{n} \mathbf{D}_i^T \mathbf{V}_i^{-1} \mathbf{S}_i \mathbf{S}_i^T \mathbf{V}_i^{-1} \mathbf{D}_i,$$

$$\Gamma_{n,12} = \frac{1}{n} \sum_{i=1}^{n} w_i \left\{(n_{i,m_i} - \mu_{i,m_i})^2 - \sigma_i^2\right\} \mathbf{D}_i^T \mathbf{V}_i^{-1} \mathbf{S}_i,$$

$$\Gamma_{n,22} = \frac{1}{n} \sum_{i=1}^{n} w_i^2 \left\{(n_{i,m_i} - \mu_{i,m_i})^2 - \sigma_i^2\right\}^2,$$

and $\Gamma_{n,21} = \Gamma_{n,12}^T$. Then if the covariance matrices V_i's specified in (2.16) are correct, one can consistently estimate the asymptotic covariance matrix of $\sqrt{n}\left(\hat{\boldsymbol{\theta}}_E - \boldsymbol{\theta}_0\right)$ by

$$\Sigma_n^{-1}(\hat{\boldsymbol{\beta}}_E^T, \hat{\boldsymbol{\alpha}}_E^T, \hat{\gamma}_E) \Gamma_n(\hat{\boldsymbol{\beta}}_E^T, \hat{\boldsymbol{\alpha}}_E^T, \hat{\gamma}_E) \Sigma_n^{-T}(\hat{\boldsymbol{\beta}}_E^T, \hat{\boldsymbol{\alpha}}_E^T, \hat{\gamma}_E).$$

In the above, $\boldsymbol{\theta}_0$ denotes the true value of $\boldsymbol{\theta}$ and Σ_n^{-T} the transpose of the inverse of the matrix Σ_n. In this case, $\hat{\gamma}_E$ is also consistent.

In general, as mentioned above, the specification given in (2.16) may not be correct. In this case, a robust estimator of the asymptotic covariance matrix of $\hat{\boldsymbol{\beta}}_E$ and $\hat{\boldsymbol{\alpha}}_E$ is given by

$$\Sigma_{n,11}^{-1}(\hat{\boldsymbol{\beta}}_E^T, \hat{\boldsymbol{\alpha}}_E^T, \hat{\gamma}_E) \Gamma_{n,11}(\hat{\boldsymbol{\beta}}_E^T, \hat{\boldsymbol{\alpha}}_E^T, \hat{\gamma}_E) \Sigma_{n,11}^{-T}(\hat{\boldsymbol{\beta}}_E^T, \hat{\boldsymbol{\alpha}}_E^T, \hat{\gamma}_E).$$

To implement both the likelihood-based and estimating equation-based procedures described above, one also needs to choose the number of partitions k and the partition points s_l's. For the selection of the s_l's, a common approach is to choose them such that they divide the observed data evenly. For k, which determines the smoothness of the baseline rate function,

Lawless and Zhan (1998) suggested the range of 4–10 if the main goal is estimation of regression parameters. On the other hand, it is apparent that if one wants a smoother estimator of the baseline rate function, some large k should be used.

2.4.3 An Illustration

To illustrate the two estimation procedures described above, we apply them to the bladder tumor data discussed in Sect. 1.2.3 and given in the data set II of Chap. 9. As mentioned before, this is a set of panel count data arising from 85 patients with superficial bladder tumors. The patients belong to two treatment groups, the placebo (47) and thiotepa (38) groups. In addition to the information on the observation times and the numbers of recurrences of bladder tumors, the observed data also include the information on two baseline covariates. They are the number of initial tumors and the size of the largest initial tumor.

Table 2.2. Estimated covariate effects for the bladder tumor data

	Method I		Method II	
	$\hat{\boldsymbol{\beta}}_L$ (SD)	$\hat{\boldsymbol{\beta}}_E$ (SD)	$\hat{\boldsymbol{\beta}}_L$ (SD)	$\hat{\boldsymbol{\beta}}_E$ (SD)
β_1	−1.2191 (0.399)	−1.1749 (0.317)	−1.2200 (0.403)	−1.2387 (0.326)
β_2	0.3792 (0.109)	0.3716 (0.086)	0.3786 (0.108)	0.3818 (0.088)
β_3	−0.0103 (0.140)	−0.0094 (0.104)	−0.0100 (0.141)	−0.0086 (0.105)

For the analysis, we first define the covariates $\boldsymbol{Z}_i = (Z_{i1}, Z_{i2}, Z_{i3})^T$ such that $Z_{i1} = 1$ if subject i is in the thiotepa treatment group and 0 otherwise, and Z_{i2} and Z_{i3} denote the number of initial tumors and the size of the largest initial tumor, respectively, $i = 1, \ldots, 85$. To apply the two estimation procedures described above, we need to partition the whole observation period. In the following, we consider two methods for this. One, which is referred to as Method I below, is to divide the period $(0, 53]$ into five intervals with the s_l's being 0, 5.5, 15.5, 25.5, 40.5 and 53. The other, referred to as Method II below, is to divide the period $(0, 53]$ into eight intervals with the s_l's equal to 0, 5.5, 10.5, 15.5, 20.5, 25.5, 30.5, 40.5 and 53.

Tables 2.2 and 2.3 present the estimated covariate effects and recurrence rates of bladder tumors, respectively, given by the two estimation procedures. One can see that the results seem to be quite consistent with respect to both the partition method and the estimation procedure. In particular, they suggest that the patients in the thiotepa group seem to have a lower recurrence rate of bladder tumors than the patients in the placebo group. That is, the thiotepa treatment had some significant effects in reducing the recurrence rate of bladder tumors. On the two baseline covariates, the results indicate

2.4 Regression Analysis with Piecewise Models

Table 2.3. Estimated recurrence rates of the bladder tumors

	Method I		Method II	
Interval	$\hat{\alpha}_L$ (SD)	$\hat{\alpha}_E$ (SD)	$\hat{\alpha}_L$ (SD)	$\hat{\alpha}_E$ (SD)
1	0.1329 (0.060)	0.1329 (0.057)	0.1341 (0.061)	0.1338 (0.059)
2	0.0790 (0.036)	0.0791 (0.040)	0.0722 (0.034)	0.0722 (0.038)
3	0.0991 (0.045)	0.0992 (0.047)	0.0895 (0.042)	0.0896 (0.054)
4	0.1053 (0.048)	0.1047 (0.051)	0.0657 (0.033)	0.0658 (0.037)
5	0.0426 (0.023)	0.0424 (0.029)	0.1424 (0.067)	0.1421 (0.073)
6			0.0798 (0.041)	0.0789 (0.042)
7			0.1176 (0.055)	0.1167 (0.061)
8			0.0430 (0.024)	0.0427 (0.029)

that the tumor recurrence rate seems to be positively related to the number of initial tumors, but has no significant correlation with the size of the largest initial tumor. With respect to the estimation of the parameter γ, all approaches suggest that γ is significantly away from zero. That is, the latent variables ν_i's indeed have non-zero variance. For example, the likelihood-based procedure gives $\hat{\gamma}_L = 2.3632$ and 2.3697 with the estimated standard errors of 0.465 and 0.528 with the use of Methods I and II, respectively.

2.4.4 Discussion

As mentioned above, the piecewise model approaches discussed in this section are essentially parametric procedures as those investigated in Sect. 2.3. On the other hand, they are usually more flexible than fully or typical parametric procedures as one can easily change the number of partition points and thus the smoothness of the baseline rate function. The flexibility of the former can also be seen in that it is often regarded as approximate parametric procedures in the sense that the piecewise model simply provides an approximation to the underlying baseline rate function. Among others, Lawless and Zhan (1998) provided some discussion on this. In particular, they showed through a simulation study that the approaches perform well and give stable results about the regression parameters and mean function with respect to the number of partitions or steps used.

Note that instead of the baseline rate function, one can alternatively and equivalently model the baseline mean function using the piecewise constant function. For example, one could start with model (2.13) and assume that $\mu_0(t)$ has the form

$$\mu_0(t) = \sum_{l=1}^{k} \alpha_l I(s_{l-1} < t \leq s_l).$$

That is, it is a step function that jumps only at the time points s_l's. For estimation of regression parameters, one can develop both likelihood-based and estimating equation-based approaches similarly as above.

With respect to the comparison of the two estimation procedures discussed above, it is apparent that the likelihood-based approach should be used if the mixed Poisson process assumption is reasonable. In general, it may be difficult to assess the assumption and thus one may prefer the estimating equation-based approach. Of course, one may also question the appropriateness of another assumption behind both approaches, the piecewise model assumption for the baseline rate function. To relax it, one way is to allow the number of partitions k to change with the sample size n and develop a data-driven procedure for the selection of k. Another general method is to leave the baseline rate function $r_0(t)$ or mean function $\mu_0(t)$ arbitrary and to develop semiparametric estimation procedures, the subject in the following chapters.

2.5 Bibliography, Discussion, and Remarks

In addition to those mentioned above, other references that investigated the problems similar to the ones discussed in this chapter include Hinde (1982) and Breslow (1984), and both considered the log-linear model for the event rate. More specifically, the former developed the maximum likelihood approach when the model error follows a normal distribution, while the latter proposed an iterative reweighted least squares approach. More on these methods can be found in Cameron and Trivedi (1998). As mentioned before, the focus of the book is not about Poisson-based models or parametric inference procedures. On the other hand, it is not difficult to generalize the methods discussed here to more complicated situations. One such situation is that there exists some truncation (Hu and Lawless, 1996), and another one is that the observation process depends on covariates or is informative about the underlying recurrent event process of interest as discussed later.

The Poisson process plays a major role in the parametric inference procedures discussed in this chapter. Some authors have also investigated nonparametric or semiparametric procedures under the Poisson process. For example, Staniswalls et al. (1997) considered the situation where the $N_i(t)$'s are mixed Poisson processes and the rate function satisfies model (2.12) with the baseline rate function $r_0(t)$ completely unspecified. For inference, they employed some smoothing techniques and the generalized profile likelihood method (Severini and Wong, 1992) for estimation of the baseline rate function and regression parameters, respectively. Also one can find some discussion about the comparison of parametric and semiparametric inference procedures in Staniswalls et al. (1997). In particular, they showed through an example that as expected, the parametric approach may not fully capture some patterns of the underlying rate function. In contrast, the semiparametric approach can

2.5 Bibliography, Discussion, and Remarks

provide substantive insights that would not be revealed by the parametric approach. More discussions on the nonparametric and semiparametric methods developed under the Poisson process assumption for the analysis of panel count data are given in both Chaps. 3 and 5.

It is worth to emphasize again that throughout the chapter, it has been assumed that the observation process or the process generating the observation times $t_{i,j}$'s is independent of the recurrent event process $N_i(t)$ of interest. As discussed before and also again in later chapters, this may not be true sometimes and in this situation, the methods described above would give biased results. In other words, some new inference procedures are needed.

3
Nonparametric Estimation

3.1 Introduction

This chapter discusses one-sample analysis of panel count data with the focus on nonparametric estimation of the mean function of the underlying recurrent event process. As discussed above, one main objective of recurrent event studies is to investigate the recurrence pattern or shape of the recurrent event of interest. Although not completely determining the underlying process, the mean function does provide some insights about the recurrence patterns or shapes. Also it can be used for a graphical presentation of the underlying process as survival functions for failure time processes. Of course, it would be ideal to estimate the corresponding intensity process, but as discussed before, this is not possible for panel count data in general without some restrictive assumptions.

Consider a recurrent event study that involves n independent subjects from a homogeneous population and in which each subject gives rise to a counting process $N_i(t)$. Suppose that only panel count data are available for the $N_i(t)$'s. Specifically, let $0 < t_{i,1} < \cdots < t_{i,m_i}$ denote the observation time points for subject i and define $n_{i,j} = N_i(t_{i,j})$, the observed value of $N_i(t)$ at time $t_{i,j}$, $j = 1, \ldots, m_i$, $i = 1, \ldots, n$. That is, subject i is observed m_i times and the observed data are

$$\{ (t_{i,j}, n_{i,j}) \, ; \, j = 1, \ldots, m_i, i = 1, \ldots, n \} \, . \tag{3.1}$$

Define $\mu(t) = E\{ N_i(t) \}$, the mean function of the processes N_i's, and suppose that the goal is to estimate $\mu(t)$. To motivate the general estimation procedures described below, first assume that we have a simple situation where $m_1 = \cdots = m_n = m$ and $t_{i,j} = s_j$ for all j and i. That is, all study subjects have the same number of observations and the same observation time points. This can occur if all subjects follow exactly a prespecified observation schedule. In this case, it is easy to see that one can estimate only the values of the mean function $\mu(t)$ at $s_1 < \cdots < s_m$ and a natural and simple estimator of $\mu(s_j)$ is given by

$$\hat{\mu}(s_j) = \frac{1}{n}\sum_{i=1}^{n} n_{i,j} = \frac{1}{n}\sum_{i=1}^{n} N_i(s_j), \qquad (3.2)$$

the sample mean at s_j, $j = 1, \ldots, m$. In reality, of course, real observation numbers and times tend to differ from subject to subject, and thus the question of interest is how to generalize the sample mean estimator described above.

In Sect. 3.2, we first discuss some likelihood-based procedures for nonparametric estimation of the mean function $\mu(t)$. In particular, we describe an estimator that is derived under the non-homogeneous Poisson process assumption. The estimator applies to more general situations and is consistent without the Poisson assumption. Section 3.3 presents an isotonic regression-based estimator, which can be seen as a direct generalization of the sample mean estimator given in (3.2) and is derived without the use of the Poisson assumption. A key advantage of the estimator is its simplicity and it can be relatively easily determined. In Sect. 3.4, we generalize the isotonic regression estimator by applying the generalized least squares method. The new class of estimators allow more flexibility and could be more efficient depending on the selection of appropriate weight functions.

In addition to estimating mean functions, sometimes one may also be interested in estimating the rate function of an underlying recurrent event process. It is well-known that the rate function could reveal some aspects of the process that cannot be seen from the mean function. Also one could directly derive an estimator of the mean function based on an estimated rate function. Section 3.5 discusses several simple procedures for nonparametric estimation of the rate function. In Sect. 3.6, we give some bibliographic notes and discuss some issues and open problems that are not touched in the previous sections. In this chapter, as in Chap. 2, we assume that the observation process or the process generating the observation times $t_{i,j}$'s is independent of the underlying recurrent event process.

3.2 Likelihood-Based Estimation of the Mean Function

Let the $N_i(t)$'s and $\mu(t)$ be defined as above and suppose that the observed data have the form (3.1). In the following, we first present the nonparametric maximum likelihood estimator of the mean function $\mu(t)$ derived under the non-homogeneous Poisson assumption on the $N_i(t)$'s. The estimator can be applied to more general situations and was first studied by Wellner and Zhang (2000). A couple of other likelihood-based estimators, also under the Poisson process assumption, are then briefly discussed.

3.2 Likelihood-Based Estimation of the Mean Function

3.2.1 Non-homogeneous Poisson Process-Based Estimator

To derive the non-homogeneous Poisson-based estimator of $\mu(t)$, we need to pretend that the $N_i(t)$'s are non-homogeneous Poisson processes. Then the resulting log full likelihood function is proportional to

$$l(\mu) = \sum_{i=1}^{n} \sum_{j=1}^{m_i} (n_{i,j} - n_{i,j-1}) \log\{\mu(t_{i,j}) - \mu(t_{i,j-1})\} - \sum_{i=1}^{n} \mu(t_{i,m_i}),$$

where $t_{i,0} = 0$ and $n_{i,0} = 0$, and it is natural to estimate $\mu(t)$ by maximizing $l(\mu)$. Let $s_1 < \ldots < s_m$ denote the ordered distinct observation times in the set $\{t_{i,j} : j = 1, \ldots, m_i, \; i = 1, \ldots, n\}$. Also let $b_l = \sum_{i=1}^{n} I(t_{i,m_i} = s_l)$ for $l = 1, \ldots, m$ and

$$\tilde{n}_{l,l'} = \sum_{i=1}^{n} \sum_{j=1}^{m_i} (n_{i,j} - n_{i,j-1}) I(t_{i,j} = s_l, t_{i,j-1} = s_{l'}),$$

for $0 \leq l' < l \leq m$, where $s_0 = 0$. Then the log likelihood function $l(\mu)$ can be rewritten as

$$l(\mu) = \sum_{l'=0}^{m-1} \sum_{l=l'+1}^{m} \tilde{n}_{l,l'} \log\{\mu(s_l) - \mu(s_{l'})\} - \sum_{l=1}^{m} b_l \mu(s_l). \qquad (3.3)$$

It is apparent that only the values of $\mu(t)$ at the s_l's can be estimated. This suggests that one can define the nonparametric maximum likelihood estimator (NPMLE) of $\mu(t)$, denoted by $\hat{\mu}_F(t)$, as the non-decreasing step function with possible jumps only at the s_l's that maximizes (3.3). Thus the maximization of $l(\mu)$ over functions $\mu(t)$ becomes maximizing $l(\mu)$ over m-dimensional parameter vectors $\boldsymbol{\mu} = (\mu_1, \ldots, \mu_m)^T$ with $\mu_1 \leq \ldots \leq \mu_m$, where $\mu_l = \mu(s_l)$, $l = 1, \ldots, m$. Of course, other definitions for $\hat{\mu}_F(t)$ between the s_l's can be used too. Also it can be easily seen that there is no closed solution for the maximizer of $l(\mu)$.

For the determination of $\hat{\mu}_F(t)$, for $l = 1, \ldots, m$, define

$$\phi_l(\boldsymbol{\mu}) = \frac{\partial l(\boldsymbol{\mu})}{\partial \mu_l}, \quad \phi_{ll}(\boldsymbol{\mu}) = \frac{\partial^2 l(\boldsymbol{\mu})}{\partial \mu_l^2}.$$

Also define

$$\Delta_{l,l'}(\boldsymbol{\mu}) = \frac{\sum_{j=l'}^{l} \{\phi_j(\boldsymbol{\mu}) - \mu_j \phi_{jj}(\boldsymbol{\mu})\}}{\sum_{j=l'}^{l} \{-\phi_{jj}(\boldsymbol{\mu})\}},$$

$1 \leq l' \leq l \leq m$. Let $\hat{\mu}_{F,l} = \hat{\mu}_F(s_l)$, $l = 1, \ldots, m$. By using the Fenchel duality theorem, it can be shown that $\hat{\boldsymbol{\mu}}_F = (\hat{\mu}_{F,1}, \ldots, \hat{\mu}_{F,m})^T$ satisfies

$$\sum_{l=1}^{m} \phi_l(\hat{\boldsymbol{\mu}}_F) \hat{\mu}_{F,l} = 0$$

and

$$\sum_{j=l}^{m} \phi_l(\hat{\boldsymbol{\mu}}_F) \leq 0$$

for all $l = 1, \ldots, m$. From these, Wellner and Zhang (2000) give the following iterative convex minorant algorithm. Let $\epsilon > 0$ be a prespecified number.
Step 1. Choose an initial estimator $\boldsymbol{\mu}_F^{(0)} = (\mu_{F,1}^{(0)}, \ldots, \mu_{F,m}^{(0)})^T$.
Step 2. At the kth iteration, obtain the updated estimator by

$$\mu_{F,l}^{(k)} = \max_{j' \leq l} \min_{j \geq l} \Delta_{j,j'}(\boldsymbol{\mu}_F^{(k-1)}), l = 1, \ldots, m,$$

where $\boldsymbol{\mu}_F^{(k-1)} = (\mu_{F,1}^{(k-1)}, \ldots, \mu_{F,m}^{(k-1)})^T$ denotes the estimator from the $(k-1)$th iteration.
Step 3. If

$$\left| \sum_{l=1}^{m} \phi_l(\boldsymbol{\mu}_F^{(k)}) \mu_{F,l}^{(k)} \right| > \epsilon$$

or

$$\max_{1 \leq l \leq m} \sum_{j=l}^{m} \phi_l(\boldsymbol{\mu}_F^{(k)}) > \epsilon,$$

return to Step 2. Otherwise stop and set $\hat{\mu}_{F,l} = \mu_{F,l}^{(k)}$.

To implement the iterative convex minorant algorithm described above, one needs to choose an initial estimator and for this, one choice is the sample mean of available observations at each observation time point. Note that although the algorithm described above works well in many applications, sometimes the resulting estimator may not be the globe maximizer. More discussion on this can be found in Wellner and Zhang (2000). As mentioned above, although the estimator $\hat{\mu}_F(t)$ is derived under the non-homogeneous Poisson process assumption, it is consistent and can be applied without the assumption. If the Poisson process assumption does hold, one can expect that the NPMLE should be efficient, but for other situations, it may not be efficient. Also it is easy to see that the determination of the NPMLE may not be easy in computation. More comments on these are given in the next section.

3.2.2 Other Likelihood-Based Estimators

As discussed above, the NPMLE has the advantage that it could be efficient if the underlying recurrent event process is indeed a non-homogeneous Poisson process. On the other hand, it does have some shortcomings. To address

3.2 Likelihood-Based Estimation of the Mean Function

these shortcomings, in this subsection, we briefly introduce two other Poisson process-based estimators of the mean function $\mu(t)$.

First as in the previous subsection, we still pretend that the $N_i(t)$'s are non-homogeneous Poisson processes. Let S_l denote the set of the indices of the subjects who are observed at s_l and define $w_l = |S_l|$, the number of elements in S_l. Instead of the log likelihood function $l(\mu)$, consider the log likelihood function

$$l_p(\mu) = \sum_{i=1}^{n} \sum_{j=1}^{m_i} \{ n_{i,j} \log \mu(t_{i,j}) - \mu(t_{i,j}) \} = \sum_{l=1}^{m} w_l \left(\bar{n}_l \log \mu_l - \mu_l \right), \quad (3.4)$$

where $\bar{n}_l = \sum_{i \in S_l} N_i(s_l)/w_l$, the average of all observations made at time s_l. It is not hard to see that $l_p(\mu)$ is not a real likelihood function, but the likelihood function if one ignores the dependency of $\{N_i(t_{ij}), j = 1, \ldots, m_i\}$ for each i. Wellner and Zhang (2000) call it the log pseudo-likelihood function of $\mu(t)$ and the resulting estimator as the nonparametric maximum pseudo-likelihood estimator (NPMPLE). It will be seen that the estimator given by $l_p(\mu)$ can be easily determined and furthermore, it actually has a closed form. The detailed discussion on this is given in the next section.

It is well-known that although it is handy, the Poisson process assumption may be restrictive in practice and it would be more realistic to relax it or employ some general processes. As discussed in Chap. 2, one such process that is commonly used is the mixed Poisson or negative binomial process. Specifically, for subject i, assume that there exists a gamma-frailty random variable $\nu_i \sim \text{Gamma}(\alpha, 1/\alpha)$, and given ν_i, $N_i(t)$ is a non-homogeneous Poisson process with the mean function

$$E\{ N_i(t) | \nu_i \} = \nu_i \mu(t).$$

It is easy to see that $E(\nu_i) = 1$ and $E\{ N_i(t) \} = \mu(t)$. To estimate $\mu(t)$ based on the panel count data (3.1), Zhang and Jamshidian (2003) suggested to treat the data as cluster data and the counts within each cluster or from the same subject being independent. Among others, Lawless (1987b) and Thall (1988) considered the same approach.

Under these assumptions, one can show that the $n_{i,j}$'s follow the negative binomial distribution and the resulting likelihood function has the form

$$L_n(\mu) = \prod_{i=1}^{n} \prod_{j=1}^{m_i} \left[\frac{\Gamma(n_{i,j} + \alpha^{-1})}{\Gamma(\alpha^{-1})} \frac{\{\alpha \mu(t_{i,j})\}^{n_{i,j}}}{n_{i,j}! \{1 + \alpha \mu(t_{i,j})\}^{n_{i,j} + \alpha^{-1}}} \right].$$

Zhang and Jamshidian (2003) proposed to estimate $\mu(t)$ by maximizing the likelihood function above and developed an EM-algorithm for the maximization. Furthermore, they show through simulation that as the NPMLE, the estimator defined above also applies to more general situations and could be more efficient than the NPMPLE. On the other hand, also as the NPMLE, the determination of the new estimator is more involved numerically than that of the NPMLE. In addition, the theoretical study of its asymptotic behavior is not easy.

3.3 Isotonic Regression-Based Estimation of the Mean Function

In this section, we present a new and different estimator, the isotonic regression estimator (IRE), of the mean function $\mu(t)$. The key idea behind the IRE is to directly generalize the sample mean estimator defined in (3.2) by applying the isotonic regression technique. Unlike the NPMLE, it does not need the Poisson process assumption and was first proposed by Sun and Kalbfleisch (1995). In the following, we first introduce the IRE and then present two illustrative examples for both the NPMLE and IRE. Some discussion on the two estimators is then followed.

3.3.1 Isotonic Regression Estimator

To describe the isotonic regression estimator, we start with a simple situation, but more general than the case discussed in Sect. 3.1. Specifically, suppose that all subjects have the same observation time points but the numbers of observations may be different. That is, we have $t_{i,j} = s_j$ for all $i = 1, \ldots, n$ and $j = 1, \ldots, m_i$ with $m_i \leq m$. This can be the case in a follow-up study in which all subjects follow exactly the prespecified observation schedule except that some may drop out of the study early. For the case, it is easy to see that a natural generalization of the estimator (3.2) is to estimate $\mu(s_l)$ by

$$\frac{\sum_{i=1}^{n} I(s_l \leq s_{m_i}) N_i(s_l)}{\sum_{i=1}^{n} I(s_l \leq s_{m_i})} = \frac{\sum_{i=1}^{n} I(s_l \leq s_{m_i}) n_{i,l}}{\sum_{i=1}^{n} I(s_l \leq s_{m_i})},$$

the sample mean of observed values of the $N_i(s_l)$'s from the subjects still under study. One can easily show that the sample mean or estimator above can be rewritten as

$$\sum_{j=1}^{l} \frac{\sum_{i=1}^{n} I(s_j \leq t_{i,m_i}) \{ N_i(s_j) - N_i(s_{j-1}) \}}{\sum_{i=1}^{n} I(s_j \leq t_{i,m_i})}$$

or

$$\int_{0}^{s_l} \frac{\sum_{i=1}^{n} I(s \leq t_{i,m_i}) \, dN_i(s)}{\sum_{i=1}^{n} I(s \leq t_{i,m_i})} . \tag{3.5}$$

The latter is the Nelson-Aalen estimator given in (1.5) (Andersen et al., 1993).

3.3 Isotonic Regression-Based Estimation of the Mean Function

Now we consider the situation where subjects may not have identical observation times. In this case, the estimator given above is not available. However, we can still define the sample mean at each time point s_l based on available observations. But, unlike the simple situation above, this approach may give an estimator that does not share the non-decreasing property of $\mu(t)$. To fix this, let w_l and $\bar{n}_l$ denote the number and mean value, respectively, of the observations made at s_l, $l = 1,\ldots,m$. The IRE, denoted by $\hat{\boldsymbol{\mu}}_I = (\hat{\mu}_{I,1},\ldots,\hat{\mu}_{I,m})^T$, of $\mu(t)$ at the s_l's is defined as $\boldsymbol{\mu} = (\mu_1,\ldots,\mu_m)^T$ that minimizes the weighted sum of squares

$$L_I(\mu) = \sum_{l=1}^m w_l\,(\bar{n}_l - \mu_l)^2 \tag{3.6}$$

subject to the order restriction $\mu_1 \leq \cdots \leq \mu_m$ (Sun and Kalbfleisch, 1995). Given $\hat{\boldsymbol{\mu}}_I$, the IRE of $\mu(t)$ denoted by $\hat{\mu}_I(t)$ can be defined as the non-decreasing step function with possible jumps only at the s_l's and $\hat{\mu}_I(s_l) = \hat{\mu}_{I,l}$, $l = 1,\ldots,m$.

The estimator $\hat{\boldsymbol{\mu}}_I$ defined above is in fact the isotonic regression of $\{\bar{n}_1,\ldots,\bar{n}_m\}$ with weights $\{w_1,\ldots,w_m\}$ (Robertson et al., 1988). It follows from the isotonic regression theory that the IRE $\hat{\boldsymbol{\mu}}_I$ actually has a closed form given by

$$\hat{\mu}_{I,l} = \max_{r \leq l} \min_{s \geq l} \frac{\sum_{v=r}^s w_v \bar{n}_v}{\sum_{v=r}^s w_v} = \min_{s \geq l} \max_{r \leq l} \frac{\sum_{v=r}^s w_v \bar{n}_v}{\sum_{v=r}^s w_v}$$

using the max-min formula (Barlow et al., 1972; Robertson et al., 1988). In practice, several algorithms such as the pool-adjacent-violators and the up-and-down algorithms can be used to determine $\hat{\boldsymbol{\mu}}_I$. Obviously if $\bar{n}_1 \leq \cdots \leq \bar{n}_m$, $\hat{\mu}_{I,l} = \bar{n}_l$, $l = 1,\ldots,m$, and for the simple situation discussed above, the IRE reduces to the Nelson-Aalen estimator (3.5).

It can be shown that the minimization of (3.6) is equivalent to the maximization of $l_p(\mu)$ given in (3.4) (Robertson et al., 1988; Wellner and Zhang, 2000). In other words, the IRE is the same as the NPMPLE. Furthermore, the IRE is also the same as the NPMLE if each subject is observed only once as in cross-sectional or some reliability studies. That is, $m_i = 1$, $i = 1,\ldots,n$, or we have current status data. In this case, it is easy to see that the two likelihood functions $l(\mu)$ and $l_p(\mu)$ are identical.

3.3.2 Illustrations

Now we illustrate the NPMLE and IRE using the two examples discussed in Sect. 1.2. First we apply the two methods to the panel count data arising from the reliability study of nuclear plants described in Sect. 1.2.1 and then the gallstone data in Sect. 1.2.2. Note that the first set of panel count data is really current status data and thus the two approaches give the same estimators.

For the reliability data, as mentioned before, they concern the loss of feedwater flow in nuclear plants and consist of 30 observations from 30 plants, one observation per plant. One can see from Table 1.3 that there are a total of 10 different observation time points, giving $m = 10$. Assume that the numbers of the losses of feedwater flow for all 30 nuclear plants follow the same counting process. To determine the IRE of the mean or average number of losses of feedwater flow based on the observed data, we first calculate the w_l's and $\bar{n}_l$'s. That is, we need to obtain the number of observations and the sample mean of the numbers of the observed losses of feedwater flow at each observation time point. Figure 3.1 presents the IRE of the average number of losses of feedwater flow given by the max-min formula. As mentioned above, for the data, the NPMLE and IRE are identical. The figure suggests that the loss of feedwater flow seems to increase linearly during the first and third 4-year periods but it does not seem to occur during the second 4-year period. For comparison and understanding the IRE, Fig. 3.1 also includes the sample means, the dots, of the numbers of observed losses ($\bar{n}_l$ vs s_l). It can be clearly seen that the IRE is obtained by pooling the $\bar{n}_l$'s according to the order restriction.

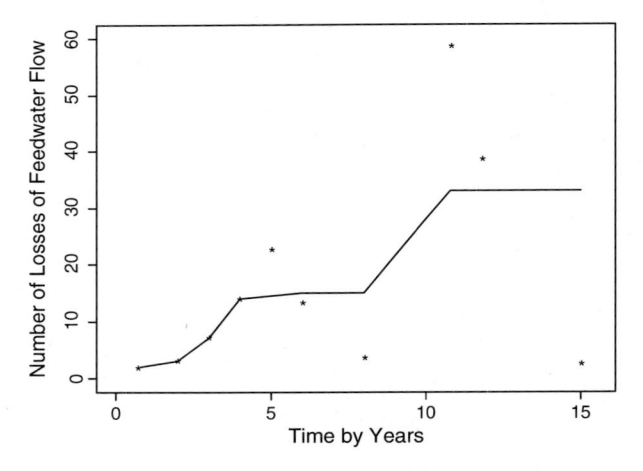

Fig. 3.1. IRE of the average number of losses of feedwater flow

Now we consider the gallstone data, and as mentioned above, one of the primary objectives of the study is to assess the impact of the treatments on the incidence of digestive symptoms commonly associated with the gallstone disease. The data contain the observed information on nausea, one of the symptoms commonly associated with the gallstone disease and whose occurrence incidences may depend on or be related to the treatment. Figure 3.2 displays the estimated average cumulative numbers of the occurrences of nausea for the patients in the placebo and high dose groups, respectively, obtained by using the NPMLE and IRE. These estimators indicate that the patients in the placebo group seem to have higher incidences of nausea than those in the high dose group over the first 40 weeks. Most of this difference seems due to an early difference over the first 10 weeks. After 40 weeks, the incidence of nausea for the patients in the high dose group seems to catch up that for those in the placebo group. A possible reason for this is that the treatment, cheno, may only have short-term effects.

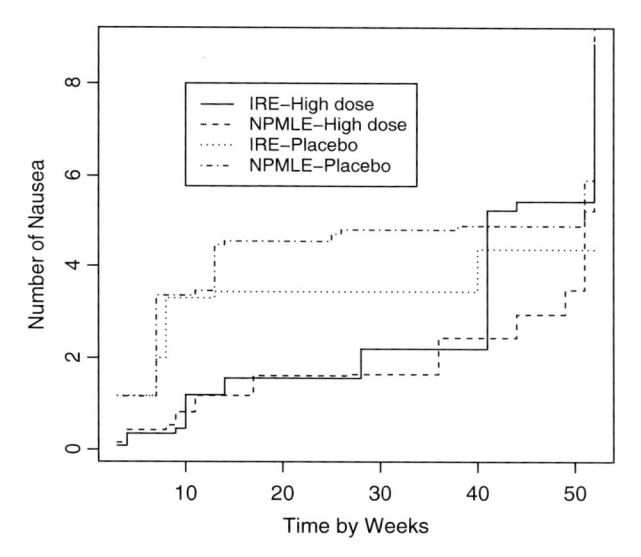

Fig. 3.2. Estimators of the average cumulative counts of episodes of nausea

It is interesting to note that for the patients in the high dose group, the NPMLE and IRE are quite close to each other, especially for the period of the first 40 weeks. In contrast, the two estimators for those in the placebo group differ and the NPMLE gives a higher estimate of the incidence of nausea. Also one can see from the figure that the incidence rate for the patients in the high dose group seems to change gradually, while the incidence rate for the patients in the placebo group seems to change relatively less. More comments on this are given below from the point of the estimated rate functions.

By looking at the data carefully, one can see that there exist several patients who seem to have experienced relatively larger numbers of nausea than the others. Specifically, there are four in the high dose group (patients 13, 25, 50 and 57) and three in the placebo group (patients 78, 89 and 109). To see their effects on the estimation, Fig. 3.3 gives the IRE of the average cumulative numbers of the occurrences of nausea for the patients in the placebo and high dose groups, respectively, based on the reduced data, the data after removing these seven patients. For comparison, it also includes the IRE based

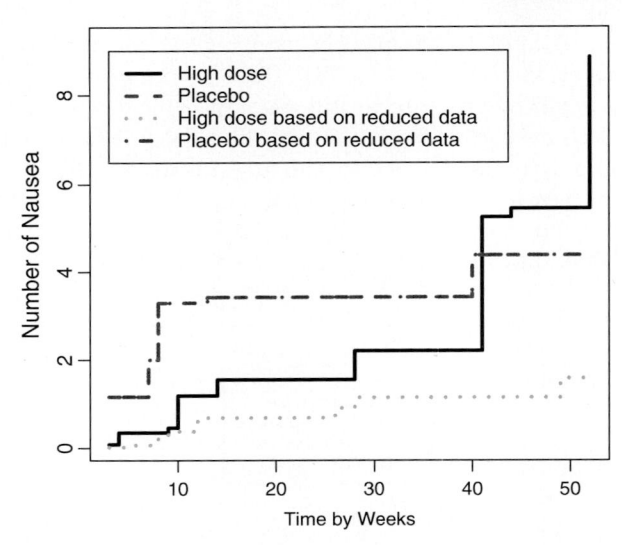

Fig. 3.3. IRE of the average cumulative counts of episodes of nausea based on reduced data

on the whole data given in Fig. 3.2. One can see that the two estimators for the placebo group are basically identical. On the other hand, the new estimator for the high dose group suggests a higher occurrence rate of nausea than the old one, although the difference may not be significant.

3.3.3 Discussion

So far we have discussed four nonparametric estimators of the mean function $\mu(t)$ of the recurrent event process of interest in this chapter and some comments and discussion on their comparison are clearly needed. As pointed out above, the NPMPLE and IRE are actually the same although they are derived from different points of view. In terms of the comparison with the IRE, the other likelihood-based estimator discussed in Sect. 3.2.2 is similar to the NPMLE and thus in the following, we focus on the NPMLE and IRE only.

If the underlying recurrent event process of interest is indeed a non-homogeneous Poisson process, it is easy to see that the NPMLE should be more efficient than the IRE in general. Wellner and Zhang (2000) show through simulation that this could be true even when the recurrent event process is some other counting processes. A disadvantage of the NPMLE is that its implementation is much more involved in terms of programming and requires much more computing time than that of the IRE. In general, one may want to use the IRE if the main interest is to have a general idea about the shape of the mean function $\mu(t)$, or when the number of observations for each subject is small. The NPMLE should be used if efficiency is the main concern.

With respect to the asymptotic properties of the NPMLE and IRE, Wellner and Zhang (2000) prove that under some regularity conditions, both estimators are consistent in L_2. Furthermore, for fixed t, both $n^{1/3}\{\hat{\mu}_F(t) - \mu(t)\}$ and $n^{1/3}\{\hat{\mu}_I(t) - \mu(t)\}$ converge in distribution to the maximum point of a two-sided Brownian motion process multiplied by some constants. Discussion about this limit distribution can be found in Groeneboom and Wellner (2001). Note that these asymptotic results do not rely on the non-homogeneous Poisson assumption. However, the asymptotic properties of the other estimator discussed in Sect. 3.2.2 are still unknown.

Finally we remark that all methods discussed above are similar in that they all directly estimate the mean function $\mu(t)$, which needs to take into account the monotonic property of $\mu(t)$. An alternative is to estimate the rate function $d\mu(t)$ first and then to estimate $\mu(t)$ by the integral of the rate function estimator. Among others, Thall and Lachin (1988) considered this approach and more discussion on this is given below.

3.4 Generalized Isotonic Regression-Based Estimation of the Mean Function

As discussed above, one of the main advantages of the IRE is its simplicity. However, it may not be efficient in general. To address this, in this section, we present a class of estimators that are generalizations of the IRE, which will be referred to as the generalized isotonic regression estimator (GIRE). The estimators were first investigated by Hu et al. (2009a), who also refer them as generalized least squares monotonic estimators.

3.4.1 Generalized Isotonic Regression Estimators

Again let the $N_i(t)$'s and $\mu(t)$ be defined as above and suppose that the observed data have the form (3.1). Also let the s_l's and S_l be defined as before. To present the GIRE, first note that we can rewrite the function $L_I(\mu)$ given in (3.6) as

$$L_I(\mu) = \sum_{l=1}^{m}\sum_{i\in S_l}\{n_{i,l} - \mu(s_l)\}^2 - \sum_{l=1}^{m}\sum_{i\in S_l}\{n_{i,l} - \bar{n}_l\}^2$$
$$= \sum_{i=1}^{n}\sum_{j=1}^{m_i}\{n_{i,j} - \mu(t_{i,j})\}^2 - \sum_{l=1}^{m}\sum_{i\in S_l}\{n_{i,l} - \bar{n}_l\}^2.$$

This suggests that the minimization of $L_I(\mu)$ is equivalent to the minimization of

$$L_I^*(\mu) = \sum_{i=1}^n \sum_{j=1}^{m_i} \{n_{i,j} - \mu(t_{i,j})\}^2 = \sum_{i=1}^n \sum_{j=1}^{m_i} \{N_i(t_{i,j}) - \mu(t_{i,j})\}^2 \,,$$

which would give the least squares estimator of $\boldsymbol{\mu} = (\mu(s_1), \ldots, \mu(s_m))^T = (\mu_1, \ldots, \mu_m)^T$ without considering the order restriction.

For estimation of $\mu(t)$ or $\boldsymbol{\mu}$, motivated by $L_I^*(\mu)$ and the weighted least squares estimation, it is natural to consider the following weighted least squares function

$$L_{GI}(\mu|\boldsymbol{W}) = \sum_{i=1}^n \sum_{j_1=1}^{m_i} \sum_{j_2=1}^{m_i} w(t_{i,j_1}, t_{i,j_2}) \{N_i(t_{i,j_1}) - \mu(t_{i,j_1})\} \{N_i(t_{i,j_2} - \mu(t_{i,j_2})\}$$

$$= \sum_{i=1}^n \sum_{j_1=1}^{m_i} \sum_{j_2=1}^{m_i} w(t_{i,j_1}, t_{i,j_2}) \{n_{i,j_1} - \mu(t_{i,j_1})\} \{n_{i,j_2} - \mu(t_{i,j_2})\} \,.$$

Here $\boldsymbol{W} = \{w(s_j, s_l)\}$ is a given $m \times m$ symmetric weight matrix or function. Let $\hat{\boldsymbol{\mu}}_{GI} = (\hat{\mu}_{GI,1}, \ldots, \hat{\mu}_{GI,m})^T$ denote the value of $\boldsymbol{\mu}$ that minimizes $L_{GI}(\mu)$ subject to the order restriction $\mu_1 \leq \cdots \leq \mu_m$. As $\hat{\mu}_I(t)$, we define the GIRE, denoted by $\hat{\mu}_{GI}(t)$, of $\mu(t)$ as the non-decreasing step function with possible jumps only at the s_l's and $\hat{\mu}_{GI}(s_l) = \hat{\mu}_{GI,l}$, $l = 1, \ldots, m$. It is apparent that if taking $\boldsymbol{W} = I_{m \times m}$, the identity matrix, we have $L_{GI}(\mu|\boldsymbol{W}) = L_I^*(\mu)$ and the GIRE $\hat{\mu}_{GI}(t)$ reduces to the IRE $\hat{\mu}_I(t)$.

The GIRE gives a class of estimators of the mean function $\mu(t)$ depending on the selection of the weight matrix $\boldsymbol{W}$ and in theory, any symmetric matrix could be used. On the other hand, it is apparent that some weight matrices yield more efficient estimators than others. To determine the weight matrix that may result in a better estimator, note that by using the identity matrix, the resulting estimator, the IRE, treats the observed counts $n_{i,j}$'s equally. Also it makes use of only the information given by the counts themselves, not the correlation or relationship among them. This suggests the following two simple choices for the weight matrix.

The first one, again motivated by the weighted least squares estimation, is to take $\boldsymbol{W} = \boldsymbol{W}_1$, where $\boldsymbol{W}_1$ is a diagonal matrix with different diagonal elements $w(s_j, s_j)$'s. In this case, $L_{GI}(\mu|\boldsymbol{W})$ becomes a weighted least squares function and a well-known choice for them is to take $w(s_j, s_j)$ to be the inverse of the variance of $n_{i,j}$ or its approximation. A specific choice is to let $w(s_j, s_j) = 1/\mu(s_j)$, motivated by the fact that $\mu(t)$ is the variance of $N_i(t)$ if $N_i(t)$ is a Poisson process. To minimize $L_{GI}(\mu|\boldsymbol{W})$ with such weight matrix, Hu et al. (2009a) suggest to use the following iterative algorithm. Given $\hat{\mu}_{GI}^{(k-1)}(t)$ from the $(k-1)$ iteration, take $w^{(k)}(s_j, s_j) = 1/\hat{\mu}_{GI}^{(k-1)}(s_j)$ and minimize $L_{GI}(\mu|\boldsymbol{W}^{(k)})$ to obtain $\hat{\mu}_{GI}^{(k)}(t)$. Then repeat this process until the convergence.

3.4 Generalized Isotonic Regression-Based Estimation of the Mean Function

Another simple choice for the weight matrix is to let $\boldsymbol{W} = \boldsymbol{W}_2 = \Sigma^T \Sigma$, where $\Sigma = (\sigma_{j,l})$ is a $m \times m$ matrix with

$$\sigma_{j,l} = \begin{cases} 1 & \text{for } l = j \text{ with } j = 1, \ldots, m, \\ -1 & \text{for } l = j-1 \text{ with } j = 2, \ldots, m, \\ 0 & \text{otherwise.} \end{cases}$$

Note that although the weight matrix $\boldsymbol{W}_1$ is not the identity matrix, it is still a diagonal matrix, and hence the resulting object function $L_{GI}(\mu|\boldsymbol{W})$ still does not take into account the correlation among the observed counts $n_{i,j}$'s from the same subject. In contrast, with the use of $\boldsymbol{W}_2$, the resulting object function depends on the observed increments $\Delta N_i(t_{i,j}) = N_i(t_{i,j}) - N_i(t_{i,j-1})$, $j = 2, \ldots, m_i$, $i = 1, \ldots, n$.

Some other weight matrices can be found in Hu et al. (2009a) and especially, they considered

$$(Cov\{ N_i(s_j), N_i(s_l) \})^{-1},$$

motivated by the construction of generalized estimating equations. Of course, the covariance involved above is generally unknown and one needs to approximate or estimate it. The selection of the optimal weight matrix is still an open question.

3.4.2 Determination of the GIRE

Now we discuss the procedure for the minimization of the weighted least squares function $L_{GI}(\mu|\boldsymbol{W})$ or the determination of $\hat{\boldsymbol{\mu}}_{GI}$ given a weight matrix $\boldsymbol{W}$. For this, define $\boldsymbol{N}_i = (N_i(s_1), \ldots, N_i(s_m))^T$ and $\delta_i(s_l) = 1$ if $t_{i,j} = s_l$ for some $j = 1, \ldots, m_i$ and 0 otherwise. Also define $\Delta_i = \text{diag}\{\delta_i(s_l)\}$, a $m \times m$ diagonal matrix, and $\boldsymbol{W}_i$ to be the $m_i \times m_i$ matrix given by parts of $\boldsymbol{W}$ corresponding to the observation times $t_{i,j}$. Then $L_{GI}(\mu|\boldsymbol{W})$ can be rewritten as

$$L_{GI}(\mu|\boldsymbol{W}) = \sum_{i=1}^n (\boldsymbol{N}_i - \boldsymbol{\mu})^T \Delta_i^T \boldsymbol{W}_i \Delta_i (\boldsymbol{N}_i - \boldsymbol{\mu}).$$

Furthermore, we can decompose $L_{GI}(\mu|\boldsymbol{W})$ as

$$L_{GI}(\mu|\boldsymbol{W}) = \sum_{i=1}^n (\boldsymbol{N}_i - \tilde{\boldsymbol{\mu}}_{GI})^T \Delta_i^T \boldsymbol{W}_i \Delta_i (\boldsymbol{N}_i - \tilde{\boldsymbol{\mu}}_{GI}) \\ + (\tilde{\boldsymbol{\mu}}_{GI} - \boldsymbol{\mu})^T B_n(\boldsymbol{W}) (\tilde{\boldsymbol{\mu}}_{GI} - \boldsymbol{\mu}), \qquad (3.7)$$

where

$$B_n(\boldsymbol{W}) = \sum_{i=1}^{n} \Delta_i^T \boldsymbol{W}_i \Delta_i \,, \; \tilde{\boldsymbol{\mu}}_{GI} = B_n^{-1}(\boldsymbol{W}) \sum_{i=1}^{n} \Delta_i^T \boldsymbol{W}_i \Delta_i \boldsymbol{N}_i \,.$$

It is easy to see from (3.7) that $\tilde{\boldsymbol{\mu}}_{GI}$ minimizes $L_{GI}(\mu|\boldsymbol{W})$ and we would have $\hat{\boldsymbol{\mu}}_{GI} = \tilde{\boldsymbol{\mu}}_{GI}$ if $\tilde{\boldsymbol{\mu}}_{GI}$ satisfies the order restriction. However, $\tilde{\boldsymbol{\mu}}_{GI}$ may not satisfy the order restriction in general. To determine $\hat{\boldsymbol{\mu}}_{GI}$, let $L_{GI}^*(\mu|\boldsymbol{W}) = L_{GI}(\mu|\boldsymbol{W})/2$ and define

$$\pi_l(\boldsymbol{\mu}) = \frac{\partial L_{GI}^*(\mu|\boldsymbol{W})}{\partial \mu_l} \,, \; \pi_{ll}(\boldsymbol{\mu}) = \frac{\partial^2 L_{GI}^*(\mu|\boldsymbol{W})}{\partial \mu_l^2} \,.$$

One can show that $B_n(\boldsymbol{W}) = d^2 L_{GI}^*(\mu|\boldsymbol{W})$ and that $\pi_l(\boldsymbol{\mu})$ and $\pi_{ll}(\boldsymbol{\mu})$ are actually the lth component of

$$dL_{GI}^*(\mu|\boldsymbol{W}) = -\sum_{i=1}^{n} \Delta_i^T \boldsymbol{W}_i \Delta_i (\boldsymbol{N}_i - \boldsymbol{\mu}) = -B_n(\boldsymbol{W})(\tilde{\boldsymbol{\mu}}_{GI} - \boldsymbol{\mu})$$

and the (l,l) element of the matrix $B_n(\boldsymbol{W})$, respectively. Also it can be shown that as $\hat{\boldsymbol{\mu}}_F$, $\hat{\boldsymbol{\mu}}_{GI}$ satisfies the following equation

$$\sum_{l=1}^{m} \pi_l(\hat{\boldsymbol{\mu}}_{GI}) \hat{\mu}_{GI,l} = 0$$

and the inequalities

$$\sum_{j=l}^{m} \pi_j(\hat{\boldsymbol{\mu}}_{GI}) \geq 0 \,.$$

It is apparent that one could determine or find $\hat{\boldsymbol{\mu}}_{GI}$ by solving the equation and inequalities above. However, this may be difficult in general. Corresponding to this and as with $\hat{\boldsymbol{\mu}}_F$, Hu et al. (2009a) give the following iterative convex minorant algorithm. Specifically, let $\boldsymbol{\mu}_{GI}^{(0)} = (\mu_{GI,1}^{(0)}, \ldots, \mu_{GI,m}^{(0)})^T$ denote the initial estimator. Then at the kth iteration, define the updated estimator $\boldsymbol{\mu}_{GI}^{(k)} = (\mu_{GI,1}^{(k)}, \ldots, \mu_{GI,m}^{(k)})^T$ as

$$\mu_{GI,l}^{(k)} = \max_{u \leq l} \min_{v \geq l} \frac{\sum_{j=u}^{v} \pi_{jj}(\mu_{GI}^{(k-1)}) \mu_{GI,j}^{(k-1)} - \pi_j(\mu_{GI}^{(k-1)})}{\sum_{j=u}^{v} \pi_{jj}(\mu_{GI}^{(k-1)})} \,, \quad (3.8)$$

$l = 1, \ldots, m$, and continue the process until convergence.

To understand the GIRE and the iterative convex minorant algorithm above, define $L_{GI}^{**}(\mu|\boldsymbol{W}) = (\tilde{\boldsymbol{\mu}}_{GI} - \boldsymbol{\mu})^T B_n(\boldsymbol{W})(\tilde{\boldsymbol{\mu}}_{GI} - \boldsymbol{\mu})/2$. Then it follows from (3.7) that the GIRE $\hat{\boldsymbol{\mu}}_{GI}$ minimizes $L_{GI}^{**}(\mu|\boldsymbol{W})$ under the order restriction. Also it can be shown that the kth step estimator $\boldsymbol{\mu}_{GI}^{(k)}$ defined in (3.8) is the left derivative of the greatest convex minorant of the cumulative sum diagram

$$\left(\sum_{j=1}^{l} b_{jj}(\boldsymbol{\mu}), \sum_{j=1}^{l} a_j(\boldsymbol{\mu}) \right) \Big|_{\boldsymbol{\mu}=\boldsymbol{\mu}_{GI}^{(k)}},$$

$l = 1, \ldots, m$. In the above, $b_{jj}(\boldsymbol{\mu})$ is the (j,j) element of the matrix $B_n(\boldsymbol{W})$ and $a_j(\boldsymbol{\mu})$ the jth component of the vector

$$B_n(\boldsymbol{W}) \tilde{\boldsymbol{\mu}}_{GI} + \{\operatorname{diag}(B_n(\boldsymbol{W})) - B_n(\boldsymbol{W})\} \boldsymbol{\mu}.$$

If $B_n(\boldsymbol{W})$ is a diagonal matrix, the GIRE $\hat{\boldsymbol{\mu}}_{GI}$ is actually the isotonic regression of $\tilde{\boldsymbol{\mu}}_{GI}$ with respect to the weights given by the diagonal elements of $B_n(\boldsymbol{W})$. In other words, $\hat{\boldsymbol{\mu}}_{GI}$ could be regarded as a generalized isotonic regression of $\tilde{\boldsymbol{\mu}}_{GI}$ with the weight matrix $B_n(\boldsymbol{W})$.

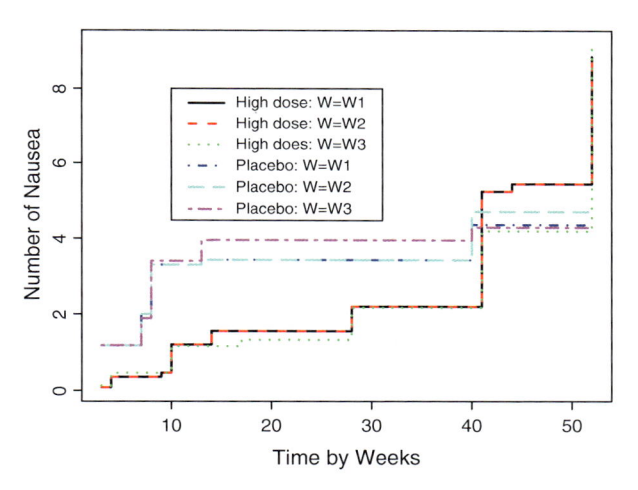

Fig. 3.4. GIRE of the average cumulative counts of episodes of nausea

3.4.3 An Illustration

For the illustration of the estimation procedure described above, we apply it to the gallstone data discussed in Sect. 3.3.2 again with the focus on comparing the recurrence rates of nausea between the two groups. For the application of the procedure, in addition to the weight matrices $\boldsymbol{W}_1$ and $\boldsymbol{W}_2$ given above, we also consider $\boldsymbol{W}_3 = \Sigma^T \Sigma$ with $\Sigma = (\sigma_{j,l})$ being a $m \times m$ matrix and

$$\sigma_{j,l} = \begin{cases} 1 & \text{for } j = l \text{ with } l = 1, \ldots, m, \\ -1 & \text{for } j = \min\{k; l < k < m, \delta_i(s_k) = 1 \text{ for some } i \in S_l\}, \\ 0 & \text{otherwise.} \end{cases}$$

Note that the motivation behind the matrix $\boldsymbol{W}_2$ is to take into account the possible correlation between the observations at two successive observation time points s_{j-1} and s_j. On the other hand, it is easy to see that for a given subject observed at s_{j-1}, the person may not be observed at s_j. This leads to the consideration of the weight matrix $\boldsymbol{W}_3$.

Figure 3.4 presents the GIRE of the average cumulative numbers of the occurrences of nausea for the patients in the placebo and high dose groups, respectively. It is interesting to see that the estimators with different weight matrices are similar to each other for both groups. Note that this may not be the case in general. Also the estimators are similar to those given in Fig. 3.2.

3.5 Estimation of the Rate Function

As discussed above, sometimes one may also be interested in estimating the rate function of the underlying recurrent event process of interest. One reason for this is that the rate function could reveal some aspects of the process that cannot be seen from the mean function. In addition, one could also use an estimator of the rate function to derive an estimator of the corresponding mean function. As with the estimation of a hazard function in failure time analysis, a raw estimator of the rate function may often be unstable or jumpy. Thus a smooth estimator may be preferred in general.

Consider a recurrent event study that consists of n independent subjects from a homogeneous population. Let the $N_i(t)$'s and $\mu(t)$ be defined as above and $r(t)$ denote the rate function of the recurrent event processes $N_i(t)$'s. That is, $r(t)\,dt = d\mu(t)$. Suppose that we observe only panel count data given in (3.1) with the s_l's denoting all ordered distinct observation time points as before. In the following, we first discuss direct or raw estimation of the rate function $r(t)$ and three simple procedures are described. The smooth estimation of $r(t)$ is then considered with the focus on the kernel estimation (Hart, 1986; Wand and Jones, 1995), which is followed by two illustrations.

3.5.1 Raw Estimators of the Rate Function

To estimate $r(t)$, let $\hat{\mu}(t)$ denote one of the estimators of $\mu(t)$ given in the previous sections of this chapter. Then by the definition of $r(t)$ and the fact that $\hat{\mu}(t)$ is a step function with jumps only at the s_l's, it is natural to define an estimator of $r(t)$ as

$$\hat{r}_1(s_l) = \Delta\hat{\mu}(s_l) = \hat{\mu}(s_l) - \hat{\mu}(s_l-)\,, \ l = 1,\ldots,m\,,$$

and $\hat{r}_1(t) = 0$ for all other $t \neq s_l$. Or it may be more natural to define

$$\hat{r}_1^*(t) = \frac{\Delta\hat{\mu}(s_l)}{s_l - s_{l-1}}\,, \text{ for } s_{l-1} < t < s_l\,,$$

3.5 Estimation of the Rate Function

$l = 1, \ldots, m$. It is easy to see that the resulting estimator of $\mu(t)$ from $\hat{r}_1(t)$ gives exactly the estimator $\hat{\mu}(t)$, but the one from $\hat{r}_1^*(t)$ does not as the latter is not a step function.

Another simple estimator of the rate function $r(t)$ is given by the empirical estimator

$$\hat{r}_2(t) = \frac{1}{\sum_{i=1}^n I(t \leq t_{i,m_i})} \sum_{i=1}^n \hat{r}_{2i}(t)$$

$$= \frac{1}{\sum_{i=1}^n I(t \leq t_{i,m_i})} \sum_{i=1}^n \sum_{j=1}^{m_i} \frac{n_{i,j} - n_{i,j-1}}{t_{i,j} - t_{i,j-1}} I(t_{i,j-1} < t \leq t_{i,j}) \quad (3.9)$$

(Thall and Lachin, 1988). Here $\hat{r}_{2i}(t)$ can be regarded as the estimated rate function from subject i and $\hat{r}_2(t)$ the average of the estimated rate functions over all subjects. One can easily show that in the case of recurrent event data, the estimator above reduces to the estimator given in (1.6) resulting from the Nelson-Aalen estimator.

Note that all estimators of both mean and rate functions described so far are essentially step functions with the jump points determined by the observed data. Motivated by this, we can employ a different but similar approach that assumes that the rate function $r(t)$ is a piecewise consistent function. Specifically, suppose that $0 = a_0 < a_1 < \ldots < a_k < \infty$ is a prespecified sequence of time points and $r(t) = \alpha_l$ for $t \in A_l = (a_{l-1}, a_l]$, where the α_l's are some parameters, $l = 1, \ldots, k$. It follows that for the corresponding mean function $\mu(t)$, we have

$$\mu(t) = \sum_{l=1}^k \left\{ \sum_{j=1}^{l-1} \alpha_j (a_j - a_{j-1}) + \alpha_l (t - a_{l-1}) \right\} I(a_{l-1} < t \leq a_l), \quad (3.10)$$

where we define $\sum_{j=1}^0 = 0$.

To estimate $r(t)$ or the α_j's, by using the relationship (3.10) given above, one could employ any of the likelihood-based estimation procedures described in the previous sections for estimation of the mean function $\mu(t)$. For example, corresponding to the NPMPLE or IRE, we can consider the log pseudo-likelihood function $l_p(\mu)$ given in (3.4). By plugging in the relationship (3.10), we obtain the following estimating equations

$$\frac{\partial l_p(\mu)}{\partial \alpha_j} = \frac{\partial l_p(\alpha_j's)}{\partial \alpha_j} = \sum_{l=1}^m w_l \left(\frac{\bar{n}_l}{\mu_l} - 1 \right) \frac{\partial \mu_l}{\partial \alpha_j} = 0, \, j = 1, \ldots, k$$

for the α_j's, where

$$\frac{\partial \mu_l}{\partial \alpha_j} = (s_l - a_{j-1}) I(a_{j-1} < s_l \leq a_j) + (a_j - a_{j-1}) I(s_l > a_j)$$

and the s_l's and μ_l's are defined as before. Given the a_j's, one can develop a Newton-Raphson or EM algorithm to solve the equations above.

For the implementation of the likelihood-based procedure described above, one needs to choose the sequence of partition points a_j's. It is apparent that the larger the number of partitions k, the closer the resulting estimator is to the nonparametric estimator of $r(t)$ such as $\hat{r}_1(t)$ or $\hat{r}_1^*(t)$. Of course, for larger k, the implementation is more time consuming too. For a given set of panel count data, it is natural and also simple to take $k = m$ and $a_j = s_j$, $j = 1, \ldots, m$. As mentioned above, instead of $l_p(\mu)$, one could use $l(\mu)$ or $L_n(\mu)$ to develop an estimation procedure for $r(t)$ similarly as with $l_p(\mu)$.

3.5.2 Smooth Estimators of the Rate Function

In this subsection, we consider the smooth estimation of a rate function $r(t)$ with the focus on kernel estimation. A kernel estimator is essentially the weighted average of an existing estimator. A major advantage of the kernel estimation approach is its simplicity and flexibility as it can be easily implemented given an existing estimator. On the other hand, the inference on kernel estimators may not be straightforward.

Let $K(t)$ be a nonnegative function symmetric about $t = 0$ and suppose that $\int_{-\infty}^{\infty} K(t)\,dt = 1$. It is usually referred to as a kernel function. Also let h be a positive parameter called the bandwidth parameter, which determines how large a neighborhood of t is used to calculate the local average. Suppose that there exists an estimator $\hat{r}(t)$ of the rate function $r(t)$ that is not equal to zero only at finite time points, a step function with finite jump points, or a discontinuous function with finite discontinuous time points. To save the notation, we use $s_1 < \ldots < s_m$ to denote these time points. Define $\hat{r}_l = \hat{r}(s_l)$,

$$w_l^*(t, h) = h^{-1} K\{(t - s_l)/h\}$$

and

$$w_l(t) = \frac{w_l^*(t, h)}{\sum_{u=1}^{m} w_u^*(t, h)},$$

$l = 1, \ldots, m$. Then given $K(t)$ and h as well as $\hat{r}(t)$, the kernel estimator of $r(t)$ is defined to be

$$\hat{r}_{K,1}(t) = \sum_{l=1}^{m} w_j(t)\hat{r}_l, \qquad (3.11)$$

the weighted averages of the $\hat{r}_l$'s.

As discussed above, the estimation of mean and rate functions can be exchangeable. The kernel estimator given above is constructed based on the direction estimation of a rate function. Similarly one could derive a kernel estimator of $r(t)$ based on the estimation of its corresponding mean

3.5 Estimation of the Rate Function

function. Specifically, let $\hat{\mu}(t)$ denote an estimator of the mean function $\mu(t) = \int_0^t r(s)\,ds$. Then a kernel estimator of $r(t)$ can be derived as

$$\hat{r}_{K,2}(t) = \frac{1}{h}\int_{t-h}^{t+h} K\left(\frac{t-s}{h}\right) d\hat{\mu}(s), \qquad (3.12)$$

the average or smooth version of the raw estimator $d\hat{\mu}(t)$ of $r(t)\,dt$.

To obtain the smooth estimator of $r(t)$ described above, one needs to choose the kernel function K and the bandwidth parameter h, which together control the degree of the smoothness of the estimator. For the kernel function, there are many choices. One simple one is

$$K_1(t) = I(|t| \leq 1)$$

and under this kernel function, the estimators $\hat{r}_{K,1}(t)$ and $\hat{r}_{K,2}(t)$ are moving average estimators. At time t, only these $\hat{r}_l$'s and the jumps of $\hat{\mu}(s_l)$ with $|s_l - t| \leq h$ contribute to their corresponding estimators, respectively. In other words, $\hat{r}_{K,1}(t)$ and $\hat{r}_{K,2}(t)$ are simply the averages of the contributing components. Another commonly used kernel function is

$$K_2(t) = (2\pi)^{-1/2} \exp(-t^2/2),$$

which is usually referred to as the Gaussian kernel. Under this function, all components $\hat{r}_l$'s and the whole function $\hat{\mu}(t)$ contribute to their resulting estimators at each time point t. The degrees of contributions depend on the closeness of each time point to the given t and the closer, the larger the contribution. More comments about these two kernel functions are given in the next subsection through illustrations.

For the selection of the bandwidth parameter h, one way is to apply the methods commonly used for kernel estimation of density functions (Bean and Tsokos, 1980; Wand and Jones, 1995). Suppose that the goal is to provide a simple, graphical presentation of the rate function. In this case, the trial and error method seems to be a natural choice. It is obvious that h cannot be too small or large, and the appropriate range for h depends on specific problems.

3.5.3 Illustrations

For the illustration of the procedures discussed above for estimation of the rate function, we consider the same two examples used in Sect. 3.3.2. First we apply them to the reliability data on the loss of feedwater flow collected from 30 nuclear plants. In this case, as mentioned before, only one observation is available for each plant and thus we have current status data. Figure 3.5 presents the estimated rate functions given by the empirical estimator (3.9) and the kernel estimator (3.12) based on the Gaussian kernel function $K_2(t)$

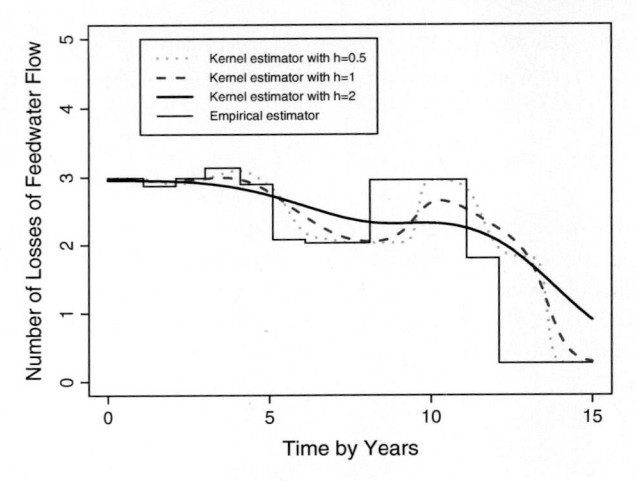

Fig. 3.5. Estimated loss rates of feedwater flow

with $h = 0.5$, 1 or 2 and the use of the IRE shown in Fig. 3.1. It is interesting to see that all four estimators suggest that the loss rate of feedwater flow seems to decrease with time and there are two peak periods about the loss rates. However, the two different procedures tell us different peak periods or points although they are close. Note that it is apparent that one may not easily see these from the estimated mean function given in Fig. 3.1. With respect to the kernel estimators, it is clear that the value of the bandwidth h determines the smoothness of the estimator.

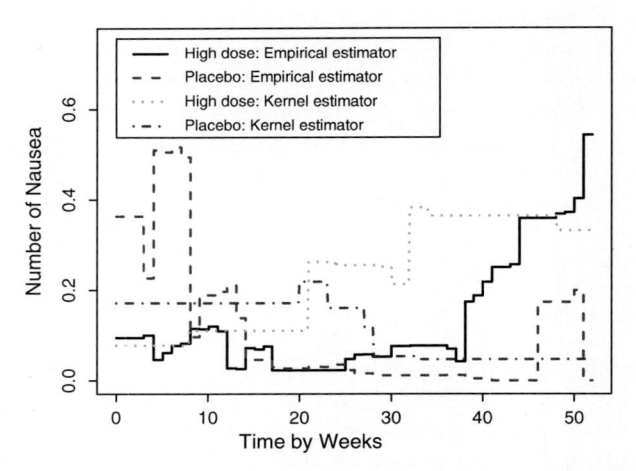

Fig. 3.6. Estimated occurrence rates of nausea based on (3.9) and (3.12) with $K_1(t)$

3.5 Estimation of the Rate Function   67

Now we apply the estimation procedures discussed above to the panel count data arising from the National Cooperative Gallstone Study. First Fig. 3.6 displays the estimated occurrence rates of nausea given by the empirical estimator (3.9) and the kernel estimator (3.12) based on the kernel function $K_1(t)$ with $h = 20$. One can easily see that both methods indicate that the occurrence rate for the placebo group was higher than that for the high-dose group initially, but the relationship reversed later. This is consistent with what one can see from the estimated mean function given before. One explanation for the higher occurrence rate in the high-dose group in the later period could be that it is due to the small number of the patients available. Note that the empirical approach seems to be more clear or give more details than the kernel approach with the kernel function $K_1(t)$ about the pattern or shape of the underlying occurrence rate. For comparison, Fig. 3.7 gives the estimated occurrence rate by the kernel approach based on the Gaussian kernel function $K_2(t)$ with $h = 0.5$. It basically tells us the same story about the patterns of the occurrence rates of nausea as the two other methods. But it is obvious that this latter method gives a much more clear picture about the shape or peaks of the underlying occurrence rate of nausea than the other two methods. Note that here as above, the IRE is used for the determination of the estimator (3.12).

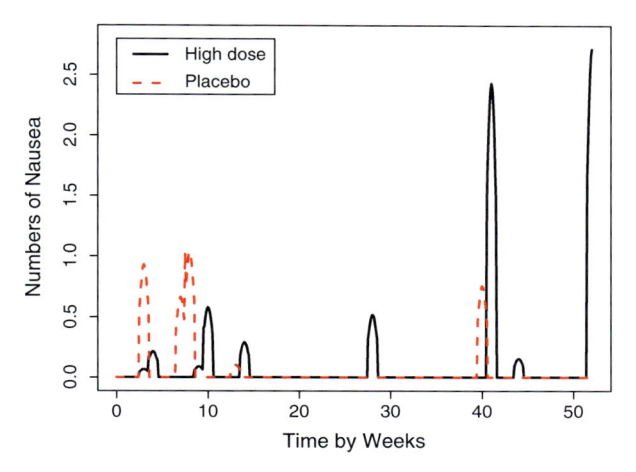

Fig. 3.7. Estimated occurrence rates of nausea based on (3.12) with $K_2(t)$

3.5.4 Discussion

As discussed above, a main advantage of kernel estimation is its simplicity and flexibility. Also it does not depend on any distribution assumption. On the other hand, if one is willing to make some assumptions such that the $N_i(t)$'s are non-homogeneous Poisson processes, then likelihood-based approaches can also be used to derive smooth estimators of the rate function $r(t)$.

Suppose that one can write the mean function $\mu(t)$ as a function of the values, denoted by the r_l's, of the rate function $r(t)$ at finite time points such as the expression (3.10). Let $l(\mu)$ denote a log likelihood function used to estimate $\mu(t)$ such as those discussed in Sect. 3.2. Then it is apparent that we can estimate the r_l's by maximizing the log likelihood function $l(r'_l s) = l(\mu)$ with replacing $\mu(t)$ by the r_l's. On the other hand, it is well-known that the resulting estimator of the r_l's or $r(t)$ is usually unstable or not smooth even if $r(t)$ is indeed a smooth function. To overcome this and obtain a smooth estimator, a common approach is to construct and maximize a penalized log likelihood function given by

$$l_g(r(t); \tau) = l(r'_l s) - \tau g\{r(t)\}.$$

In the above, g is a known penalty function measuring the roughness of the rate function and $\tau\ (>0)$ is an unknown parameter that controls the amount of smoothing. If $\tau = 0$, $l_g(r(t); \tau) = l(r'_l s)$ and there is no smoothing.

Suppose that $r(t)$ is a smooth function. Instead of employing the penalized likelihood approach, an alternative is to directly model the rate function. For example, one such model is to assume that $r(t)$ has the form

$$r(t) = \sum_{j=1}^{p} \exp(\alpha_j) B_j(t), \qquad (3.13)$$

where $\{\alpha_j\,;\,j = 1,\ldots p\,\}$ are unknown parameters and $\{B_j(t)\,;\,j = 1,\ldots p\,\}$ are some known smooth functions. Then for estimation of $r(t)$ or the α_j's, it is natural to maximize the log likelihood function

$$l(\alpha'_j s) = l\left\{\mu(t) = \int_0^t \sum_{j=1}^{p} \exp(\alpha_j) B_j(s)\,ds\right\}.$$

In practice, instead of modeling $r(t)$ directly, sometimes one may prefer to model the log rate function such as

$$\log r(t) = \sum_{j=1}^{p} \alpha_j B_j(t). \qquad (3.14)$$

Here the α_j's and $B_j(t)$'s are the same as defined in (3.13). In this case, the estimation can be carried out similarly by plugging (3.14) into the log likelihood function $l(\mu)$ instead of (3.13).

For the selection of the smooth functions $B_j(t)$'s, there are many choices. A simple one is to take them to be power functions. Another choice, which may be more commonly used, is to let them be some spline functions such as B-splines or M-splines (Rosenberg, 1995). Of course, one can also take them to be the base functions of a function space.

Note that the penalized likelihood approach described above is to employ a penalty function to enforce the smoothness of the resulting estimator of a rate function. Another related approach is first to model the rate function and then to apply the penalized likelihood approach. That is, one can combine the two approaches described above together. The local likelihood method is another likelihood-based approach for smooth estimation, which was proposed by Tibishirani and Hastie (1987) for smooth estimation of covariate effects in the context of regression analysis. The method is an extension of the local fitting technique used in scatterplot smoothing (Cleveland, 1979). To implement the method, one needs to preselect a set of intervals and to approximate the rate function by a linear function of time over each interval. The parameters in the linear function are estimated using the local likelihood contributed by the data related to the interval over which the linear model is defined.

As a final remark, it should be noted that the likelihood-based procedures discussed above can be applied only if the assumed distribution can be completely determined by the mean function, or with some assumptions. Otherwise, no likelihood function is available.

3.6 Bibliography, Discussion, and Remarks

Nonparametric estimation of recurrent event processes has been discussed by many authors. However, most of the existing literature is on recurrent event data and the discussion on the case of panel count data is relatively limited. For the former situation, there exist two types of research. One is on estimation of the intensity or cumulative intensity process of the underlying recurrent event process (Andersen et al., 1993), while the other is on estimation of the mean and rate functions of the recurrent event process (Cook and Lawless, 2007; Lawless and Nadeau, 1995; Lin et al., 2000). For the panel count data situation, as discussed above, the majority of the existing work is on the mean and rate functions of the recurrent event process.

One of the early work on nonparametric estimation based on panel count data is given by Thall and Lachin (1988), who gave a simple empirical estimator of the rate function. Sun and Kalbfleisch (1995) developed a simple isotonic regression-based estimator, the IRE, of the mean function and investigated the consistency of the estimator. Following them, Wellner and Zhang (2000) considered two likelihood-based estimators, the NPMLE and NPMPLE, of the mean function and established their asymptotic properties. In particular, the NPMPLE is the same as the IRE. A likelihood-based estimator of the mean function was also proposed in Zhang and Jamshidian (2003). The difference between these estimators is that the former was derived by using Poisson processes, while the latter employed mixed Poisson processes. Also following Sun and Kalbfleisch (1995),

Hu et al. (2009a) proposed a class of generalized isotonic regression-based estimators, GIRE, of the mean function by using the weighted least squares criterion.

Other authors who considered nonparametric estimation of the mean or rate function of the recurrent event process based on panel count include Lu et al. (2007) and Hu et al. (2009b). The former studied likelihood-based procedures like those discussed above but with the use of the monotone cubic I-splines to approximate the mean function. The latter presented two estimation procedures by using two types of self-consistency estimating equations and by expressing the mean function as a summation of the values of the rate function at finite time points. In other words, the procedures essentially estimate the mean function by estimating the rate function. Also one of the procedures is based on the log likelihood function $l(\mu)$ given in (3.3) and the resulting estimator is actually the NPMLE. In addition, one could also apply the procedure given by Hu and Lagakos (2007), who investigated the same problem for a general response process that includes the recurrent event process as a special case.

It is clear that more research remains to be done for nonparametric estimation with panel count data. One such direction or area is that in all discussion so far, it has been assumed that the observation process is independent of the underlying recurrent event process of interest. In practice, as discussed before, this may not be true sometimes as, for example, the former may contain relevant information about or depend on the latter. Some discussion on this is given below in the context of regression analysis. Another area that is difficult and has not been studied much is the asymptotic behavior of the various estimators discussed in this chapter. A relatively easy problem is the variance or covariance estimation of these estimators. Also it is useful to develop some criteria for the optimal weight selection for the GIRE.

4
Nonparametric Comparison of Point Processes

4.1 Introduction

This chapter discusses nonparametric or distribution-free comparison of several point or recurrent event processes when one observes only panel count data. As commented above, in the case of panel count data, it is very difficult or impossible to estimate the intensity process and in consequence, one usually focuses on the rate or mean functions of the underlying recurrent event processes of interest. For the same reason, with respect to the comparison of the processes, it is common and also convenient to formulate the null hypothesis using the mean functions.

In the following, we consider three situations for the comparison of mean functions of several recurrent event processes. First we discuss in Sect. 4.2 the two-sample situation where study subjects come from two different populations or are given two different treatments. For the comparison, two nonparametric procedures are discussed. The first procedure is constructed by treating each subject coming from its own treatment. As a result, it can also be applied to the situation where there exist more than two samples or treatments that can be characterized by a scale variable such as animal dose studies. In comparison, the second procedure is constructed for a general two treatment comparison problem and thus applies to more general two-sample situations than the first procedure. Section 4.3 investigates the second situation, the general p-sample comparison. For the problem, two types of nonparametric procedures are discussed. One is based on the use of the IRE or NPMPLE and the other on the use of the NPMLE. Section 4.4 gives some numerical comparisons and an illustration of the procedures described in Sects. 4.2 and 4.3.

As discussed above and also below, in the case of panel count data, one faces an additional observation process in addition to the underlying recurrent event process of interest. All nonparametric comparison procedures described in Sects. 4.2 and 4.3 assume that the observation processes for subjects in all populations or different treatment groups are identical. It is well-known that

J. Sun and X. Zhao, *Statistical Analysis of Panel Count Data*, Statistics for Biology and Health 80, DOI 10.1007/978-1-4614-8715-9_4,
© Springer Science+Business Media New York 2013

this may not be true in reality and it has been shown (Sun, 1999; Zhao et al., 2011a) that without taking this into account, the analysis can yield biased or misleading results. Section 4.5 discusses this situation and presents a class of nonparametric test procedures that allow different observation processes for the subjects in different treatment groups. Section 4.6 concludes with some bibliographical notes and some future research directions related to the comparison of recurrent event processes.

4.2 Two-Sample Comparison of Cumulative Mean Functions

Consider a recurrent event study that consists of n independent subjects and yields only panel count data. For subject i, as in Chap. 3, let $N_i(t)$ denote the point process representing the total number of the occurrences of the recurrent events up to time t and $0 < t_{i,1} < \cdots < t_{i,m_i}$ the observation times on $N_i(t)$. Define $n_{i,j} = N_i(t_{i,j})$, the observed value of $N_i(t)$ at time $t_{i,j}$, $j = 1,\ldots,m_i$, $i = 1,\ldots,n$. Suppose that all subjects come from two populations or are given one of two treatments, and the goal is to test if there is treatment difference based on the observed panel count data.

Let $\mu_1(t)$ and $\mu_2(t)$ denote the mean functions of the $N_i(t)$'s corresponding to the subjects given treatments 1 and 2, respectively. Then the null hypothesis of interest can be expressed as $H_0 : \mu_1(t) = \mu_2(t)$ for all t. In the following, we describe two different nonparametric procedures for testing H_0.

4.2.1 Nonparametric Test Procedure I

To present the first nonparametric test procedure, for subject i, define Z_i to be the treatment indicator, being 0 if given treatment 1 and 1 otherwise, $i = 1,\ldots,n$. Let $\hat{\mu}_I(t)$ denote the IRE of $\mu_1(t)$ and $\mu_2(t)$ under the null hypothesis H_0. Then to test H_0, by following the log-rank test for right-censored failure time data (Kalbfleisch and Prentice, 2002), it is natural to use the statistic

$$U_{SF} = \frac{1}{\sqrt{n}} \sum_{i=1}^{n} Z_i \sum_{j=1}^{m_i} \{ n_{i,j} - \hat{\mu}_I(t_{i,j}) \}$$

(Sun and Fang, 2003). It is easy to see that U_{SF} represents the summation of the differences between the observed numbers of the recurrent event of interest and the estimated numbers of the event over the treatment group with $Z_i = 1$.

To further look at the statistic U_{SF}, let $\hat{\mu}_{I,1}(t)$ denote the IRE of $\mu_1(t)$ based on the data from the subjects with $Z_i = 0$. Also let the $s_l^{(1)}$'s and

4.2 Two-Sample Comparison of Cumulative Mean Functions

$w_l^{(1)}$'s denote the time points and weights associated with $\hat{\mu}_{I,1}(t)$ and the s_l's and w_l's the time points and weights associated with $\hat{\mu}_I(t)$. Then one can rewrite U_{SF} as

$$U_{SF} = \frac{1}{\sqrt{n}} \int w^{(1)}(t) \{\hat{\mu}_{I,1}(t) - \hat{\mu}_I(t)\} \, d\bar{N}^{(1)}(t), \qquad (4.1)$$

where $w^{(1)}(t)$ denotes the step function that jumps only at the $s^{(1)}$'s with $w^{(1)}(s_l^{(1)}) = w_l^{(1)}$ and $\bar{N}^{(1)}(t) = \sum_l I(t \geq s_l^{(1)})$. That is, U_{SF} represents the integrated weighted difference between an individual treatment group estimator $\hat{\mu}_{I,1}(t)$ and the overall estimator $\hat{\mu}_I(t)$ of the common mean function of the $N_i(t)$'s under the null hypothesis H_0.

Note that in the case of current status data, we have $m_i = 1$ and the statistic U_{SF} reduces to

$$\frac{1}{\sqrt{n}} \sum_{i=1}^{n} Z_i \{n_{i,1} - \hat{\mu}_I(t_{i,1})\}, \qquad (4.2)$$

first discussed in Sun and Kalbfleisch (1993). If we further assume that $t_{i,1} = t_0$, then the statistic has the form

$$\frac{1}{\sqrt{n}} \left\{ \sum_{i:Z_i=1} N_i(t_0) - \bar{Z} \sum_{i=1}^{n} N_i(t_0) \right\},$$

where $\bar{Z} = \sum_{i=1}^{n} Z_i/n$. It is worth to note that if the $N_i(t)$'s are Poisson processes with the mean functions $E\{N_i(t) \mid Z_i\} = \mu_0(t) \exp(\beta Z_i)$, then the hypothesis H_0 is equivalent to $\beta = 0$, and the statistic in (4.2) is exactly the score statistic for testing $\beta = 0$. Here $\mu_0(t)$ denotes the true mean function of the $N_i(t)$'s under H_0 and β an unknown parameter.

Suppose that the treatment indicators Z_i's can be regarded as independent and identically distributed random variables asymptotically. Note that this is often true in, for example, clinical trials in which randomization is used to assign study subjects to different groups. Then under some regularity conditions, Sun and Fang (2003) show that under H_0 and as $n \to \infty$, the statistic U_{SF} has a normal distribution with mean 0 and the variance that can be consistently estimated by

$$\hat{\sigma}_{SF}^2 = \frac{1}{n} \sum_{i=1}^{n} \left[(Z_i - \bar{Z}) \sum_{j=1}^{m_i} \{n_{i,j} - \hat{\mu}_I(t_{i,j})\} \right]^2.$$

Thus for large n, one can carry out the testing of the null hypothesis H_0 using the statistic $U_{SF}^* = U_{SF}/\hat{\sigma}_{SF}$ based on the standard normal distribution.

We remark that the discussion and result given above are actually valid for any asymptotically independent and identically distributed random variables

Z_i's. In other words, the test procedure described above is applicable to these situations. One of such situations is the animal dose study that involves several doses of certain chemicals and where one is interested in testing the dose effect on tumor growth. In this case, the Z_i's can be defined as the quantities of the dose given to the animals.

4.2.2 Nonparametric Test Procedure II

Now we describe another statistic for testing the hypothesis H_0. For this, let $\hat{\mu}_{I,2}(t)$ denote the IRE of the mean function $\mu_2(t)$ based on the data from the subjects with $Z_i = 1$. To motivate the new statistic, note that the procedure given in the previous subsection requires that the treatment indicators Z_i's can be treated as independent and identically distributed random variables. It is apparent that this may not be true in some situations. Also as commented above, the statistic U_{SF} compares the individual estimator to the overall estimator of the same mean function. An alternative to this that may be more powerful is to compare directly the two individual estimators of the two mean functions under the study. These suggest to use the statistic

$$U_{PSZ} = \sqrt{\frac{n_1 n_2}{n}} \int_0^\tau W_n(t) \{ \hat{\mu}_{I,1}(t) - \hat{\mu}_{I,2}(t) \} \, dG_n(t).$$

In the above, n_1 and n_2 denote the numbers of subjects in treatment groups 1 and 2, respectively, τ denotes the largest observation time, $W_n(t)$ is a bounded weight process that may depend on the observed data, and

$$G_n(t) = \frac{1}{n} \sum_{i=1}^n \sum_{j=1}^{m_i} I(t_{i,j} \leq t),$$

the empirical observation process.

By plugging $G_n(t)$ into U_{PSZ}, we have

$$U_{PSZ} = \sqrt{\frac{n_1 n_2}{n^3}} \sum_{i=1}^n \sum_{j=1}^{m_i} W_n(t_{i,j}) \{ \hat{\mu}_{I,1}(t_{i,j}) - \hat{\mu}_{I,2}(t_{i,j}) \}.$$

That is, U_{PSZ} is a Wilcoxon-type statistic. Similar statistics are often used in the analysis of repeated measurement data (Davis and Wei, 1988). Suppose that there exists a bounded weight process $W(t)$ such that

$$\sup_n E \int_0^\tau | \sqrt{n} \{ W_n(t) - W(t) \} |^2 \, dG_n(t) < \infty. \qquad (4.3)$$

Also suppose that $n_1/n \to p_1$ and $n_2/n \to p_2$ as $n \to \infty$, where $0 < p_1, p_2 < 1$ and $p_1 + p_2 = 1$. Then Park et al. (2007) show that under some

4.2 Two-Sample Comparison of Cumulative Mean Functions

regularity conditions and H_0, the distribution of U_{PSZ} can be asymptotically approximated by the normal distribution with mean zero and the variance

$$\hat{\sigma}^2_{PSZ} = \frac{n_2}{n} \hat{\sigma}^2_1 + \frac{n_1}{n} \hat{\sigma}^2_2 .$$

In the above,

$$\hat{\sigma}^2_l = \frac{1}{n_l} \sum_{i \in S_l} \left[\sum_{j=1}^{m_i} W_n(t_{i,j}) \{N_i(t_{i,j}) - \hat{\mu}_{I,l}(t_{i,j})\} \right]^2$$

with S_l denoting the set of indices of the subjects belonging to treatment group l, $l = 1, 2$. Thus it follows as above that the test of the null hypothesis H_0 can be performed by using the statistic $U^*_{PSZ} = U_{PSZ}/\hat{\sigma}_{PSZ}$ based on the standard normal distribution.

To apply the test procedure above, one needs to choose the weight process $W_n(t)$. For this, a simple and natural choice is clearly $W_n^{(1)}(t) = 1$. Another natural choice is $W_n^{(2)}(t) = Y_n(t) = n^{-1} \sum_{i=1}^{n} I(t \leq t_{i,m_i})$ and in this case, the weights are proportional to the number of the subjects still under follow-up. A third choice, which is commonly used in both failure time data and recurrent event data analyses (Cook and Lawless, 2007; Kalbfleisch and Prentice, 2002), is

$$W_n^{(3)}(t) = \frac{Y_{n,1}(t) Y_{n,2}(t)}{Y_n(t)} .$$

Here $Y_{n,1}(t)$ and $Y_{n,2}(t)$ are defined as $Y_n(t)$ but with the summation being over the subjects only within treatment groups 1 and 2, respectively.

4.2.3 Discussion

To test H_0, in addition to the two procedures described above, one may also apply the procedures proposed in Li et al. (2010) and Thall and Lachin (1988). The former discussed the current status data situation and suggested to apply the test statistic

$$\sum_{i=1}^{n} (Z_i - \bar{Z}) \{n_{i,1} - \hat{\mu}_I(t_{i,1})\}$$

instead the one given in (4.2). Furthermore, they show numerically that the newly resulting procedure could be more powerful. In the parametric procedure given in Thall and Lachin (1988), it transforms the comparison problem to a multivariate comparison problem and then applies a multivariate Wilcoxon-like rank test. For the transformation, however, one needs to partition the whole study period into several fixed, consecutive and non-overlapping intervals. It is apparent that the test result may depend on these grouping intervals.

Note that in the construction of U_{PSZ} as well as U_{SF}, the IRE of the mean function is employed. Instead of using the IRE, one could develop some nonparametric test procedures similarly by using other estimators of the mean functions discussed in Chap. 3 such as the NPMLE. A possible advantage of using the NPMLE could be the gain of efficiency since it can be more efficient than the IRE. On the other hand, as discussed in Chap. 3, the NPMLE is much more complicated both theoretically and computationally than the IRE. In particular, the former has no closed-form expression. In consequence, the asymptotic distributions of the statistics U_{SF} and U_{PSZ} with the IRE replaced by the NPMLE are still unknown. Alternatively to make use of the NPMLE of the mean function, Balakrishnan and Zhao (2010a) suggest to use the statistic

$$\frac{1}{\sqrt{n}} \sum_{i=1}^{n} Z_i \left[\sum_{j=1}^{m_i-1} \hat{\mu}_F(t_{i,j}) \left\{ \frac{\Delta n_{i,j+1}}{\Delta \hat{\mu}_F(t_{i,j+1})} - \frac{\Delta n_{i,j}}{\Delta \hat{\mu}_F(t_{i,j})} \right\} \right. \\
\left. + \hat{\mu}_F(t_{i,m_i}) \left\{ 1 - \frac{\Delta n_{i,m_i}}{\Delta \hat{\mu}_F(t_{i,m_i})} \right\} \right]. \tag{4.4}$$

In the above, $\hat{\mu}_F(t)$ denotes the NPMLE of the common mean function of the $N_i(t)$'s under the hypothesis H_0, $\Delta n_{i,j} = n_{i,j} - n_{i,j-1}$, and $\Delta \hat{\mu}_F(t_{i,j}) = \hat{\mu}_F(t_{i,j}) - \hat{\mu}_F(t_{i,j-1})$. Furthermore, they give the asymptotic distribution of the statistic above under the hypothesis H_0. More discussion about this statistic is given below.

Note that the statistic U_{PSZ} represents the integrated weighted difference between the estimators of $\mu_1(t)$ and $\mu_2(t)$ and is expected to be sensitive especially to stochastically ordered mean functions. Sometimes one may be more interested in other types of the difference between the two mean functions such as the absolute difference. To address this, instead of U_{PSZ}, one may want to consider the test statistic

$$\sqrt{\frac{n_1 n_2}{n}} \int_0^\tau W_n(t) \left\{ \hat{\mu}_{I,1}(t) - \hat{\mu}_{I,2}(t) \right\}^2 dG_n(t)$$

or

$$\sqrt{\frac{n_1 n_2}{n}} \int_0^\tau W_n(t) \left| \hat{\mu}_{I,1}(t) - \hat{\mu}_{I,2}(t) \right| dG_n(t).$$

However, it may be difficult to derive the asymptotic distributions of these two statistics.

4.3 General p-Sample Comparison of Cumulative Mean Functions

Now we discuss the general p-sample comparison of recurrent event processes based on panel count data. Specifically, we consider the same set-up and use the same notation defined in the previous section, but assume that study subjects come from p different populations or are given p different treatments. Let $\mu_l(t)$ and n_l denote the mean function of the $N_i(t)$'s corresponding to and the number of the subjects given treatment l and S_l the set of indices of these subjects, $l = 1, \ldots, p$. Suppose that the goal of interest is to test the null hypothesis $H_0^* : \mu_1(t) = \cdots = \mu_p(t)$ for all t.

To test H_0^*, in the following, we discuss two classes of test statistics, which give two types of nonparametric test procedures. The first class of test statistics make use of the IRE or NPMPLE of the mean function of recurrent event processes and are generalizations of the test statistic U_{PSZ}. In contrast, the second class of test statistics rely on the NPMLE of the mean function of recurrent event processes and can be regarded as generalizations of the test statistic given in (4.4).

4.3.1 NPMPLE-Based Nonparametric Procedures

In this subsection, we generalize the test procedure based on the statistic U_{PSZ} to the general p-sample situation. For this, let $\hat{\mu}_{I,l}(t)$ denote the IRE of the mean function $\mu_l(t)$ based only on the observed data from the subjects given treatment l, $l = 1, \ldots, p$. Then a natural generalization of U_{PSZ} is given by $U_{BZ1} = (U_{BZ1,2}, \ldots, U_{BZ1,p})^T$, where

$$U_{BZ1,l} = \sqrt{n} \int_0^\tau W_{n,l}(t) \left\{ \hat{\mu}_{I,1}(t) - \hat{\mu}_{I,l}(t) \right\} dG_n(t),$$

$l = 2, \ldots, p$. In the above, τ and $G_n(t)$ are defined as in the previous section and the $W_{n,l}(t)$'s are bounded weight processes that may depend on the observed data.

It is obvious that U_{BZ1} is equivalent to U_{PSZ} if $p = 2$ and one can rewrite $U_{BZ1,l}$ as

$$U_{BZ1,l} = \frac{1}{\sqrt{n}} \sum_{i=1}^n \sum_{j=1}^{m_i} W_{n,l}(t_{i,j}) \left\{ \hat{\mu}_{I,1}(t_{i,j}) - \hat{\mu}_{I,l}(t_{i,j}) \right\}.$$

For the selection of the weight process $W_{n,l}(t)$, a simple choice is to take $W_{n,l}(t) = W_n^{(1)}(t)$ or $W_n^{(2)}(t)$, defined in the previous section. In corresponding to $W_n^{(3)}(t)$ given in the previous section, one could use $W_{n,l}(t) = g\{Y_{n,1}(t), Y_{n,l}(t)\}$, where g is a fixed function and $Y_{n,l}(t) = n_l^{-1} \sum_{i \in S_l} I(t \leq t_{i,m_i})$, $l = 1, \ldots, p$.

Define $\tilde{H}_i(t) = \sum_{j=1}^{m_i} I(t \geq t_{i,j})$, the observation process on subject i, $i = 1,\ldots,n$. As before, we assume that the $\tilde{H}_i(t)$'s follow the same probability law and $n_l/n \to p_l$ as $n \to \infty$, where $0 < p_l < 1$ and $p_1 + \cdots + p_p = 1$. Also suppose that there exists a bounded function $W(t)$ such that

$$\left[\int_0^\tau \{W_{n,l}(t) - W(t)\}^2 \, dG(t)\right]^{1/2} = o_p(n^{-1/6}), \, l = 2,\ldots,p, \quad (4.5)$$

where $G(t) = E\{\tilde{H}_i(t)\}$. Then Balakrishnan and Zhao (2010b) show that under some regularity conditions and H_0^*, U_{BZ1} asymptotically follows the multivariate normal distribution with mean zero and the covariance matrix that can be consistently estimated by

$$\hat{\Sigma}_{BZ1} = H \, \mathrm{diag}(\hat{\sigma}_{1,1}^2, \hat{\sigma}_{1,2}^2, \ldots, \hat{\sigma}_{1,p}^2) \, H^T.$$

In the above,

$$H = \begin{pmatrix} -\sqrt{\frac{n}{n_1}} & \sqrt{\frac{n}{n_2}} & 0 & \cdots & 0 \\ -\sqrt{\frac{n}{n_1}} & 0 & \sqrt{\frac{n}{n_3}} & \cdots & 0 \\ \cdots & \cdots & \cdots & \cdots & \cdots \\ -\sqrt{\frac{n}{n_1}} & 0 & 0 & \cdots & \sqrt{\frac{n}{n_p}} \end{pmatrix} \quad (4.6)$$

and

$$\hat{\sigma}_{1,l}^2 = \frac{1}{n_l} \sum_{i \in S_l} \left[\sum_{j=1}^{m_i} W_{n,l}(t_{i,j}) \{N_i(t_{i,j}) - \hat{\mu}_{I,l}(t_{i,j})\}\right]^2, \, l = 1,\ldots,p,$$

where $W_{n,1}(t)$ is a specified weight process as the others.

Note that for $p = 2$, the condition (4.5) is more general than the condition (4.3). That is, the latter implies the former. Based on the result above, one can test the null hypothesis H_0^* by using the statistic $U_{BZ1}^* = U_{BZ1}^T \hat{\Sigma}_{BZ1}^{-1} U_{BZ1}$ based on the χ^2-distribution with $(p-1)$ degrees of freedom.

4.3.2 NPMLE-Based Nonparametric Procedures

As commented before, for any statistical or specially test procedure based on the IRE or NPMPLE of the mean function of recurrent event processes, it is natural to consider the same or similar procedure based on the NPMLE of the mean function. In this subsection, we discuss one such class of nonparametric procedures for testing the null hypothesis H_0^*. Also as remarked above, due to the different structures of the two types of estimators, the corresponding test statistics take different forms. Specifically, to test H_0^* and similar to the statistic given in (4.4), Balakrishnan and Zhao (2009) suggest to use the statistic $U_{BZ2} = (U_{BZ2,2}, \ldots, U_{BZ2,p})^T$, where

4.3 General p-Sample Comparison of Cumulative Mean Functions

$$U_{BZ2,l} = \frac{1}{\sqrt{n}} \sum_{i=1}^{n} \left[\sum_{j=1}^{m_i-1} W_{n,l}(t_{i,j}) \hat{\mu}_F(t_{i,j}) \left\{ \left(\frac{\Delta \hat{\mu}_{F,1}(t_{i,j+1})}{\Delta \hat{\mu}_F(t_{i,j+1})} - \frac{\Delta \hat{\mu}_{F,1}(t_{i,j})}{\Delta \hat{\mu}_F(t_{i,j})} \right) \right. \right.$$
$$\left. - \left(\frac{\Delta \hat{\mu}_{F,l}(t_{i,j+1})}{\Delta \hat{\mu}_F(t_{i,j+1})} - \frac{\Delta \hat{\mu}_{F,l}(t_{i,j})}{\Delta \hat{\mu}_F(t_{i,j})} \right) \right\}$$
$$+ W_{n,l}(t_{i,m_i}) \hat{\mu}_F(t_{i,m_i}) \left\{ \left(1 - \frac{\Delta \hat{\mu}_{F,1}(t_{i,m_i})}{\Delta \hat{\mu}_F(t_{i,m_i})} \right) - \left(1 - \frac{\Delta \hat{\mu}_{F,l}(t_{i,m_i})}{\Delta \hat{\mu}_F(t_{i,m_i})} \right) \right\} \right],$$

$l = 2, \ldots, p$. In the above, as before, $\Delta H(t_{i,j}) = H(t_{i,j}) - H(t_{i,j-1})$ for any function $H(t)$ and the $W_{n,l}(t)$'s are some bounded weight processes. Also $\hat{\mu}_F(t)$ and $\hat{\mu}_{F,l}(t)$ denote the NPMLE of the common mean function of the $N_i(t)$'s under H_0^* based on all samples and $\mu_l(t)$ based only on the sample from the subjects in treatment group l, respectively.

It is apparent that as the one given in (4.4), the test statistics $U_{BZ2,l}$'s are much more complicated than those based on the NPMPLE of mean functions. On the other hand, all test statistics discussed above have similar meanings as some summations of differences between two estimators of the same function. In particular, $U_{BZ2,l}$ represents the integrated weighted difference between the rates of the increases of the estimators $\hat{\mu}_F(t)$ and $\hat{\mu}_{F,l}(t)$ over the observation period. Also the construction of all test statistics discussed above actually results from some forms of the functional of either the NPMPLE or NPMLE that have asymptotic normal distributions (Balakrishnan and Zhao, 2009). For example, the characteristic of the NPMLE $\hat{\mu}_F(t)$ that plays a key role in the asymptotic normality of the functional of $\hat{\mu}_F(t)$ and motivates the test statistics $U_{BZ2,l}$'s is

$$\sum_{i=1}^{n} \left[\sum_{j=1}^{m_i-1} \hat{\mu}_F(t_{i,j}) \left\{ \frac{\Delta n_{i,j+1}}{\Delta \hat{\mu}_F(t_{i,j+1})} - \frac{\Delta n_{i,j}}{\Delta \hat{\mu}_F(t_{i,j})} \right\} \right.$$
$$\left. + \hat{\mu}_F(t_{i,m_i}) \left\{ 1 - \frac{\Delta n_{i,m_i}}{\Delta \hat{\mu}_F(t_{i,m_i})} \right\} \right] = 0.$$

Suppose that the weight processes $W_{n,l}(t)$'s satisfy the condition (4.5) and

$$\max_{1 \leq i \leq n} E \left[\sum_{j=1}^{m_i} \{ W_{n,l}(t_{i,j}) - W(t_{i,j}) \}^2 \right] \longrightarrow 0$$

for $l = 1, \ldots, p$. Also suppose that $n_l/n \to p_l$ as $n \to \infty$ as before, where $0 < p_l < 1$ and $p_1 + \cdots + p_p = 1$. Balakrishnan and Zhao (2009) show that as U_{BZ1}, under some regularity conditions and H_0^*, the distribution of U_{BZ2} can be asymptotically approximated by the multivariate normal distribution with mean zero and the covariance matrix

$$\hat{\Sigma}_{BZ2} = H \operatorname{diag}(\hat{\sigma}_{2,1}^2, \hat{\sigma}_{2,2}^2, \ldots, \hat{\sigma}_{2,p}^2) H^T.$$

In the above, H is defined as in (4.6) and

$$\hat{\sigma}_{2,l}^2 = \frac{1}{n}\sum_{i=1}^{n}\left[\sum_{j=1}^{m_i-1} W_{n,l}(t_{i,j})\,\hat{\mu}_F(t_{i,j})\left\{\frac{\Delta n_{i,j+1}}{\Delta\hat{\mu}_F(t_{i,j+1})} - \frac{\Delta n_{i,j}}{\Delta\hat{\mu}_F(t_{i,j})}\right\}\right.$$
$$\left. + W_{n,l}(t_{i,m_i})\,\hat{\mu}_F(t_{i,m_i})\left\{1 - \frac{\Delta n_{i,m_i}}{\Delta\hat{\mu}_F(t_{i,m_i})}\right\}\right]^2,$$

$l = 1,\ldots,p$. It follows that the null hypothesis H_0^* can be tested by using the statistic $U_{BZ2}^* = U_{BZ2}^T \hat{\Sigma}_{BZ2}^{-1} U_{BZ2}$ based on the χ^2-distribution with $(p-1)$ degrees of freedom.

As with U_{BZ1}, the use of U_{BZ2} needs the selection of the weight processes $W_{n,l}(t)$'s and it is apparent that the discussion on this given in the previous subsection applies here. In addition, some other choices for $W_{n,l}(t)$ include

$$Y_{n,l}(t)\,,\quad \frac{Y_{n,l}(t)}{Y_n(t)}\,,\quad \frac{Y_{n,1}(t)\,Y_{n,l}(t)}{Y_n(t)}\,,$$

or

$$1 - Y_{n,l}(t)\,,\quad \frac{1 - Y_{n,l}(t)}{1 - Y_n(t)}\,,\quad \frac{\{1 - Y_{n,1}(t)\}\{1 - Y_{n,l}(t)\}}{1 - Y_n(t)}.$$

4.3.3 Discussion

There exist a couple of other test statistics similar to either U_{BZ1} or U_{BZ2} that have been investigated for testing the null hypothesis H_0^*. One, similar to $U_{BZ1,l}$, is

$$\sqrt{n}\int_0^{\tau} W_{n,l}(t)\left\{\hat{\mu}_I(t) - \hat{\mu}_{I,l}(t)\right\}dG_n(t)$$

(Balakrishnan and Zhao, 2010b), where $\hat{\mu}_I(t)$ denotes the IRE of the common mean function of the $N_i(t)$'s under H_0^* based on all observed data as before. Instead of comparing individual estimators of the same mean function under different conditions as in $U_{BZ1,l}$, the statistic above compares the individual estimator to the overall estimator. Also it is apparent that the statistic above is similar to and can be regarded as a generalization of the statistic U_{SF} given in (4.1). Some discussion on the statistic U_{BZ1} can also be found in Zhang (2006) for the situation where the weight processes $W_{n,l}(t)$'s are taken to be identical.

To test H_0^*, instead of and similar to $U_{BZ2,l}$, Balakrishnan and Zhao (2009) also suggest to use the statistic

$$\frac{1}{\sqrt{n}} \sum_{i=1}^{n} \left[\sum_{j=1}^{m_i-1} W_{n,l}(t_{i,j})\, \hat{\mu}_F(t_{i,j}) \left\{ \frac{\Delta \hat{\mu}_{F,l}(t_{i,j+1})}{\Delta \hat{\mu}_F(t_{i,j+1})} - \frac{\Delta \hat{\mu}_{F,l}(t_{i,j})}{\Delta \hat{\mu}_F(t_{i,j})} \right\} \right.$$
$$\left. + W_{n,l}(t_{i,m_i})\, \hat{\mu}_F(t_{i,m_i}) \left\{ 1 - \frac{\Delta \hat{\mu}_{F,l}(t_{i,m_i})}{\Delta \hat{\mu}_F(t_{i,m_i})} \right\} \right].$$

It can be shown that the statistic above has a similar meaning to $U_{BZ2,l}$ and its asymptotic distribution can be similarly established. In addition, it is apparent that one can develop a test procedure by using the statistic given in (4.4) with replacing Z_i by a vector of treatment indicators.

In terms of comparison about the test statistics or procedures described above, the comments given in Chap. 3 about the comparison between the NPMPLE and NPMLE of the mean function of recurrent event processes apply. More specifically, a major difference between the two types of procedures is that the ones based on the NPMPLE are much simpler and can be easily carried out, while the ones based on the NPMLE could be more efficient. More comments on this are given in the next section through some numerical comparison and an illustration.

Note that as the test procedures discussed in the previous section, all nonparametric procedures described in this section assume that the underlying point processes generating observation times $t_{i,j}$'s are identical. That is, the observation processes $\tilde{H}_i(t)$'s follow the same probability law. It is obvious that this may not be true in reality. One simple such example is that the patients receiving a placebo treatment may have more or less clinical visits than the patients given some effective treatments. As remarked above, if such difference exists, the test procedure that ignores it can yield misleading or wrong conclusions. Section 4.5 gives a class of nonparametric procedures that take such differences into account.

4.4 Numerical Comparison and Illustration

In this section, we compare and illustrate the four nonparametric test procedures, based on the test statistics U_{SF}, U_{PSZ}, U_{BZ1} and U_{BZ2}, respectively, discussed in the previous two sections. First we apply them to the gallstone data arising from the National Cooperative Gallstone Study discussed in Sect. 1.2.2. A comparison based on simulated data is then presented and followed by some general comments. Note that for the gallstone data, there exist only two treatments and thus we have $p = 2$. Also in this case, the two test procedures based on U_{PSZ} and U_{BZ1} are equivalent and thus only the latter is considered.

4.4.1 Analysis of National Cooperative Gallstone Study

As described before, this study is a 10-year, multicenter, double-blinded, placebo-controlled clinical trial on the use of cheno for the dissolution of cholesterol gallstones. The original study consists of three treatments groups, placebo, low dose, and high dose of cheno, and one of the main objectives of the study is to compare the treatment groups in terms of the incidence or occurrence rates of nausea. Also as before, for the analysis here and below, we confine ourselves to the panel count data observed during the first 52 weeks on the 113 patients in the placebo and high dose groups.

Table 4.1. Test results for the floating gallstone data

Statistic	U_{SF}	U_{BZ1}				U_{BZ2}			
Weight process		$W_n^{(1)}$	$W_n^{(2)}$	$W_n^{(3)}$	$W_n^{(4)}$	$W_n^{(1)}$	$W_n^{(2)}$	$W_n^{(3)}$	$W_n^{(4)}$
p-value	0.143	0.454	0.417	0.413	0.891	0.861	0.000	0.000	0.000

Table 4.1 presents the p-values given by the three test procedures based on U_{SF}, U_{PSZ} and U_{BZ2}, respectively, for testing the no treatment difference between the placebo and high dose groups. Here for the procedures based on U_{BZ1} and U_{BZ2}, four weight processes are used with the first three being those discussed in Sect. 4.2.2 and $W_n^{(4)}(t) = 1 - W_n^{(2)}(t)$. One can see from the table that the procedures based on U_{SF} and U_{BZ1} as well as the one based on U_{BZ2} with $W_n^{(1)}(t)$ suggest no significant difference between the two groups. On the other hand, the procedure based on U_{BZ2} with other three weight processes suggests that the treatment effect was significant. To explain the difference between the test results here, it is worth noting from Figs. 3.2 and 3.4 that the estimated mean functions between the two groups cross each other. As commented below, this makes the selection of weight processes difficult. In general, one can try to explain the difference from the use of either different procedures or different weight processes, or both. Some general comments on the selection of the procedures above are given below. With respect to the four weight processes used here, note that in comparison with $W_n^{(1)}(t)$, all other three emphasize the difference between the estimated mean functions during the middle period of the follow-up. Figures 3.2 and 3.4 indicate that this happens to be the period where the estimated mean functions for the two groups have the largest difference.

4.4.2 Numerical Comparison of the Test Procedures

As seen from the example above, for the treatment comparison, a difficult question that can occur in practice is the selection of an appropriate test procedure as well as an appropriate weight process. To address this, we conduct a

4.4 Numerical Comparison and Illustration

Table 4.2. Empirical size and power with non-crossing mean functions

β	U_{SF}	U_{BZ1}				U_{BZ2}			
		$W_n^{(1)}$	$W_n^{(2)}$	$W_n^{(3)}$	$W_n^{(4)}$	$W_n^{(1)}$	$W_n^{(2)}$	$W_n^{(3)}$	$W_n^{(4)}$
				$n_1 = 40, n_2 = 60$					
0.0	0.045	0.049	0.047	0.048	0.048	0.050	0.057	0.053	0.050
0.1	0.090	0.069	0.069	0.068	0.080	0.109	0.090	0.090	0.107
0.2	0.191	0.154	0.153	0.155	0.160	0.246	0.213	0.213	0.174
0.3	0.357	0.309	0.302	0.302	0.297	0.447	0.411	0.414	0.334
				$n_1 = 80, n_2 = 120$					
0.0	0.042	0.044	0.041	0.041	0.046	0.052	0.051	0.050	0.052
0.1	0.112	0.097	0.094	0.095	0.093	0.140	0.138	0.138	0.124
0.2	0.320	0.282	0.282	0.283	0.282	0.377	0.358	0.355	0.280
0.3	0.643	0.620	0.616	0.615	0.605	0.735	0.687	0.691	0.578

Table 4.3. Empirical power with crossing mean functions

β	U_{SF}	U_{BZ1}				U_{BZ2}			
		$W_n^{(1)}$	$W_n^{(2)}$	$W_n^{(3)}$	$W_n^{(4)}$	$W_n^{(1)}$	$W_n^{(2)}$	$W_n^{(3)}$	$W_n^{(4)}$
				$n_1 = 40, n_2 = 60$					
3	0.402	0.462	0.394	0.394	0.718	0.849	0.323	0.310	0.989
5	0.061	0.079	0.059	0.058	0.298	0.411	0.065	0.066	0.945
8	0.138	0.115	0.140	0.141	0.047	0.059	0.265	0.272	0.766
				$n_1 = 80, n_2 = 120$					
3	0.668	0.708	0.604	0.601	0.957	0.993	0.491	0.476	1.000
5	0.084	0.104	0.062	0.061	0.472	0.669	0.063	0.064	0.999
8	0.205	0.179	0.237	0.237	0.061	0.083	0.471	0.484	0.968

general comparison by using simulated data with the focus on the two-sample situation and the three test procedures used in the previous subsection.

To generate panel count data, we assume that $N_i(t)$ is a mixed Poisson process with the mean function $\mu(t|\nu_i)$ given ν_i, where the ν_i's are independent and identically distributed random variables from Gamma(2, 1/2). With respect to observation times, we first generate m_i from the uniform distribution $U\{1,\ldots,10\}$ and then take $t_{i,1} < \cdots < t_{i,m_i}$ to be the order statistics of m_i random variables again from the uniform distribution $U\{1,\ldots,10\}$. For $\mu(t|\nu_i)$, we consider two cases. One is to let $\mu(t|\nu_i) = \nu_i\, t\, \exp(\beta Z_i)$, where Z_i is the treatment indicator taking value 0 or 1 and β represents the treatment difference. The other is to take $\mu(t|\nu_i) = \nu_i t$ for the subjects with $Z_i = 0$ and $\mu(t|\nu_i) = \nu_i \sqrt{\beta t}$ otherwise. Note that for the first case, the two mean functions do not overlap, while the two mean functions for the latter case cross over each other.

Tables 4.2 and 4.3 present the empirical size and power of the three test procedures based on the simulated panel count data. Here the same four weight processes as those used in the previous subsection are considered and the sample sizes between the two groups are assumed to be different, being 40 and 60 or 80 and 120. Note that in Table 4.3, only the empirical power of the test procedures is included. One can see from Table 4.2 that when the underlying mean functions do not overlap, all procedures perform reasonably well and their performance does not seem to depend on the weight process. As expected, the NPMLE-based procedure (U_{BZ2}) shows larger power than the NPMPLE-based procedures (U_{SF} and U_{BZ1}) in general.

Table 4.3 shows that when the underlying mean functions cross over each other, the selection of both test procedure and weight process is much more complicated. One key point in this case is that the NPMPLE-based procedures could have better power in some situations than the NPMLE-based procedure. Also the results in Table 4.3 and from other simulation studies indicate that the performance or power of a test procedure can heavily depend on the shapes of mean functions. It is well-known that in practice, it may not be possible to know the shapes of true mean functions. It is apparent that for the problem here, an ideal solution is to develop an approach that automatically selects the appropriate procedure and weight process. On the other hand, this may be very difficult or impossible. The same issue exists in other fields too such as failure time data analysis.

4.5 Comparison of Cumulative Mean Functions with Different Observation Processes

This section discusses the same problem as that considered in the previous sections. However, unlike in the previous sections, it is assumed that the processes generating observation times, or the observation processes, may be different for the study subjects in different treatment groups. In other words, the observation process may depend on the treatment and sometimes this is also referred to as with unequal observation processes (Zhao and Sun, 2011). In the following, we use the same notation as those used in the previous sections and assume that the goal is to test the null hypothesis H_0^*. A class of new statistics is first presented and then followed by an illustration.

4.5.1 Test Statistics

To present the new test statistics for the hypothesis H_0^*, for $l = 1, \ldots, p$, let $p_l = n_l/n$, π_l be the limit of p_l, and

$$G_l(t) = \mathrm{E}\left\{\tilde{H}_i(t)\right\} \text{ for } i \in S_l \,, \; G^*(t) = \sum_{l=1}^{p} \pi_l \, G_l(t) \,.$$

4.5 Comparison of Cumulative Mean Functions ...

Define
$$g_l(t) = G'_l(t), \ g(t) = G'(t), \ \nu_l(t) = g(t)/g_l(t),$$
and
$$G_{n,l}(t) = \frac{1}{n_l} \sum_{i \in S_l} \sum_{j=1}^{m_i} I(t_{i,j} \leq t),$$

the empirical observation process for the subjects in treatment group l. Then it is apparent that we have

$$G_n(t) = \sum_{l=1}^{p} p_l \, G_{n,l}(t),$$

which is the overall empirical observation process. Also define

$$\hat{\sigma}_l^2 = \frac{1}{n_l} \sum_{i \in S_l} \left[\sum_{j=1}^{m_i} \Lambda_l(t_{i,j}) \{ N_i(t_{i,j}) - \hat{\mu}_{I,l}(t_{i,j}) \} \right]^2,$$

and
$$\Psi_{n,l} = \int_0^\tau W_n(t) \, \hat{\mu}_{I,l}(t) \, d\, G_n(t),$$

where $W_n(t)$ is a bounded weight process and

$$\Lambda_l(t) = \sum_{j=1}^{p} \frac{n_j}{n} W_n(t) \frac{G_{n,j}(t) - G_{n,j}(t-)}{G_{n,l}(t) - G_{n,l}(t-)},$$

$l = 1, \ldots, p$. It is easy to see that the statistic $\Psi_{n,l}$ can be regarded as a measure of the summary of the observed information related to treatment l.

To test the hypothesis H_0^*, Zhao and Sun (2011) suggest to apply the statistic

$$U_{ZS} = \sum_{l=1}^{p} c_l \left(\Psi_{n,l} - \bar{\Psi}_n \right)^2,$$

where $c_l = n_l / \hat{\sigma}_l^2$ and $\bar{\Psi}_n = \sum_{l=1}^{p} \alpha_l \Psi_{n,l}$ with $\alpha_l = c_l \left(\sum_{j=1}^{p} c_j \right)^{-1}$. Furthermore, they show that under some regularity conditions and H_0^*, U_{ZS} asymptotically follows the χ^2-distribution with $(p-1)$ degrees of freedom if there exists a bounded function $W(t)$ such that

$$\int_0^\tau \{ W_n(t) - W(t) \}^2 \, dG_l(t) = o_p(n^{-1/3})$$

and
$$\max_{i \in S_l} E \left[\sum_{j=1}^{m_i} \{ W_n(t_{i,j}) - W(t_{i,j}) \}^2 \right] \to 0$$

for all $l = 1, \ldots, p$.

It is easy to see that the test statistic U_{ZS} has similar meanings to those given in the previous sections and constructed based on the IRE or NPMPLE of the mean function of recurrent event processes, especially the statistic U_{SF}. More specifically, U_{ZS} represents the integrated weighted difference among the estimated mean functions $\hat{\mu}_{I,l}(t)$'s. Actually it is not difficult to show that the test statistic $U_{BZ1,l}$ with the same weight processes can be expressed as the difference between $\Psi_{n,1}$ and $\Psi_{n,l}$. For the selection of the weight process $W_n(t)$, some simple choices include $W_n^{(1)}(t)$ and $W_n^{(2)}(t)$ given in Sect. 4.2 as well as $1 - W_n^{(2)}(t)$.

4.5.2 An Application

Now we illustrate the test procedure described above using the bladder tumor data discussed in Sect. 1.2.3 and given in the data set II of Chap. 9. As mentioned before, the data include the clinical visit or observation times and the numbers of recurrent bladder tumors that occurred between the visit or observation times from 85 patients who had superficial bladder tumors. There exist two treatment groups, placebo (47 patients) and thiotepa (38 patients), and one objective of the study is to compare the recurrence rates of bladder tumors between the groups.

To compare the two groups, we first investigate the observation process corresponding to each of the two groups. For this, note that for the patients in the placebo and thiotepa groups, the average numbers of clinical visits or observations are 8.66 and 13.50, respectively. That is, the patients in the placebo group seem to have the smaller numbers of visits or observations than those in the treatment group. To give a more complete picture on this, Fig. 4.1 presents the separate Nelson-Aalen estimators, given by (1.5), of the cumulative intensity functions of the observation processes corresponding to the two groups. It is apparent that the patients in the placebo group indeed seem to have a significantly lower observation rate, which suggests that one should apply the test procedure discussed in this section.

Table 4.4 gives the p-values yielded by the application of the test statistic U_{ZS} discussed above with the use of three weight processes, $W_n^{(1)}(t)$, $W_n^{(2)}(t)$ and $1 - W_n^{(2)}(t)$. Although they are not close, the results indicate that the two groups seem to have different recurrence rates of bladder tumors. To further look at this, Fig. 4.2 gives the separate IRE of the mean functions of the underlying recurrence processes of bladder tumors corresponding to the patients in the two groups. One can easily see that the recurrence rates indeed seem to be different, and the patients in the thiotepa treatment group had a lower recurrence rate than those in the placebo group. In other words, the thiotepa treatment seems to be effective in reducing the recurrence rate of bladder tumors. More discussions on this data set are given below.

4.5 Comparison of Cumulative Mean Functions ...   87

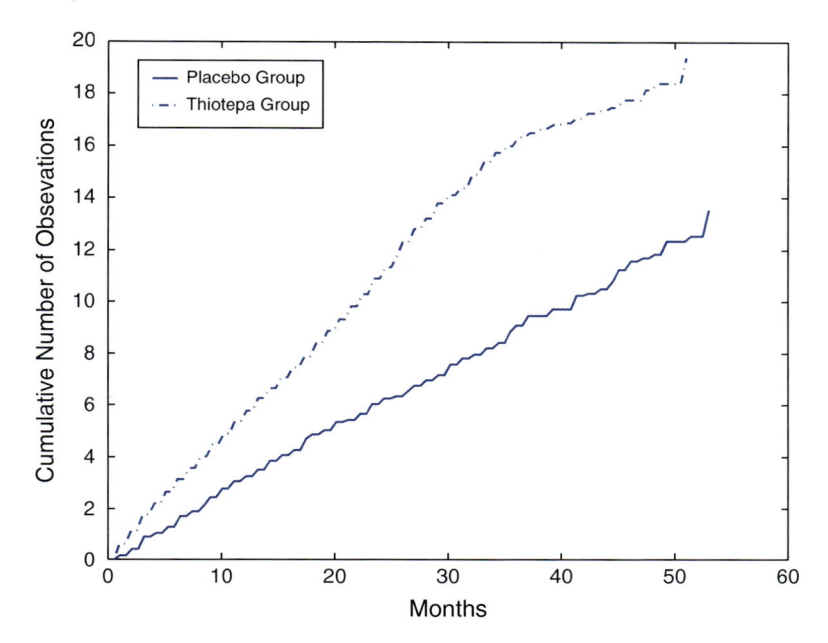

Fig. 4.1. The Nelson-Aalen estimators for the observation processes

Table 4.4. Test results based on U_{ZS} for the bladder tumor data

Weight process	$W_n^{(1)}$	$W_n^{(2)}$	$1 - W_n^{(2)}$
p-value	0.0477	0.0861	0.00004

4.5.3 Discussion

For the situation discussed in this section, two practical questions naturally arise. One is how the test procedure given in this section differs from the procedures given in Sects. 4.2 and 4.3. The other is if one can still apply the nonparametric procedures discussed in the previous sections to the current situation. To answer the first one, note that as discussed before, all test statistics are constructed as some kinds of differences among different groups. For the statistics introduced in the previous sections, the difference is about the estimated mean functions of the underlying recurrent event processes given the observation processes. In other words, the difference does not involve or use the information involved in the observation processes (assumed to be identical). In contrast, the quantity used to measure the difference in the test statistic U_{ZS} can be seen as a summary measure of the whole system that involves both the underlying recurrent event process and the observation process.

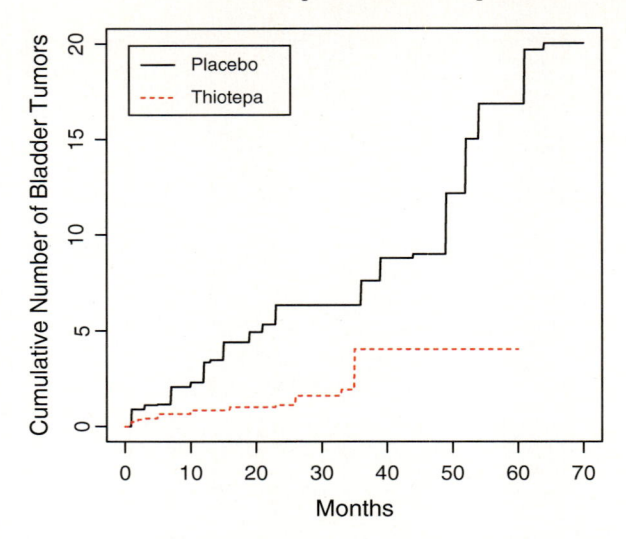

Fig. 4.2. IRE of the cumulative average numbers of bladder tumors

To answer the second question above, Zhao and Sun (2011) conducted a simulation study to compare the two test procedures based on the test statistics U_{BZ1} and U_{ZS}, respectively. They show that the procedures perform similarly when observation processes are the same, but if the observation processes differ between treatment groups, the former tends to inflate the test size and power. In other words, in the presence of the difference among the observation processes, it is necessary or essential to apply the test procedure discussed in this section to obtain valid results. More comments on this are given in later chapters.

As discussed in Sect. 4.3, it is not difficult to see that one can construct some test statistics similar to U_{ZS} by replacing the used IRE or NPMPLE with the NPMLE of the mean function of recurrent event processes. Again one would face the same problem discussed before. That is, the structure of the resulting test statistics may have to be different from that of U_{ZS} and the derivation of the null distribution of the new statistics would not be easy. By still using the IRE, in the case of two treatment groups and instead of using the test statistic U_{ZS}, Zhang (2006) suggested the test statistic

$$\int_0^\tau \left\{ \hat{g}_1^{-1}(t)\,\hat{\mu}_{I,1}(t)\,dG_{n,1}(t) - \hat{g}_2^{-1}(t)\,\hat{\mu}_{I,2}(t)\,dG_{n,2}(t) \right\},$$

where $\hat{g}_1(t)$ and $\hat{g}_2(t)$ are kernel estimators of $g_1(t)$ and $g_2(t)$, respectively. Note that the statistic above involves estimation of $g_1(t)$ and $g_2(t)$, which may not be easy. More importantly, its null distribution is unknown.

4.6 Bibliography, Discussion, and Remarks

The majority of the existing nonparametric test procedures for comparing recurrent event processes based on panel count data can be classified into two types with respect to the estimator of the mean function of the processes used in test statistics. One is these constructed based on the NPMPLE or IRE (Balakrishnan and Zhao, 2010b; Li et al., 2010; Park, 2005; Park et al., 2007; Sun and Fang, 2003; Sun and Kalbfleisch, 1993; Zhang, 2006; Zhao and Sun, 2011), and the other is these constructed based on the NPMLE (Balakrishnan and Zhao, 2009, 2010a). As discussed above, the main difference between the two is that the former may be less powerful than the latter, but the latter is much more complicated both computationally and theoretically than the former. In addition to those mentioned above, other authors who investigated the comparison of recurrent event processes in the case of panel count data include Sun and Rai (2001) and Thall and Lachin (1988). The former is commented below and the latter gives a parametric procedure as discussed above. In addition, Zhao et al. (2013c) gave a class of nonparametric test procedures for multivariate panel count data and more on it is discussed in Chap. 7.

The focus in this chapter has been on the situation where observation processes are identical or different for the subjects in different treatment groups. In other words, they are independent of the recurrent event processes of interest completely or given treatments. As remarked above and also below, sometimes the observation process and the recurrent event process of interest may be correlated. In this case, the test procedures that do not take the relationship into account can yield biased or misleading results. In other words, one needs different and new test procedures for the comparison of recurrent event processes.

As seen in the discussion above and also is true in general, the inclusion of some weight functions or processes is a technique commonly used in the construction of test statistics. It allows investigators to put different emphases on different treatment groups or time periods. For a given alternative hypothesis, a proper selection of them could also improve the power of the resulting test procedure. On this aspect, a natural question is how or if one can choose an optimal one or develop some guideline for their selections given a practical problem. Unfortunately, there does not seem to exist such a procedure or guideline even for recurrent event data. Another issue on the test procedures discussed above for which there does not seem to exist any literature is the investigation of the properties of them under alternative hypotheses. In consequence, they are not ready to be used for sample size calculations.

Finally we remark again that the focus of this chapter and also the literature on the treatment comparison based on panel count data has been on the hypothesis formulated by mean functions. This leads to the fact that most of the existing nonparametric test procedures are based on the comparison of different estimated mean functions. Of course it is natural to ask if one can or could formulate the hypothesis using intensity functions or processes and develop corresponding test procedures. Sun and Rai (2001) discussed this under a simple set-up where all study subjects have asymptotically the same observation times. As discussed in Chap. 3 on nonparametric estimation based on panel count data and in this chapter on the test procedures based on the NPMLE, one can easily see that the task would be very difficult or close to impossible. It is worth noting that the way used to develop test statistics here is actually the same as that used for the case of recurrent event data (Cook and Lawless, 2007) and also similar for the case of failure time data (Kalbfleisch and Prentice, 2002). In the latter case, the null hypothesis is usually formulated by using the hazard or survival function, and the test statistics are commonly constructed by comparing the estimated hazard or survival functions. Also as with recurrent event data and failure time data, instead of applying the procedures discussed above, an alternative for comparing different treatment groups is to apply some regression techniques. Discussions on this are given in later chapters.

5
Regression Analysis of Panel Count Data I

5.1 Introduction

This chapter discusses regression analysis of panel count data. As discussed before, unlike recurrent event data, panel count data involve an extra observation process and this observation process may be independent of or could be related to the underlying recurrent event process of interest. In this chapter, we consider the situation where the two processes are independent of each other completely or conditionally given covariates. The situation where the two processes are related is investigated in the next chapter.

To perform regression analysis of recurrent event data, as remarked above, it is common to model the intensity process as well as the rate or mean function of the underlying recurrent event process of interest (Andersen et al., 1993; Cook and Lawless, 2007). On the other hand, for regression analysis of panel count data, only the rate or mean function is usually used to model the effects of covariates on the recurrent event process. In this latter case, of course, one can fit the data to parametric Poisson processes or mixed parametric Poisson processes as discussed on Chap. 2. Another parametric approach is to treat the data as longitudinal count data and to use the generalized estimating equation approach (Diggle et al., 1994). A main drawback of all parametric methods is that it is often difficult to determine or find an appropriate parametric model for a given problem and the data. In this chapter, we discuss semiparametric approaches with the focus on the effects of covariates on the mean function of the underlying recurrent event process.

Consider a recurrent event study and let $N(t)$ denote the underlying recurrent event process of interest as before. Assume that there exists a vector of covariates denoted by Z and the main goal of the study is to estimate the effects of Z on $N(t)$. For this, in the following, we begin with considering the situation where the effects can be described by model (1.4), the proportional mean model, and discuss two types of inference procedures for estimation of the regression parameter β. Section 5.2 first describes some likelihood-based procedures with the use of some assumptions on the counting process $N(t)$. In particular, we consider the resulting procedure if $N(t)$ can be regarded as a non-homogeneous Poisson process as in Sect. 3.2. Note that a disadvantage of the likelihood-based approach is that it usually involves nonparametric estimation of unknown functions. This makes its implementation often difficult and also its validity may require large sample sizes. Corresponding to these, Sects. 5.3 and 5.4 present two types of estimating equation approaches, which do not rely on any distribution assumption on $N(t)$ and also do not require estimation of unknown functions.

Note that the proportional mean model implies that the mean functions associated with any two sets of covariate values are proportional over time. It is not hard to see that this restriction could be too strong in practice as with the proportional hazards model in failure time data analysis (Lin et al., 2001). Corresponding to this, in Sect. 5.5, we consider a class of semiparametric transformation models that include model (1.4) as a special case and also allow $\boldsymbol{Z}(t)$ to be time-dependent. For estimation of regression parameters, some estimating equation procedures are described and in addition, a procedure is given for testing the goodness-of-fit of the semiparametric transformation model. In Sect. 5.6, an illustrative example is provided by applying the described methods to the gallstone data discussed and analyzed in Sects. 1.2.2 and 4.4.1. Section 5.7 concludes with some bibliographical notes and remarks on some issues not discussed in the previous sections.

5.2 Analysis by the Likelihood-Based Approach

Consider a recurrent event study that involves n independent subjects and let $N_i(t)$ and $\boldsymbol{Z}_i$ be defined as above but associated with subject i, $i = 1, \ldots, n$. In this section, we assume that the $\boldsymbol{Z}_i$'s are time-independent. Suppose that the mean function $\mu_Z(t) = E\{N_i(t)|\boldsymbol{Z}_i\}$ of $N_i(t)$ given $\boldsymbol{Z}_i$ can be described by the proportional mean model (1.4) and one observes panel count data. Let the $t_{i,j}$'s, $n_{i,j}$'s, and s_l's be defined as in the previous chapters and then the observed data have the form

$$\{\,(t_{i,j}, n_{i,j}, \boldsymbol{Z}_i)\,;\, j = 1, \ldots, m_i, i = 1, \ldots, n\,\}\,. \qquad (5.1)$$

In the following, for estimation of regression parameter $\boldsymbol{\beta}$ in model (1.4), we first describe in details two non-homogeneous Poisson process-based procedures. Some discussions are then given about some other similar procedures.

5.2.1 A Semiparametric Maximum Pseudo-likelihood Estimation Procedure

To estimate the regression parameter $\boldsymbol{\beta}$, following the discussion in Sect. 3.2, we first assume that the $N_i(t)$'s are non-homogeneous Poisson processes. Then as with $l_p(\mu)$ given in (3.4), we can similarly derive the following log pseudo-likelihood function

$$l_p(\mu_0, \boldsymbol{\beta}) = \sum_{i=1}^{n} \sum_{j=1}^{m_i} \left\{ n_{i,j} \log \mu_0(t_{i,j}) + n_{i,j} \boldsymbol{\beta}^T \boldsymbol{Z}_i - \mu_0(t_{i,j}) \exp(\boldsymbol{\beta}^T \boldsymbol{Z}_i) \right\} \tag{5.2}$$

by ignoring the dependence of $\{N_i(t_{i,j}), j = 1, \ldots, m_i\}$ for each i. Thus it is natural to estimate $\boldsymbol{\beta}$ by maximizing $l_p(\mu_0, \boldsymbol{\beta})$ over $\mu_0(t)$ and $\boldsymbol{\beta}$ together.

For the maximization of $l_p(\mu_0, \boldsymbol{\beta})$, let the w_l's and $\bar{n}_l$'s be defined as in Sect. 3.3. Also define

$$\bar{a}_l(\boldsymbol{\beta}) = \frac{1}{w_l} \sum_{i=1}^{n} \sum_{j=1}^{m_i} \exp(\boldsymbol{\beta}^T \boldsymbol{Z}_i) \, I(t_{i,j} = s_l)$$

and

$$\bar{b}_l(\boldsymbol{\beta}) = \frac{1}{w_l} \sum_{i=1}^{n} \sum_{j=1}^{m_i} n_{i,j} \boldsymbol{\beta}^T \boldsymbol{Z}_i \, I(t_{i,j} = s_l)$$

for given $\boldsymbol{\beta}$, $l = 1, \ldots, m$. Then the log pseudo-likelihood function $l_p(\mu_0, \boldsymbol{\beta})$ can be rewritten as

$$l_p(\mu_0, \boldsymbol{\beta}) = \sum_{l=1}^{m} w_l \left\{ \bar{n}_l \log \mu_0(s_l) - \bar{a}_l(\boldsymbol{\beta}) \mu_0(s_l) + \bar{b}_l(\boldsymbol{\beta}) \right\}.$$

It is easy to see that as with the estimation of $\mu(t)$ in Chap. 3, only the values of $\mu_0(t)$ at the s_l's can be estimated. Let $\hat{\mu}_{PL}(t)$ and $\hat{\boldsymbol{\beta}}_{PL}$ denote the estimators of $\mu_0(t)$ and $\boldsymbol{\beta}$, respectively, given by the maximization of $l_p(\mu_0, \boldsymbol{\beta})$ with $\hat{\mu}_{L0}(t)$ being a non-decreasing step function with possible jumps only at the s_l's. Then their determination is equivalent to maximizing $l_p(\mu_0, \boldsymbol{\beta}) = l_p(\boldsymbol{\mu}, \boldsymbol{\beta})$ over the $(m + p)$ unknown parameters $\boldsymbol{\mu} = (\mu_1, \ldots, \mu_m)^T$ and $\boldsymbol{\beta}$ under the restriction $\mu_1 \leq \ldots \leq \mu_m$, where p denotes the dimension of $\boldsymbol{\beta}$ as before and $\mu_l = \mu_0(s_l)$, $l = 1, \ldots, m$.

For the determination of $\hat{\mu}_{PL}(t)$ and $\hat{\boldsymbol{\beta}}_{PL}$ or the maximization of $l_p(\boldsymbol{\mu}, \boldsymbol{\beta})$, one way is to use a two-step iterative algorithm that maximizes l_p over $\boldsymbol{\mu}$ and $\boldsymbol{\beta}$ alternatively. Specifically, for fixed $\boldsymbol{\beta}$, note that the maximization of l_p over $\boldsymbol{\mu}$ is equivalent to maximizing

$$\sum_{l=1}^{m} w_l \, \bar{a}_l(\boldsymbol{\beta}) \left\{ \frac{\bar{n}_l}{\bar{a}_l(\boldsymbol{\beta})} \log \mu_l - \mu_l \right\},$$

which is similar to the log likelihood function given in (3.4). This shows that for given $\boldsymbol{\beta}$, the $\hat{\mu}_{PL}(s_l)$'s are the IRE of $\{\bar{n}_1/\bar{a}_1(\boldsymbol{\beta}), \ldots, \bar{n}_m/\bar{a}_m(\boldsymbol{\beta})\}$ with weights $\{w_1\bar{a}_1(\boldsymbol{\beta}), \ldots, w_m\bar{a}_m(\boldsymbol{\beta})\}$. Thus they have the closed form

$$\hat{\mu}_{PL}(s_l; \boldsymbol{\beta}) = \max_{r \leq l} \min_{s \geq l} \frac{\sum_{v=r}^{s} w_v \bar{n}_v}{\sum_{v=r}^{s} w_v \bar{a}_v(\boldsymbol{\beta})} = \min_{s \geq l} \max_{r \leq l} \frac{\sum_{v=r}^{s} w_v \bar{n}_v}{\sum_{v=r}^{s} w_v \bar{a}_v(\boldsymbol{\beta})}$$

given by the max-min formula of the IRE (Barlow et al., 1972; Robertson et al., 1988). As discussed in Sect. 3.3 with the IRE, in practice, several algorithms such as the pool-adjacent-violators and up-and-down algorithms can be used to determine the $\hat{\mu}_{PL}(s_l; \boldsymbol{\beta})$'s. If $\bar{n}_1/\bar{a}_1(\boldsymbol{\beta}) \leq \ldots \leq \bar{n}_m/\bar{a}_m(\boldsymbol{\beta})$, then we have $\hat{\mu}_{PL}(s_l; \boldsymbol{\beta}) = \bar{n}_l/\bar{a}_l(\boldsymbol{\beta})$, $l = 1, \ldots, m$.

For given $\mu_0(t)$ or $\boldsymbol{\mu}$, one can simply use the Newton-Raphson algorithm for estimation of $\boldsymbol{\beta}$. It can be easily shown that the log pseudo-likelihood function $l_p(\boldsymbol{\mu}, \boldsymbol{\beta})$ is a concave function of $\boldsymbol{\beta}$ for given $\mu_0(t)$ and its value increases after each iteration (Zhang, 2002). The two-step algorithm described above can be summarized as follows.

Step 1. Choose an initial estimator $\boldsymbol{\beta}^{(0)}$ of $\boldsymbol{\beta}$.
Step 2. At the kth iteration, determine the updated estimator $\hat{\boldsymbol{\mu}}_{PL}^{(k)} = (\hat{\mu}_{PL}^{(k)}(s_1; \boldsymbol{\beta}), \ldots, \hat{\mu}_{PL}^{(k)}(s_m; \boldsymbol{\beta}))^T$ of $\boldsymbol{\mu}$ by

$$\hat{\mu}_{PL}^{(k)}(s_l; \boldsymbol{\beta}) = \max_{r \leq l} \min_{s \geq l} \frac{\sum_{v=r}^{s} w_v \bar{n}_v}{\sum_{v=r}^{s} w_v \bar{a}_v(\boldsymbol{\beta}^{(k-1)})} = \min_{s \geq l} \max_{r \leq l} \frac{\sum_{v=r}^{s} w_v \bar{n}_v}{\sum_{v=r}^{s} w_v \bar{a}_v(\boldsymbol{\beta}^{(k-1)})},$$

$l = 1, \ldots, m$.
Step 3. Determine the updated estimator, denoted by $\hat{\boldsymbol{\beta}}^{(k)}$, of $\boldsymbol{\beta}$ by maximizing $l_p(\boldsymbol{\mu}_{PL}^{(k)}, \boldsymbol{\beta})$ with respect to $\boldsymbol{\beta}$ using the Newton-Raphson algorithm.
Step 4. Repeat Steps 2 and 3 until convergence.

To check the convergence, one criterion that one can use is

$$\left| \frac{l_p(\hat{\boldsymbol{\mu}}_{PL}^{(k+1)}, \hat{\boldsymbol{\beta}}^{(k+1)}) - l_p(\hat{\boldsymbol{\mu}}_{PL}^{(k)}, \hat{\boldsymbol{\beta}}^{(k)})}{l_p(\hat{\boldsymbol{\mu}}_{PL}^{(k)}, \hat{\boldsymbol{\beta}}^{(k)})} \right| \leq \epsilon$$

for a given positive number ϵ. Another commonly used criterion is to check the relative difference between the estimators $\hat{\boldsymbol{\mu}}_{PL}^{(k+1)}$ and $\hat{\boldsymbol{\beta}}^{(k+1)}$ and the estimators $\hat{\boldsymbol{\mu}}_{PL}^{(k)}$ and $\hat{\boldsymbol{\beta}}^{(k)}$.

Note that in the above, we have assumed that the $N_i(t)$'s are nonhomogeneous Poisson processes for the derivation of the estimators $\hat{\mu}_{PL}(t)$ and $\hat{\boldsymbol{\beta}}_{PL}$. In general, on the other hand, Zhang (2002) shows that the two-step iterative algorithm described above is actually robust and seems always to converge. He also shows that under some regularity conditions, the estimators $\hat{\mu}_{PL}(t)$ and $\hat{\boldsymbol{\beta}}_{PL}$ are consistent in L_2 and the consistency result does

5.2 Analysis by the Likelihood-Based Approach

not depend on the Poisson process assumption. For the variance estimation of $\hat{\boldsymbol{\beta}}_{PL}$, Zhang (2002) suggests to employ the bootstrap procedure. It should be noted, however, that the procedure could be slow in computation as we are dealing with a semiparametric maximization problem.

5.2.2 A Semiparametric Spline-Based Maximum Likelihood Estimation Procedure

As discussed above, the log pseudo-likelihood function $l_p(\mu_0, \boldsymbol{\beta})$ is not really a true likelihood function. Under the non-homogeneous Poisson process assumption, the true log likelihood function is proportional to

$$l(\mu_0, \boldsymbol{\beta}) = \sum_{l'=0}^{m-1} \sum_{l=l'+1}^{m} \tilde{n}_{l,l'} \log\{\mu_0(s_l) - \mu_0(s_{l'})\} - \sum_{l=1}^{m} b_l(\boldsymbol{\beta}) \mu_0(s_l)$$
$$+ \sum_{i=1}^{n} n_{i,m_i} \boldsymbol{\beta}^T \boldsymbol{Z}_i.$$

Here $b_l(\boldsymbol{\beta}) = \sum_{i=1}^{n} I(t_{i,m_i} = s_l) \exp(\boldsymbol{\beta}^T \boldsymbol{Z}_i)$ and the $\tilde{n}_{l,l'}$'s are defined as in Sect. 3.2.1. Thus it is natural that instead of maximizing $l_p(\mu_0, \boldsymbol{\beta})$, one could and may want to estimate $\boldsymbol{\beta}$ by maximizing $l(\mu_0, \boldsymbol{\beta})$ given above, and it is easy to see that for current status data, the two log likelihood functions are identical. In general, on the other hand, the relationship between the two maximization procedures is actually similar to that between the NPMLE and IRE discussed in Chap. 3. In particular, although the maximization of $l(\mu_0, \boldsymbol{\beta})$ may yield more efficient estimators of regression parameters than the maximization of $l_p(\mu_0, \boldsymbol{\beta})$, the former is much more complicated than the latter (Lu et al., 2009; Wellner and Zhang, 2007). Also both procedures need a great deal of computing effort.

To reduce the computing burden and give a relatively easy estimation procedure, in this subsection, we describe an approximate semiparametric maximum likelihood estimation procedure, developed by Lu et al. (2009). The basic idea behind the new procedure is that it employs monotone cubic B-splines (Schumaker, 1981) to approximate the log baseline mean function. Specifically, assume that $\mu_0(t)$ in the log scale can be approximated by

$$\log\{\mu_0(t)\} = \sum_{l=1}^{K_n} \alpha_l B_l(t)$$

with $\alpha_1 \leq \cdots \leq \alpha_{K_n}$. Here the α_l's are unknown parameters, the $\{B_j(t)\}_{j=1}^{K_n}$ are the B-spline basis functions, and K_n denotes the number of basis functions that depends on the data. Under the approximation above, model (1.4) becomes

$$E\{N(t)|\mathbf{Z}\} = \exp\left\{\sum_{j=1}^{K_n} \alpha_j B_j(t) + \boldsymbol{\beta}^T \mathbf{Z}\right\},$$

and the log pseudo-likelihood function $l_p(\mu_0, \boldsymbol{\beta})$ has the form

$$l_p(\alpha_l's, \boldsymbol{\beta}) = \sum_{i=1}^{n} \sum_{j=1}^{m_i} \left[n_{i,j} \sum_{l=1}^{K_n} \alpha_l B_l(t_{i,j}) + n_{i,j} \boldsymbol{\beta}^T \mathbf{Z}_i \right.$$
$$\left. - \exp\left\{\sum_{j=1}^{K_n} \alpha_j B_j(t) + \boldsymbol{\beta}^T \mathbf{Z}_i\right\} \right].$$

Let the $\hat{\alpha}_l$'s and $\hat{\boldsymbol{\beta}}_{SL}$ denote the maximum likelihood estimators of the α_l's and $\boldsymbol{\beta}$ resulting from the maximization of $l_p(\alpha_l's, \boldsymbol{\beta})$ given above. Define $\hat{\mu}_{SL}(t) = \exp\{\sum_{l=1}^{K_n} \hat{\alpha}_l B_l(t)\}$, the resulting estimator of the baseline mean function $\mu_0(t)$, and assume that the number of basis functions K_n goes to infinity when n goes to infinity. Then Lu et al. (2009) show that under some regularity conditions, $\hat{\mu}_{SL}(t)$ and $\hat{\boldsymbol{\beta}}_{SL}$ are consistent and $\hat{\boldsymbol{\beta}}_{SL}$ asymptotically follows a normal distribution. In particular, $\hat{\boldsymbol{\beta}}_{SL}$ is asymptotically equivalent to $\hat{\boldsymbol{\beta}}_{PL}$ given in the previous subsection. For the determination of the $\hat{\alpha}_l$'s and $\hat{\boldsymbol{\beta}}_{SL}$, Lu et al. (2009) suggest to employ the generalized Rosen algorithm discussed in Jamshidian (2004) and Zhang and Jamshidian (2004). In practice, the number of basis functions K_n is usually set to be smaller than the number of the different observation time points m or the dimension of $\boldsymbol{\mu}$ defined in the previous subsection. In consequence, the maximization of $l_p(\alpha_l's, \boldsymbol{\beta})$ can be much easier than that of $l_p(\mu_0, \boldsymbol{\beta})$.

5.2.3 Discussion

As mentioned above, instead of maximizing the log pseudo-likelihood function $l_p(\mu_0, \boldsymbol{\beta})$, one can maximize the true log likelihood function $l(\mu_0, \boldsymbol{\beta})$ for estimation of model (1.4). The same is true about the procedure described in Sect. 5.2.2. That is, instead of maximizing the approximate log pseudo-likelihood function $l_p(\alpha_l's, \boldsymbol{\beta})$, one can maximize the approximate true log likelihood function $l(\alpha_l's, \boldsymbol{\beta})$ given by replacing $\mu_0(t)$ in $l(\mu_0, \boldsymbol{\beta})$ with the monotone cubic B-spline approximation. Lu et al. (2009) show that as $\hat{\boldsymbol{\beta}}_{SL}$, the resulting estimators of regression parameters from this latter approach is also asymptotically equivalent to the maximum likelihood estimator of the regression parameters given by $l(\mu_0, \boldsymbol{\beta})$. In other words, with respect to estimation of regression parameters in model (1.4), the resulting estimators with and without using the smooth function approximation have the same asymptotic properties. On the other hand, the methods based on the mono-

5.3 Analysis by the Estimating Equation Approach I

tone cubic B-splines have the advantage of the computer efficiency, which makes the bootstrap procedure more feasible in practice. In addition, the estimation of the baseline mean function with the use of B-splines can also have a better convergence rate than that without the use of B-splines if the true baseline mean function is sufficiently smooth (Lu et al., 2009).

Note that as discussed in Sect. 3.2.2, a drawback of the Poisson process assumption is that it could be too restrictive in practice and instead, one may consider the mixed Poisson process. Specifically, assume that the $N_i(t)$'s are non-homogeneous Poisson processes with the mean function

$$E\{N_i(t)|\mathbf{Z}_i, \nu_i\} = \nu_i \mu_0(t) \exp(\boldsymbol{\beta}^T \mathbf{Z}_i)$$

given $\mathbf{Z}_i$ and a latent variable ν_i, where the ν_i's follow the gamma distribution with mean one. Then it can be shown that the $n_{i,j}$'s follow the negative binomial distribution and the resulting likelihood function has the form

$$L_n(\mu_0, \boldsymbol{\beta}) = \prod_{i=1}^{n} \prod_{j=1}^{m_i} \left[\frac{\Gamma(n_{i,j}+\alpha^{-1})}{\Gamma(\alpha^{-1})} \frac{\{\alpha\mu(t_{i,j})\exp(\boldsymbol{\beta}^T \mathbf{Z}_i)\}^{n_{i,j}}}{n_{i,j}!\{1+\alpha\mu(t_{i,j})\exp(\boldsymbol{\beta}^T \mathbf{Z}_i)\}^{n_{i,j}+\alpha^{-1}}} \right].$$

As with the estimators $\hat{\boldsymbol{\beta}}_{PL}$ and $\hat{\boldsymbol{\beta}}_{SL}$, one could define an estimator of $\boldsymbol{\beta}$ by maximizing either the likelihood function $L_n(\mu_0, \boldsymbol{\beta})$ or $L_n(\mu_0, \boldsymbol{\beta})$ with $\mu_0(t)$ replaced by the monotone cubic B-spline approximation used above.

Also note that all estimation procedures discussed above involve the estimation of either an unknown function or many extra parameters in addition to regression parameters. Thus in general, their implementations are usually expensive in computation. Also it is difficult to study the asymptotic properties of the resulting estimators, and sometimes one has to employ the bootstrap procedure for the variance estimation of the resulting estimators. In these cases, no formal inference about $\boldsymbol{\beta}$ can be carried out based on these estimators. In the next three sections, the estimating equation approach is employed to derive estimators of the regression parameter $\boldsymbol{\beta}$. One can see that the resulting estimation procedures are free of the estimation of unknown functions or extra parameters, and the asymptotic properties of the resulting estimators can be relatively easily established.

5.3 Analysis by the Estimating Equation Approach I

To motivate the estimating equation approach given below, note that one feature of the estimation procedures discussed in the previous section is that they are conditional approaches with respect to observation processes. In other words, they condition on observation times or treat them as fixed. The focus of this chapter is on estimation of the effects of covariates on the underlying recurrent event process of interest. In the meantime, the same covariates may have some effects on observation processes too although the latter may not be of main interest. As an alternative to the conditional approach, sometimes it may be convenient or useful to directly model the two processes together and to make unconditional inference about covariate effects.

This section considers the same problem as in the previous section but takes the unconditional approach that models together both the process of interest and the observation process marginally. In addition, the approach allows one to directly model the possible effects of covariates on the censoring or follow-up time too. In the following, we first describe the assumptions and models needed for the estimation procedure to be derived. The estimating equations are then presented for estimation of all possible effects of covariates on both the recurrent event process of interest and the observation process as well as on the follow-up time or process. Finally we consider a special case where covariates have no effect on the follow-up process.

5.3.1 Assumptions and Models

Consider a recurrent event study that yields panel count data and let the $N_i(t)$'s, $t_{i,j}$'s, $n_{i,j}$'s, and s_l's be defined as in the previous section. Also let $\tilde{H}_i(t)$ denote the underlying observation process representing the potential number of observations up to time t on subject i, $i = 1, \ldots, n$. In addition, for subject i, assume that there exists a censoring or follow-up time denoted by C_i and define $H_i(t) = \tilde{H}_i\{\min(t, C_i)\} = \sum_{j=1}^{m_i} I(t_{i,j} \leq t)$, the real observation process on the subject. Then $N_i(t)$ is observed only at the time points where $H_i(t)$ jumps, $i = 1, \ldots, n$. The observed data consist of the independent and identically distributed $\{\, H_i(t), N_i(t) dH_i(t), C_i, \boldsymbol{Z}_i\,;\, t \geq 0, i = 1, \ldots, n\,\}$ or have the form

$$\{\,(t_{i,j}, n_{i,j}, C_i, \boldsymbol{Z}_i)\,;\, j = 1, \ldots, m_i, i = 1, \ldots, n\,\}. \tag{5.3}$$

In the following, we assume that $N_i(t)$, $\tilde{H}_i(t)$, C_i and $\boldsymbol{Z}_i$ may be dependent, but given $\boldsymbol{Z}_i$, $N_i(t)$, $\tilde{H}_i(t)$ and C_i are independent. Also we assume that the mean function of $N_i(t)$ is given by model (1.4) as in the previous section.

To model the dependence of $\tilde{H}_i(t)$ on covariates $\boldsymbol{Z}_i$, as for $N_i(t)$, it is assumed that the mean function of $\tilde{H}_i(t)$ has the form

$$\tilde{\mu}_{Z_i}(t) = E\{\,\tilde{H}_i(t)\,|\,\boldsymbol{Z}_i\,\} = \tilde{\mu}_0(t)\,\exp(\boldsymbol{\gamma}^T \boldsymbol{Z}_i) \tag{5.4}$$

given $\boldsymbol{Z}_i$. In the model above, $\tilde{\mu}_0(t)$ is a completely unspecified function as $\mu_0(t)$ and $\boldsymbol{\gamma}$ is a p-dimensional vector of regression parameters representing the effects of covariates on $\tilde{H}_i(t)$. As mentioned above, the covariates $\boldsymbol{Z}_i$ may have effects on C_i too. For this, we suppose that given $\boldsymbol{Z}_i$, the hazard function $\lambda_i^*(t)$ of C_i satisfies the following proportional hazards (PH) model

5.3 Analysis by the Estimating Equation Approach I

$$\lambda_i^*(t;\boldsymbol{Z}_i) = \lambda_0^*(t)\exp(\boldsymbol{\tau}^T\boldsymbol{Z}_i) \quad (5.5)$$

(Cox, 1972; Kalbfleisch and Prentice, 2002). Here $\lambda_0^*(t)$ is a completely unspecified baseline hazard function and $\boldsymbol{\tau}$ is a p-dimensional vector of regression parameters denoting the effects of covariates on C_i. Note that here C_i is always observable unlike in the case of right-censored failure time data. In the following, for simplicity of presentation, it is assumed that the $\boldsymbol{Z}_i$'s are centered around zero. Otherwise, one can simply replace $\boldsymbol{Z}_i$ by $\boldsymbol{Z}_i - \bar{\boldsymbol{Z}}_n$, where $\bar{\boldsymbol{Z}}_n = \sum_{i=1}^n \boldsymbol{Z}_i/n$.

For estimation of regression parameters $\boldsymbol{\beta}$, $\boldsymbol{\gamma}$ and $\boldsymbol{\tau}$, we first discuss the general situation where all these parameters are unknown and need to be estimated. The special case where $\boldsymbol{\tau} = 0$ is then discussed, implying that the C_i's follow the same distribution.

5.3.2 Estimation of All Regression Parameters

This subsection considers the estimation of all regression parameters $\boldsymbol{\beta}$, $\boldsymbol{\gamma}$ and $\boldsymbol{\tau}$ together. To motivate the estimating equations derived below, first consider a simple situation where $m_i = 1$ and $\boldsymbol{\gamma} = \boldsymbol{\tau} = 0$, $i = 1,\ldots,n$. That is, one has current status data and the $\tilde{H}_i(t)$'s and C_i's have the same mean and hazard functions, respectively. Note that in this case, under model (1.4), we have the following fact that the quantity

$$E\left\{\exp(-\boldsymbol{\beta}^T\boldsymbol{Z}_i)\,N_i(t_{i,1})|\boldsymbol{Z}_i\right\} = E\left\{\exp(-\boldsymbol{\beta}^T\boldsymbol{Z}_i)\int N_i(t)\,dH_i(t)|\boldsymbol{Z}_i\right\}$$

is independent of subject index i. This suggests that for given $\boldsymbol{\beta}$ and if one is interested in testing model (1.4), a natural method is to use the following Wilcoxon-type statistic

$$U_0^*(\boldsymbol{\beta}) = \sum_{i=1}^n \sum_{j=1}^n (\boldsymbol{Z}_i - \boldsymbol{Z}_j)\left\{\exp(-\boldsymbol{\beta}^T\boldsymbol{Z}_i)\int N_i(t)\,dH_i(t)\right.$$
$$\left. - \exp(-\boldsymbol{\beta}^T\boldsymbol{Z}_j)\int N_j(t)\,dH_j(t)\right\}$$
$$= 2n\sum_{i=1}^n\left\{\boldsymbol{Z}_i\exp(-\boldsymbol{\beta}^T\boldsymbol{Z}_i)\int N_i(t)\,dH_i(t)\right\}.$$

It thus follows that a natural estimating equation for estimation of $\boldsymbol{\beta}$ is given by

$$U_0(\boldsymbol{\beta}) = (2n)^{-1}U_0^*(\boldsymbol{\beta}) = 0.$$

Note that if $m_i \geq 1$, we have $\int N_i(t)\,dH_i(t) = \sum_{j=1}^{m_i} N_i(t_{i,j})$. Thus it is easy to see that in this case, $U_0(\boldsymbol{\beta})$ is still an unbiased estimating function under model (1.4) and can be used for estimation of $\boldsymbol{\beta}$ with $\boldsymbol{\gamma} = \boldsymbol{\tau} = 0$.

Now we consider the general case where γ and τ may not be zero. Let $S_0(t) = \exp\left\{-\int_0^t \lambda_0^*(s)\,ds\right\}$ and define

$$d\tilde{M}_i(t) = dH_i(t) - I(C_i \geq t)\exp(\gamma^T \boldsymbol{Z}_i)\,d\tilde{\mu}_0(t),$$

which has mean zero, $i = 1, \ldots, n$. Then one has

$$\int N_i(t)dH_i(t) = \int N_i(t)d\tilde{M}_i(t) + \int N_i(t)\exp(\gamma^T \boldsymbol{Z}_i)\,I(C_i \geq t)\,d\tilde{\mu}_0(t),$$

and under model (5.4) and conditional on $\boldsymbol{Z}_i$, we have

$$E\left\{\int N_i(t)dH_i(t)\right\} = \exp\left\{(\boldsymbol{\beta}+\boldsymbol{\gamma})^T \boldsymbol{Z}_i\right\}\int \mu_0(t)\,S_i(t)\,d\tilde{\mu}_0(t), \quad (5.6)$$

where $S_i(t) = P(C_i \geq t) = \{S_0(t-)\}^{\exp(\boldsymbol{\tau}^T \boldsymbol{Z}_i)}$ under model (5.5). The equation above shows that $U_0(\boldsymbol{\beta})$ is biased under the situation considered and needs to be adjusted.

To have an unbiased estimating function similar to $U_0(\boldsymbol{\beta})$, it follows from (5.6) that one could consider the quantity

$$\int N_i(t)\,\{S_0(t-)\}^{-\exp(\boldsymbol{\tau}^T \boldsymbol{Z}_i)}\,dH_i(t)$$

instead of $\int N_i(t)dH_i(t)$. Under model (5.5), this quantity has the expectation

$$\exp\left\{(\boldsymbol{\beta}+\boldsymbol{\gamma})^T \boldsymbol{Z}_i\right\}\int \mu_0(t)\,d\tilde{\mu}_0(t).$$

This motivates the estimating function

$$U_I(\boldsymbol{\beta},\boldsymbol{\gamma},\boldsymbol{\tau}) = \sum_{i=1}^n \boldsymbol{Z}_i \exp\left\{-(\boldsymbol{\beta}+\boldsymbol{\gamma})^T \boldsymbol{Z}_i\right\}$$

$$\times \int N_i(t)\,\{\hat{S}_0(t-;\boldsymbol{\tau})\}^{-\exp(\boldsymbol{\tau}^T \boldsymbol{Z}_i)}\,dH_i(t) \quad (5.7)$$

for $\boldsymbol{\beta}$ with fixed $\boldsymbol{\gamma}$ and $\boldsymbol{\tau}$, where

$$\hat{S}_0(t;\boldsymbol{\tau}) = \exp\left\{-\int_0^t \frac{d\bar{N}(s)}{\sum_{i=1}^n I(C_i \geq s)\exp\{\boldsymbol{\tau}^T \boldsymbol{Z}_i\}}\right\},$$

$\bar{N}(s) = \sum_{i=1}^n \bar{N}_i(s)$ and $\bar{N}_i(s) = I(C_i \leq s)$. It can be easily shown that asymptotically, $U_I(\boldsymbol{\beta},\boldsymbol{\gamma},\boldsymbol{\tau})$ has expectation zero under the true values of the parameters (Sun and Wei, 2000).

5.3 Analysis by the Estimating Equation Approach I

To estimate γ in model (5.4), a common approach is to use the estimating equation $U_\gamma(\gamma) = \partial L(\gamma)/\partial \gamma = 0$ (Lawless and Nadeau, 1995), where

$$L(\gamma) = \int \sum_{i=1}^n \left[\gamma^T Z_i - \log\left\{ \sum_{l=1}^n I(C_l \geq t) \exp(\gamma^T Z_i) \right\} \right] dH_i(t). \quad (5.8)$$

For estimation of τ, one can use the partial likelihood score function

$$U_\tau(\tau) = \sum_{i=1}^n \int \left\{ Z_i - \frac{\sum_{l=1}^n I(C_l \geq t) \exp\{\tau^T Z_l\} Z_l}{\sum_{l=1}^n I(C_l \geq t) \exp\{\tau^T Z_l\}} \right\} d\bar{N}_i(t) \quad (5.9)$$

(Kalbfleisch and Prentice, 2002). Let $\hat{\gamma}$ and $\hat{\tau}$ denote the estimators of γ and τ given by the solutions to $U_\gamma(\gamma) = 0$ and $U_\tau(\tau) = 0$, respectively. Then one can estimate β by the solution, denoted by $\hat{\beta}_I$, to $U_I(\beta, \hat{\gamma}, \hat{\tau}) = 0$.

Let $\theta = (\beta^T, \gamma^T, \tau^T)^T$ and $\hat{\theta} = (\hat{\beta}_I^T, \hat{\gamma}^T, \hat{\tau}^T)^T$. Sun and Wei (2000) show that the estimators $\hat{\beta}_I$, $\hat{\gamma}$ and $\hat{\tau}$ are consistent and unique. For their asymptotic distributions, let

$$A(\theta) = -\frac{\partial U_I(\theta)}{\partial \beta}, \quad B(\gamma) = -\frac{\partial U_\gamma(\gamma)}{\partial \gamma}, \quad G(\tau) = -\frac{\partial U_\tau(\tau)}{\partial \tau}, \quad P(\theta) = -\frac{\partial U_I(\theta)}{\partial \tau}.$$

Define

$$R(t; \theta) = \frac{1}{n} \sum_{i=1}^n Z_i \exp\{-(\beta + \gamma - \tau)^T Z_i\} \int_t^\infty \frac{N_i(s)}{\{\hat{S}_0(s; \tau)\}^{\exp(\tau^T Z_i)}} dH_i(s),$$

and

$$S^{(j)}(t; \gamma) = \frac{1}{n} \sum_{i=1}^n I(C_i \geq t) \exp\{\gamma^T Z_i\} Z_i^{(j)},$$

where $j = 0, 1$, $Z_i^{(0)} = 1$, and $Z_i^{(1)} = Z_i$, $i = 1, \ldots, n$. Also define

$$\tilde{a}_i(\theta) = Z_i \exp\{-(\beta + \gamma)^T Z_i\} \int \frac{N_i(t)}{\{\hat{S}_0(t; \tau)\}^{\exp(\tau^T Z_i)}} dH_i(t),$$

$$\tilde{b}_i(\theta) = \int \frac{R(t, \theta)}{S^{(0)}(t; \tau)} \left\{ d\bar{N}_i(t) - \frac{I(C_i \geq t) \exp\{\tau^T Z_i\}}{n S^{(0)}(t; \tau)} d\bar{N}(t) \right\},$$

$$\tilde{d}_i(\gamma) = \int_0^\infty \left\{ Z_i - \frac{S^{(1)}(t; \gamma)}{S^{(0)}(t; \gamma)} \right\} \left\{ dH_i(t) - \frac{I(C_i \geq t) \exp\{\gamma^T Z_i\}}{n S^{(0)}(t; \gamma)} dH(t) \right\},$$

and

$$\tilde{d}_i(\boldsymbol{\tau}) = \int_0^\infty \left\{ \boldsymbol{Z}_i - \frac{S^{(1)}(t;\boldsymbol{\tau})}{S^{(0)}(t;\boldsymbol{\tau})} \right\} \left\{ d\bar{N}_i(t) - \frac{I(C_i \geq t)\exp\{\boldsymbol{\tau}^T \boldsymbol{Z}_i\}}{n\,S^{(0)}(t;\boldsymbol{\tau})} d\bar{N}(t) \right\},$$

where $H(t) = \sum_{i=1}^n H_i(t)$, $i = 1,\ldots,n$. Sun and Wei (2000) show that for large n, the distribution of $\hat{\boldsymbol{\beta}}_I - \boldsymbol{\beta}_0$ can be approximated by a normal distribution with mean zero and the covariance matrix $D(\hat{\boldsymbol{\theta}})\,\Gamma(\hat{\boldsymbol{\theta}})\,D'(\hat{\boldsymbol{\theta}})$. Here $\boldsymbol{\beta}_0$ denotes the true value of $\boldsymbol{\beta}$,

$$D(\boldsymbol{\theta}) = \left(A^{-1}(\boldsymbol{\theta}), -B^{-1}(\boldsymbol{\gamma}), -A^{-1}(\boldsymbol{\theta})\,P(\boldsymbol{\theta})\,G^{-1}(\boldsymbol{\tau}) \right),$$

and

$$\Gamma(\boldsymbol{\theta}) = \sum_{i=1}^n \begin{pmatrix} \tilde{a}_i(\boldsymbol{\theta}) + \tilde{b}_i(\boldsymbol{\theta}) \\ \tilde{d}_i(\boldsymbol{\gamma}) \\ \tilde{d}_i(\boldsymbol{\tau}) \end{pmatrix} \left(\tilde{a}_i^T(\boldsymbol{\theta}) + \tilde{b}_i^T(\boldsymbol{\theta}),\ \tilde{d}_i^T(\boldsymbol{\gamma}),\ \tilde{d}_i^T(\boldsymbol{\tau}) \right).$$

Let $\boldsymbol{\gamma}_0$ and $\boldsymbol{\tau}_0$ denote the true values of $\boldsymbol{\gamma}$ and $\boldsymbol{\tau}$, respectively. Then it can be easily shown that for large n, the distributions of $\hat{\boldsymbol{\gamma}} - \boldsymbol{\gamma}_0$ and $\hat{\boldsymbol{\tau}} - \boldsymbol{\tau}_0$ can also be approximated by the normal distributions with mean zero and the covariance matrices

$$B^{-1}(\hat{\boldsymbol{\gamma}}) \left\{ \sum_{i=1}^n \tilde{d}(\hat{\boldsymbol{\gamma}})\,\tilde{d}^T(\hat{\boldsymbol{\gamma}}) \right\} B^{-1}(\hat{\boldsymbol{\gamma}})$$

and

$$G^{-1}(\hat{\boldsymbol{\tau}}) \left\{ \sum_{i=1}^n \tilde{d}(\hat{\boldsymbol{\tau}})\,\tilde{d}^T(\hat{\boldsymbol{\tau}}) \right\} G^{-1}(\hat{\boldsymbol{\tau}}),$$

respectively (Lawless and Nadeau, 1995; Sun and Wei, 2000).

5.3.3 Estimation with Same Follow-Up Times

Sometimes it may be reasonable to assume that the C_i's are independent and identically distributed, that is, $\boldsymbol{\tau} = 0$. A simple situation where this holds is that $C_i = c_0$ for all i, where c_0 is a prespecified time point. That is, all subjects are followed the same length. In this case, of course, one can still employ the estimation procedure given above, but it is apparent that it may be less efficient. Instead, one can develop an estimation procedure similar to, but simpler than the one given above. To see this, note that under the current situation, $S_i(t)$ in (5.6) is independent of subject index i. This suggests an unbiased estimating function

$$U_{I,1}(\boldsymbol{\beta},\boldsymbol{\gamma}) = \sum_{i=1}^n \boldsymbol{Z}_i \exp\left\{ -(\boldsymbol{\beta}+\boldsymbol{\gamma})^T \boldsymbol{Z}_i \right\} \int N_i(t)\,dH_i(t)$$

for estimation of $\boldsymbol{\beta}$ with given $\boldsymbol{\gamma}$.

Let $\hat{\boldsymbol{\beta}}_{I,1}$ denote the estimator of $\boldsymbol{\beta}$ given by the solution to $U_{I,1}(\boldsymbol{\beta}, \hat{\boldsymbol{\gamma}}) = 0$. It can be easily shown that $\hat{\boldsymbol{\beta}}_{I,1}$ is consistent and unique (Sun and Wei, 2000). Furthermore, for large n, one can approximate the distribution of $\hat{\boldsymbol{\beta}}_{I,1} - \boldsymbol{\beta}_0$ by the normal distribution with mean zero and the covariance matrix

$$\left(A_1^{-1}(\hat{\boldsymbol{\beta}}_{I,1} + \hat{\boldsymbol{\gamma}}), -B^{-1}(\hat{\boldsymbol{\gamma}})\right) \hat{\Gamma}_1 \left(A_1^{-1}(\hat{\boldsymbol{\beta}}_{I,1} + \hat{\boldsymbol{\gamma}}), -B^{-1}(\hat{\boldsymbol{\gamma}})\right)^T.$$

In the above, $A_1(\boldsymbol{\beta}) = -\partial U_0(\boldsymbol{\beta})/\partial \boldsymbol{\beta}$ and

$$\hat{\Gamma}_1 = \begin{pmatrix} \sum_{i=1}^{n} \boldsymbol{Z}_i \boldsymbol{Z}_i^T e_i^{*2} e_i^2, & \sum_{i=1}^{n} \boldsymbol{Z}_i \tilde{d}_i^T(\hat{\boldsymbol{\gamma}}) e_i^* e_i \\ \sum_{i=1}^{n} \tilde{d}_i(\hat{\boldsymbol{\gamma}}) \boldsymbol{Z}_i^T e_i^* e_i, & \sum_{i=1}^{n} \tilde{d}_i(\hat{\boldsymbol{\gamma}}) \tilde{d}_i^T(\hat{\boldsymbol{\gamma}}) \end{pmatrix},$$

where $e_i = \int N_i(t) dH_i(t)$ and $e_i^* = \exp\{-(\hat{\boldsymbol{\beta}}_{I,1} + \hat{\boldsymbol{\gamma}})^T \boldsymbol{Z}_i\}$, $i = 1, \ldots, n$. It is easy to see that in the simple situation where $C_i = c_0$ for all i, the estimating function $U_I(\boldsymbol{\beta}, \boldsymbol{\gamma}, \boldsymbol{\tau})$ given in (5.7) reduces to $U_{I,1}(\boldsymbol{\beta}, \boldsymbol{\gamma})$. That is, the two estimators $\hat{\boldsymbol{\beta}}_I$ and $\hat{\boldsymbol{\beta}}_{I,1}$ are identical.

5.4 Analysis by the Estimating Equation Approach II

As discussed above, compared to the likelihood-based estimation procedures discussed in Sect. 5.2, one major advantage of the estimating equation approach described in Sect. 5.3 is that it does not depend on any distribution assumption. Also for the latter, the asymptotic properties of the resulting estimator can be easily established and its implementation is quite easy. On the other hand, the latter may be less efficient. In this section, we describe two other estimating equation approaches, which may not be as easy in implementation as the one given in Sect. 5.3 but could be more efficient. First we discuss a conditional method that treats observation times as constants or fixed. An unconditional method is then given which, as the method given in Sect. 5.3, models both the recurrent event process of interest and the observation process together. It is followed by some discussion on the comparison of the three estimating equation approaches.

5.4.1 A Conditional Estimating Equation Procedure

Let the $N_i(t)$'s, $t_{i,j}$'s, $n_{i,j}$'s, s_l's, $\tilde{H}_i(t)$'s, $H_i(t)$'s and C_i's be defined as in Sect. 5.3. Also as in Sect. 5.3, suppose that the observed data consist of independent and identically distributed $\{H_i(t), N_i(t)dH_i(t), C_i, \boldsymbol{Z}_i; t \geq 0, i = 1, \ldots, n\}$ or have the form (5.3). Furthermore, assume that $N_i(t)$, $\tilde{H}_i(t)$, C_i and $\boldsymbol{Z}_i$ may be dependent, but given $\boldsymbol{Z}_i$, $N_i(t)$, $\tilde{H}_i(t)$ and C_i are independent. Suppose that the main goal is to make inference about the regression parameter $\boldsymbol{\beta}$ in model (1.4).

To motivate the new estimating function, note that the estimating function U_I given in (5.7) is essentially constructed based on the summary statistic $\int N_i(t)\,dH_i(t)$. Corresponding to this, we consider a new process defined as

$$\tilde{N}_i(t) = \int_0^t N_i(s)\,dH_i(s)\,,\quad t \geq 0\,,$$

which is expected to contain more information than the summary statistic above, $i = 1,\ldots,n$. It is easy to see that $\tilde{N}_i(t)$ has possible jumps only at the observation time points $t_{i,j}$'s with respective jump sizes $N_i(t_{i,j})$'s. Furthermore, we actually have recurrent event data on the $\tilde{N}_i(t)$'s and one can show that

$$E\{\,d\tilde{N}_i(t)|H_i(s), 0 < s \leq t; \boldsymbol{Z}_i\,\} = \mu_0(t)\exp(\boldsymbol{\beta}^T\boldsymbol{Z}_i)dH_i(t)\,. \qquad (5.10)$$

That is, the $\tilde{N}_i(t)$'s satisfy the proportional rate model (1.3) and one can employ the estimation approach developed for recurrent event data.

For each i, define $h_i(t) = H_i(t) - H_i(t-)$, indicating whether subject i has an observation at time t, $i = 1,\ldots,n$. In the following, we use τ to denote the longest follow-up time and assume $E\{\,h_i(t)\,\} = p(t) > 0$ for $t \in \mathcal{T}$, where $\mathcal{T}$ is a subset of $(0,\tau]$ including all observation times. The assumption ensures that for any time point in $\mathcal{T}$, there is more than one subject having observation when the study size n is large enough. Also define

$$S_C^{(j)}(t;\boldsymbol{\beta}) = \frac{\sum_{i=1}^n I(C_i \geq t)\,\boldsymbol{Z}_i^{\otimes j}\,\exp(\boldsymbol{\beta}^T\boldsymbol{Z}_i)\,h_i(t)}{\sum_{i=1}^n h_i(t)}$$

for t with $\sum_{i=1}^n h_i(t) > 0$ and $j = 0, 1, 2$. Then for estimation of the regression parameter $\boldsymbol{\beta}$, by following the idea discussed in Lawless and Nadeau (1995) among others, a natural estimating function is

$$U_{II}^C(\boldsymbol{\beta};w) = \sum_{i=1}^n \int_0^\tau w(t)\,I(C_i \geq t)\,\{\boldsymbol{Z}_i - \bar{\boldsymbol{Z}}_C(t;\boldsymbol{\beta})\}\,d\tilde{N}_i(t)\,. \qquad (5.11)$$

Here $w(t)$ is a known weight function and $\bar{\boldsymbol{Z}}_C(t;\boldsymbol{\beta}) = S_C^{(1)}(t;\boldsymbol{\beta})/S_C^{(0)}(t;\boldsymbol{\beta})$, which is defined only for $t \in [0,\tau]$ with $\sum_{i=1}^n h_i(t) > 0$. Note that since $\mathcal{T}$ is finite, the integral in (5.11) and all similar integrals below are finite summations.

One can show that for any counting process satisfying (5.10), the estimating function $U_{II}^C(\boldsymbol{\beta};w)$ given in (5.11) has mean zero. Thus we can estimate $\boldsymbol{\beta}$ by the solution, denoted by $\hat{\boldsymbol{\beta}}_{II}^C$, to $U_{II}^C(\boldsymbol{\beta};w) = 0$. For the simple situation where all subjects have just one observation at the same time point $t_0 < \tau$ with $C_i = \tau$ for all i and $w(t) = 1$, the estimating function $U_{II}^C(\boldsymbol{\beta};w)$ reduces to

5.4 Analysis by the Estimating Equation Approach II

$$U_{II}^C(\boldsymbol{\beta}; 1) = \sum_{i=1}^n \boldsymbol{Z}_i N_i(t_0) - \left\{ \sum_{i=1}^n \int_0^{t_0} \frac{1}{\sum_{j=1}^n \exp(\boldsymbol{\beta}^T \boldsymbol{Z}_j)} dN_i(t) \right\}$$
$$\times \left\{ \sum_{i=1}^n \boldsymbol{Z}_i \exp(\boldsymbol{\beta}^T \boldsymbol{Z}_i) \right\}.$$

To understand the estimating function above, note that

$$E\left\{ \sum_{i=1}^n \boldsymbol{Z}_i N_i(t_0) | \boldsymbol{Z}_i's \right\} = \mu_0(t) \sum_{i=1}^n \boldsymbol{Z}_i \exp(\boldsymbol{\beta}^T \boldsymbol{Z}_i).$$

Thus $U_{II}^C(\boldsymbol{\beta}; 1)$ represents the quantity $\sum_{i=1}^n \boldsymbol{Z}_i N_i(t_0)$ minus its estimated expectation given by replacing $\mu_0(t)$ with the Breslow estimator (Fleming and Harrington, 1991).

Let $\boldsymbol{\beta}_0$ denote the true value of $\boldsymbol{\beta}$ as above. Define

$$\hat{\mu}_0^C(t; \boldsymbol{\beta}) = \frac{\sum_{i=1}^n I(C_i \geq t) N_i(t) h_i(t)}{\sum_{i=1}^n I(C_i \geq t) \exp(\boldsymbol{\beta}^T \boldsymbol{Z}_i) h_i(t)}$$

and

$$\hat{M}_i^C(t; \boldsymbol{\beta}) = \int_0^t I(C_i \geq s) \left\{ N_i(s) - \hat{\mu}_0^C(s; \boldsymbol{\beta}) \exp(\boldsymbol{\beta}^T \boldsymbol{Z}_i) \right\} dH_i(s)$$

for $t \in [0, \tau]$. Note that as $\bar{\boldsymbol{Z}}_C$, $\hat{\mu}_0^C(t; \boldsymbol{\beta})$ is also defined only for $t \in [0, \tau]$ with $\sum_{i=1}^n h_i(t) > 0$. For the easy of notation, in the remaining of this subsection, we assume that $w(t) = 1$ and it is straightforward to generalize the results given below to the situation with any other deterministic weight function. Hu et al. (2003) show that the estimator $\hat{\boldsymbol{\beta}}_{II}^C$ defined above is consistent and the distribution of $\sqrt{n}(\hat{\boldsymbol{\beta}}_{II}^C - \boldsymbol{\beta}_0)$ can be asymptotically approximated by the normal distribution with mean zero and the covariance matrix $\hat{\Sigma}_{II}^C = A_C(\hat{\boldsymbol{\beta}}_{II}^C)^{-1} B_C(\hat{\boldsymbol{\beta}}_{II}^C) A_C^{-1}(\hat{\boldsymbol{\beta}}_{II}^C)$. Here

$$A_C(\boldsymbol{\beta}) = \frac{1}{n} \frac{\partial U_{II}^C(\boldsymbol{\beta}; 1)}{\partial \boldsymbol{\beta}}$$
$$= -\frac{1}{n} \sum_{i=1}^n \int_0^\tau I(C_i \geq t) \left\{ \frac{S_C^{(2)}(t; \boldsymbol{\beta})}{S_C^{(0)}(t; \boldsymbol{\beta})} - \bar{\boldsymbol{Z}}_C(t; \boldsymbol{\beta})^{\otimes 2} \right\} d\tilde{N}_i(t)$$

and

$$B_C(\boldsymbol{\beta}) = \frac{1}{n} \left[\sum_{i=1}^n \int_0^\tau \{\boldsymbol{Z}_i - \bar{\boldsymbol{Z}}_C(t; \boldsymbol{\beta})\} d\hat{M}_i^C(t; \boldsymbol{\beta}) \right]^{\otimes 2}.$$

Note that the estimation approach described above requires $E\{h_i(t)\} = p(t) > 0$ for $t \in \mathcal{T}$. Sometimes this may not hold such as in continuous time situations and to apply the approach in this case, a simple way is to discretize the time scale or perform some grouping.

5.4.2 An Unconditional Estimating Equation Procedure

Now we discuss an unconditional estimating equation approach based on the processes $\tilde{N}_i(t)$'s that is similar to the one described in Sect. 5.3. For this, we assume that the observation processes $\tilde{H}_i(t)$'s follow the proportional rate model

$$E\{\,d\tilde{H}_i(t)|\mathbf{Z}_i\,\} = \exp(\boldsymbol{\gamma}^T \mathbf{Z}_i)\,d\tilde{\mu}_0(t)\,, \qquad (5.12)$$

where $\tilde{\mu}_0(t)$ and $\boldsymbol{\gamma}$ are defined as in model (5.4). It then follows from models (1.4) and (5.12) that we have

$$E\{\,d\tilde{N}_i(t)|\mathbf{Z}_i\,\} = \exp(\tilde{\boldsymbol{\beta}}^T \mathbf{Z}_i)\,d\tilde{\mu}_0^*(t)\,,$$

where $\tilde{\boldsymbol{\beta}} = \boldsymbol{\beta} + \boldsymbol{\gamma}$ and $\tilde{\mu}_0^*(t) = \int_0^t \mu_0(s)\,d\tilde{\mu}_0(s)$.

To estimate $\boldsymbol{\beta}$ as well as $\boldsymbol{\gamma}$, define

$$S_M^{(j)}(t; \tilde{\boldsymbol{\beta}}) = \frac{1}{n} \sum_{i=1}^{n} I(C_i \geq t)\,\mathbf{Z}_i^{\otimes j} \exp(\tilde{\boldsymbol{\beta}}^T \mathbf{Z}_i)$$

for $j = 0, 1, 2$ and $\bar{\mathbf{Z}}_M(t; \tilde{\boldsymbol{\beta}}) = S_M^{(1)}(t; \tilde{\boldsymbol{\beta}})/S_M^{(0)}(t; \tilde{\boldsymbol{\beta}})$. Then similar to the estimating function $U_{II}^C(\boldsymbol{\beta}; w)$, a natural estimating function is given by

$$U_{II}^M(\tilde{\boldsymbol{\beta}}; w) = \sum_{i=1}^{n} \int_0^{\tau} w(t)\,I(C_i \geq t)\,\left\{ \mathbf{Z}_i - \bar{\mathbf{Z}}_M(t; \tilde{\boldsymbol{\beta}}) \right\} d\tilde{N}_i(t)\,,$$

where $w(t)$ is a weight function as before. If we take $w(t) = 1$ and assume $C_i = \tau$ for all i, then the estimating function above reduces to

$$U_{II,1}^M(\tilde{\boldsymbol{\beta}}; 1) = \sum_{i=1}^{n} \mathbf{Z}_i \int_0^{\tau} N_i(t)\,dH_i(t) - \left\{ \sum_{i=1}^{n} \mathbf{Z}_i \exp(\boldsymbol{\beta}^T \mathbf{Z}_i) \right\}$$
$$\times \int_0^{\tau} \frac{\sum_{l=1}^{n} N_l(t)\,dH_l(t)}{\sum_{j=1}^{n} \exp(\boldsymbol{\beta}^T \mathbf{Z}_j)}\,.$$

Let $\hat{\boldsymbol{\gamma}}$ denote the estimator defined in Sect. 5.3 based on the function defined in (5.8) and $\hat{\tilde{\boldsymbol{\beta}}}$ the estimator of $\tilde{\boldsymbol{\beta}}$ given by the solution to the equation $U_{II}^M(\tilde{\boldsymbol{\beta}}; w) = 0$ for a given $w(t)$. Then it is natural to estimate $\boldsymbol{\beta}$ by the estimator $\hat{\boldsymbol{\beta}}_{II}^M = \hat{\tilde{\boldsymbol{\beta}}} - \hat{\boldsymbol{\gamma}}$.

5.4 Analysis by the Estimating Equation Approach II

To describe the properties of $\hat{\boldsymbol{\beta}}_{II}^{M}$, again we take $w(t) = 1$ for the easy of notation as above. It is straightforward to generalize the results below to situations with general deterministic weight functions. Let $U_\gamma(\gamma)$ be defined as in Sect. 5.3 based on the function given in (5.8) and define

$$a_i^{11}(\tilde{\boldsymbol{\beta}}, \gamma) = \int_0^\tau I(C_i \geq t) \left\{ \frac{S_M^{(2)}(t; \tilde{\boldsymbol{\beta}})}{S_M^{(0)}(t; \tilde{\boldsymbol{\beta}})} - \bar{\boldsymbol{Z}}_M(t; \tilde{\boldsymbol{\beta}})^{\otimes 2} \right\} d\tilde{N}_i(t),$$

and

$$a_i^{22}(\tilde{\boldsymbol{\beta}}, \gamma) = \int_0^\tau I(C_i \geq t) \left\{ \frac{S_M^{(2)}(t; \gamma)}{S_M^{(0)}(t; \gamma)} - \bar{\boldsymbol{Z}}_M(t; \gamma)^{\otimes 2} \right\} dH_i(t)$$

for $i = 1, \ldots, n$. Also define

$$\hat{M}_i^M(t; \tilde{\boldsymbol{\beta}}) = \int_0^t I(C_i \geq s) \left\{ d\tilde{N}_i(s) - \exp(\tilde{\boldsymbol{\beta}}^T \boldsymbol{Z}_i) d\hat{\tilde{\mu}}_0^*(s; \tilde{\boldsymbol{\beta}}) \right\},$$

and

$$\hat{M}_i^H(t; \gamma) = \int_0^t I(C_i \geq s) \left\{ dH_i(s) - \exp(\gamma^T \boldsymbol{Z}_i) d\hat{\tilde{\mu}}_0(s; \gamma) \right\}.$$

In the above, $\hat{\tilde{\mu}}_0^*(t; \tilde{\boldsymbol{\beta}})$ and $\hat{\tilde{\mu}}_0(t; \gamma)$ denote the estimators of $\tilde{\mu}_0^*(t)$ and $\tilde{\mu}_0(t)$ given by (1.10) based on the processes $\tilde{N}_i(t)$'s and $H_i(t)$'s, respectively. Note that as mentioned before, for both processes, we have recurrent event data. Hu et al. (2003) show that the estimator $\hat{\boldsymbol{\beta}}_{II}^{M}$ is consistent and the distribution of $\sqrt{n}(\hat{\boldsymbol{\beta}}_{II}^{M} - \boldsymbol{\beta}_0)$ can be asymptotically approximated by the normal distribution with mean zero and the covariance matrix

$$\hat{\Sigma}_{II}^M = (\boldsymbol{I}_p, -\boldsymbol{I}_p) A_M^{-1}(\hat{\tilde{\boldsymbol{\beta}}}, \hat{\gamma}) B_M(\hat{\tilde{\boldsymbol{\beta}}}, \hat{\gamma}) A_M^{-1}(\hat{\tilde{\boldsymbol{\beta}}}, \hat{\gamma}) (\boldsymbol{I}_p, -\boldsymbol{I}_p)^T.$$

In the above, $\boldsymbol{I}_p$ denotes the $p \times p$ identity matrix,

$$A_M(\tilde{\boldsymbol{\beta}}, \gamma) = \frac{1}{n} \frac{\partial \left(U_{II,1}^M(\tilde{\boldsymbol{\beta}}; 1)^T, U_\gamma(\gamma)^T \right)^T}{\partial(\tilde{\boldsymbol{\beta}}, \gamma)} = -\frac{1}{n} \sum_{i=1}^n \mathrm{diag}\left(a_i^{11}(\tilde{\boldsymbol{\beta}}, \gamma), a_i^{22}(\tilde{\boldsymbol{\beta}}, \gamma) \right),$$

and

$$B_M(\tilde{\boldsymbol{\beta}}, \gamma) = \frac{1}{n} \sum_{i=1}^n \left[\begin{array}{c} \int_0^\tau \{\boldsymbol{Z}_i - \bar{\boldsymbol{Z}}_M(t; \tilde{\boldsymbol{\beta}})\} d\hat{M}_i^M(t; \tilde{\boldsymbol{\beta}}) \\ \int_0^\tau \{\boldsymbol{Z}_i - \bar{\boldsymbol{Z}}_M(t; \gamma)\} d\hat{M}_i^H(t; \gamma) \end{array} \right]^{\otimes 2}.$$

5.4.3 Discussion

Given the three estimating equation-based estimators of the regression parameter $\boldsymbol{\beta}$ described above, a natural question is how different they are. It is clear that each has its own advantages and disadvantages and one basic difference among them is how the observation process is treated. The estimator $\hat{\boldsymbol{\beta}}_{II}^{C}$ does not require the modeling of the observation process, while the estimators $\hat{\boldsymbol{\beta}}_{I}$ and $\hat{\boldsymbol{\beta}}_{II}^{M}$ do need one to specify some models for the observation process. Also $\hat{\boldsymbol{\beta}}_{II}^{C}$ does not require the knowledge of the follow-up times C_i's, while the other two estimators need the values of the C_i's. In consequence, the former estimator is readily applicable to situations with time-dependent covariates. In contrast, the latter two, if extended to time-dependent covariate cases, need the values of the covariate processes $\boldsymbol{Z}_i(t)$'s at all observation time points. On the other hand, $\hat{\boldsymbol{\beta}}_{II}^{C}$ can be applied only to the situation where $E\{h_i(t)\} > 0$ for t in at least a finite time point set, but $\hat{\boldsymbol{\beta}}_{I}$ and $\hat{\boldsymbol{\beta}}_{II}^{M}$ do not have the same restriction.

Another basic difference among the three estimators is their constructions. The estimator $\hat{\boldsymbol{\beta}}_{I}$ is derived based on the summary statistic $\int N_i(t)\,dH_i(t)$, while the estimators $\hat{\boldsymbol{\beta}}_{II}^{C}$ and $\hat{\boldsymbol{\beta}}_{II}^{M}$ are derived based on the processes $\tilde{N}_i(t)$'s. The former estimator is relatively simple and easy to be determined and allows one to model the effect of covariates on the follow-up times C_i's, but the latter two estimators are expected to be more efficient. The estimator $\hat{\boldsymbol{\beta}}_{II}^{C}$ has another restriction in that for its asymptotic properties described above to be valid, the distribution, say $G(t)$, of the follow-up times C_i's has to satisfy $\lim_{t \uparrow \tau} G(t) < 1$. That is, $G(t)$ has a mass at the maximum time point τ. To deal with this in practice, one could artificially choose a finite time point that is close to but smaller than the maximum of all follow-up times, and use the point to approximate the follow-up times beyond it or set τ equal to this point.

Note that all three estimators discussed above are derived under the proportional mean model (1.4). Of course, this model assumption may not hold in practice and to deal with this, one way is to develop and apply some model checking techniques as discussed in the next section. Another way is to consider a more general model. Actually, the proposed methods, with little modification, apply to the situation in which the conditional mean function of $N_i(t)$ has the form

$$E\{N_i(t)|\boldsymbol{Z}_i\} = \mu_0(t)\,\phi(\boldsymbol{\beta};\boldsymbol{Z}_i)\,, \tag{5.13}$$

where ϕ is a known and positive function. It is apparent that the model above includes model (1.4) as a special case. In the next section, we consider another general class of models for $E\{N_i(t)|\boldsymbol{Z}_i\}$. With respect to generalization, one could also generalize model (5.12) to

$$E\{\,d\tilde{H}_i(t)|Z_i\,\} \;=\; \psi(\gamma;Z_i)\,d\tilde{\mu}_0(t) \tag{5.14}$$

and show that the estimation approaches above with little modification are valid under models (5.13) and (5.14). In the above, as ϕ, ψ is also a known and positive function.

For both estimators $\hat{\boldsymbol{\beta}}_{II}^{C}$ and $\hat{\boldsymbol{\beta}}_{II}^{M}$, one issue of practical interest that has not been discussed is how to choose an appropriate weight function $w(t)$ or the optimal weight function for a given set of panel count data. As in many cases, this is not an easy problem and also it is apparent that the weight function may not necessarily have to be deterministic. Related to this, one could also consider to add some weight functions to the estimating functions $U_\gamma(\boldsymbol{\gamma})$ and $U_\tau(\boldsymbol{\tau})$ defined based on (5.8) and (5.9), respectively. In this case, it is similar and straightforward to derive some estimators of $\boldsymbol{\beta}$ and establish their asymptotic properties as above.

5.5 Analysis with Semiparametric Transformation Models

This section discusses the same problem as in the preceding sections. However, instead of using model (1.4) to describe the effects of covariates on the recurrent event process of interest, we now consider a class of semiparametric transformation models. As mentioned above, the proportional mean model implies that the mean functions associated with any two sets of covariate values are proportional over time, which may be too restrictive in practice (Lin et al., 2001). To relax this, a new class of semiparametric transformation models is first presented in the following. They include model (1.4) as a special case. For estimation of regression parameters, as in the previous sections, a class of estimating equation-based estimators are derived. In addition, a procedure is given for testing the goodness-of-fit of the semiparametric transformation model and followed by some discussions.

5.5.1 Assumptions and Models

Consider a recurrent event study that yields panel count data and let the $N_i(t)$'s, $t_{i,j}$'s, $n_{i,j}$'s, s_l's, $\tilde{H}_i(t)$'s, $H_i(t)$'s and C_i's be defined as in Sect. 5.4. Then similarly as in Sect. 5.4, the observed data are given by independent and identically distributed $\{\,H_i(t), N_i(t)dH_i(t), C_i, \boldsymbol{Z}_i(t)\,;\, t \geq 0,\, i = 1,\ldots,n\,\}$ or have the form

$$\{\,(t_{i,j}, n_{i,j}, C_i, \boldsymbol{Z}_i(t))\,;\, j = 1,\ldots,m_i, i = 1,\ldots,n\,\}.$$

Note that here we assume that the covariates $\boldsymbol{Z}_i(t)$'s may be time-dependent.

To characterize the relationship between the recurrent event process $N_i(t)$ of interest and the covariate process $\boldsymbol{Z}_i(t)$, we assume that given $\boldsymbol{Z}_i(t)$, the conditional mean function of $N_i(t)$ has the form

$$E\{\, N_i(t)|\, \boldsymbol{Z}_i(t)\,\} = g\{\mu_0(t)\, \exp(\boldsymbol{\beta}^T \boldsymbol{Z}_i(t))\,\}. \tag{5.15}$$

In the above, $g(\cdot)$ is a known twice continuously differentiable and strictly increasing function, and $\mu_0(t)$ and $\boldsymbol{\beta}$ are defined as in model (1.4), an unspecified smooth function of t and the vector of unknown regression parameters, respectively.

Model (5.15) is often referred to as the semiparametric transformation model (Lin et al., 2001) and includes many commonly used models as special cases. For example, it gives model (1.4) with $g(x) = x$. If taking g to be the commonly referred Box-Cox transformation, we have

$$E\{\, N_i(t)|\, \boldsymbol{Z}_i(t)\,\} = \frac{[\,\mu_0(t)\, \exp\{\boldsymbol{\beta}^T \boldsymbol{Z}_i(t)\,\} + 1\,]^\rho - 1}{\rho},$$

where ρ is a constant. In particular, by letting $\rho = 0$, the model above gives

$$E\{\, N_i(t)|\, \boldsymbol{Z}_i(t)\,\} = \log\left[\mu_0(t)\, \exp\{\boldsymbol{\beta}^T \boldsymbol{Z}_i(t)\} + 1\right].$$

Among others, Lin et al. (2001) investigate model (5.15) for regression analysis of recurrent event data.

To estimate the regression parameter $\boldsymbol{\beta}$ in model (5.15), we adopt the unconditional approach used in Sect. 5.4.2. For this, we assume that the observation processes $\tilde{H}_i(t)$'s are non-homogeneous Poisson processes following the proportional rate model

$$E\{\, d\tilde{H}_i(t)|\, \boldsymbol{Z}_i(t)\,\} = \exp\{\boldsymbol{\gamma}^T \boldsymbol{Z}_i(t)\}\, d\tilde{\mu}_0(t), \tag{5.16}$$

$i = 1, \ldots, n$. In the above, both $\boldsymbol{\gamma}$ and $\tilde{\mu}_0(t)$ are defined as in model (5.12) and it is obvious that models (5.12) and (5.16) are same if the $\boldsymbol{Z}_i(t)$'s are time-independent. In the next subsection, a class of estimators is derived for estimation of both $\boldsymbol{\beta}$ and $\boldsymbol{\gamma}$.

5.5.2 Estimation Procedure

To derive the estimation procedure for regression parameters $\boldsymbol{\beta}$ and $\boldsymbol{\gamma}$, define $Y_i(t) = I(C_i \geq t)$ and

$$\begin{aligned}M_i(t; \boldsymbol{\beta}, \boldsymbol{\gamma}) = &\int_0^t Y_i(u)\, N_i(u)\, dH_i(u) - \int_0^t g\{\mu_0(u)\, \exp(\boldsymbol{\beta}^T \boldsymbol{Z}_i(u))\} \\ &\times Y_i(u)\, \exp\{\boldsymbol{\gamma}^T \boldsymbol{Z}_i(u)\}\, d\tilde{\mu}_0(u),\end{aligned} \tag{5.17}$$

5.5 Analysis with Semiparametric Transformation Models

$i = 1, \ldots, n$. Note that under models (5.15) and (5.16), one can easily show that

$$E\{Y_i(t) N_i(t) dH_i(t)\} = E[E\{Y_i(t) N_i(t) dH_i(t) | \mathbf{Z}_i(t)\}]$$
$$= E\left[Y_i(t) g\left\{\mu_0(t) \exp(\boldsymbol{\beta}^T \mathbf{Z}_i(t))\right\} \exp\{\boldsymbol{\gamma}^T \mathbf{Z}_i(t)\} d\tilde{\mu}_0(t)\right].$$

It then follows that we have $E\{M_i(t; \boldsymbol{\beta}, \boldsymbol{\gamma})\} = 0$. That is, the $M_i(t; \boldsymbol{\beta}, \boldsymbol{\gamma})$'s are zero-mean stochastic processes. This suggests that if $\boldsymbol{\beta}$, $\boldsymbol{\gamma}$ and $\tilde{\mu}_0(t)$ are known, one can estimate $\mu_0(t)$ by the solution to

$$\sum_{i=1}^{n} dM_i(t; \boldsymbol{\beta}, \boldsymbol{\gamma}) = \sum_{i=1}^{n} \Big[Y_i(t) N_i(t) dH_i(t)$$
$$- Y_i(t) g\left\{\mu_0(t) \exp(\boldsymbol{\beta}^T \mathbf{Z}_i(t))\right\} \exp\{\boldsymbol{\gamma}^T \mathbf{Z}_i(t)\} d\tilde{\mu}_0(t)\Big] = 0 \quad (5.18)$$

for $0 \leq t \leq \tau$. For estimation of $\boldsymbol{\beta}$, define

$$U_T(\boldsymbol{\beta}, \boldsymbol{\gamma}) = \sum_{i=1}^{n} \int_0^{\tau} W(t) \mathbf{Z}_i(t) dM_i(t; \boldsymbol{\beta}, \boldsymbol{\gamma}) = \sum_{i=1}^{n} \int_0^{\tau} W(t) \mathbf{Z}_i(t)$$
$$\times \Big[Y_i(t) N_i(t) dH_i(t) - Y_i(t) g\left\{\mu_0(t) \exp(\boldsymbol{\beta}^T \mathbf{Z}_i(t))\right\} \exp\{\boldsymbol{\gamma}^T \mathbf{Z}_i(t)\} d\tilde{\mu}_0(t)\Big], \quad (5.19)$$

where $W(t)$ is a possibly data-dependent weight function. Then it is easy to show that $E\{U_T(\boldsymbol{\beta}, \boldsymbol{\gamma})\} = 0$, which suggests that one can estimate $\boldsymbol{\beta}$ by using the estimating equation $U_T(\boldsymbol{\beta}, \boldsymbol{\gamma}) = 0$ given $\boldsymbol{\gamma}$.

Note that in general, $\boldsymbol{\gamma}$ and $\tilde{\mu}_0(t)$ are unknown, but we do have recurrent event data on the $\tilde{H}_i(t)$'s as mentioned before. Thus one can estimate $\boldsymbol{\gamma}$ by the consistent estimator given by the solution, say $\hat{\boldsymbol{\gamma}}_T$, to the estimating equation

$$\sum_{i=1}^{n} \int_0^{\tau} \{\mathbf{Z}_i(t) - \bar{\mathbf{Z}}(t; \boldsymbol{\gamma})\} Y_i(t) dH_i(t) = 0 \quad (5.20)$$

(Andersen et al., 1993; Cook and Lawless, 2007). In the above, $\bar{\mathbf{Z}}(t; \boldsymbol{\gamma}) = S_1(t; \boldsymbol{\gamma})/S_0(t; \boldsymbol{\gamma})$ with

$$S_k(t; \boldsymbol{\gamma}) = \frac{1}{n} \sum_{i=1}^{n} Y_i(t) \mathbf{Z}_i^k(t) \exp\{\boldsymbol{\gamma}^T \mathbf{Z}_i(t)\},$$

$k = 0, 1$. Furthermore, $\tilde{\mu}_0(t)$ can be estimated by

$$\hat{\tilde{\mu}}_0(t; \boldsymbol{\gamma}) = \sum_{i=1}^{n} \int_0^{t} \frac{Y_i(u) dH_i(u)}{n S_0(u; \boldsymbol{\gamma})} \quad (5.21)$$

with replacing $\boldsymbol{\gamma}$ by $\hat{\boldsymbol{\gamma}}_T$.

Given $\hat{\boldsymbol{\gamma}}_T$ and $\hat{\tilde{\mu}}_0(t;\boldsymbol{\gamma})$, define the estimators, denoted by $\hat{\boldsymbol{\beta}}_T$ and $\hat{\mu}_0(t)$, of $\boldsymbol{\beta}$ and $\mu_0(t)$ to be the solutions to the estimating equations $U_T(\boldsymbol{\beta},\boldsymbol{\gamma}) = 0$ and (5.18) with replacing $\boldsymbol{\gamma}$ and $\tilde{\mu}_0(t)$ by $\hat{\boldsymbol{\gamma}}_T$ and $\hat{\tilde{\mu}}_0(t;\hat{\boldsymbol{\gamma}}_T)$, respectively. Li et al. (2010) show that for large n, both $\hat{\boldsymbol{\beta}}_T$ and $\hat{\mu}_0(t)$ always exist and are unique and consistent. To describe the asymptotic distribution, define $\hat{M}_i(t)$ to be $M_i(t;\boldsymbol{\beta},\boldsymbol{\gamma})$ defined in (5.17) with all unknown parameters and functions replaced by their estimators,

$$\hat{M}_i^*(t) = \int_0^t Y_i(u)\,dH_i(u) - \int_0^t Y_i(u)\,\exp\{\hat{\boldsymbol{\gamma}}_T^T \boldsymbol{Z}_i(u)\}\,d\hat{\tilde{\mu}}_0(u;\hat{\boldsymbol{\gamma}}_T)\,,$$

$$\hat{E}_Z(t) = \frac{\sum_{i=1}^n Y_i(t)\boldsymbol{Z}_i(t)\dot{g}\{\hat{\mu}_0(t)\exp(\hat{\boldsymbol{\beta}}_T^T\boldsymbol{Z}_i(t))\}\exp\{\hat{\boldsymbol{\beta}}_T^T\boldsymbol{Z}(t)+\hat{\boldsymbol{\gamma}}_T^T\boldsymbol{Z}_i(t)\}}{\sum_{i=1}^n Y_i(t)\,\dot{g}\{\hat{\mu}_0(t)\exp(\hat{\boldsymbol{\beta}}_T^T\boldsymbol{Z}_i(t))\}\exp\{\hat{\boldsymbol{\beta}}_T^T\boldsymbol{Z}(t)+\hat{\boldsymbol{\gamma}}_T^T\boldsymbol{Z}_i(t)\}}\,,$$

$$\hat{R}(t) = \frac{1}{n}\sum_{i=1}^n \left\{ \boldsymbol{Z}_i(t) - \hat{E}_Z(t)\right\} Y_i(t) g\left\{\hat{\mu}_0(t)\exp(\hat{\boldsymbol{\beta}}_T^T\boldsymbol{Z}(t))\right\}\exp\{\hat{\boldsymbol{\gamma}}_T^T\boldsymbol{Z}_i(t)\}\,,$$

$$\hat{D} = \frac{1}{n}\sum_{i=1}^n \int_0^\tau \left\{\boldsymbol{Z}_i(t) - \bar{\boldsymbol{Z}}(t;\hat{\boldsymbol{\gamma}}_T)\right\}^{\otimes 2} Y_i(t)\,dH_i(t)\,,$$

and

$$\hat{P} = \frac{1}{n}\sum_{i=1}^n \int_0^\tau W(t)\,Y_i(t)\,g\left\{\hat{\mu}_0(t)\exp(\hat{\boldsymbol{\beta}}_T^T\boldsymbol{Z}(t))\right\}\,\exp\{\hat{\boldsymbol{\gamma}}_T^T\boldsymbol{Z}_i(t)\}$$
$$\times \left\{\boldsymbol{Z}_i(t) - \hat{E}_Z(t)\right\}\left\{\boldsymbol{Z}_i(t) - \bar{\boldsymbol{Z}}(t;\hat{\boldsymbol{\gamma}}_T)\right\}^T d\hat{\tilde{\mu}}_0(t;\hat{\boldsymbol{\gamma}}_T)\,.$$

In the above, $\dot{g}(t) = dg(t)/dt$. Li et al. (2010) show that as $n \to \infty$, $n^{1/2}(\hat{\boldsymbol{\beta}}_T - \boldsymbol{\beta}_0)$ asymptotically follows a multivariate normal distribution with mean zero and the covariance matrix that can be consistently estimated by $\hat{\Sigma}_T = A_T^{-1} B_T A_T^{-1}$. Here

$$A_T = \frac{1}{n}\sum_{i=1}^n \int_0^\tau W(t)\,Y_i(t)\,\dot{g}\left\{\hat{\mu}_0(t)\exp(\hat{\boldsymbol{\beta}}_T^T\boldsymbol{Z}(t))\right\}\left\{\boldsymbol{Z}_i(t) - \hat{E}_Z(t)\right\}^{\otimes 2}$$
$$\times \exp\left\{\hat{\boldsymbol{\beta}}_T^T\boldsymbol{Z}(t) + \hat{\boldsymbol{\gamma}}_T^T\boldsymbol{Z}_i(t)\right\} \hat{\mu}_0(t)\,d\hat{\tilde{\mu}}_0(t;\hat{\boldsymbol{\gamma}}_T)\,,$$

and

$$B_T = \frac{1}{n}\sum_{i=1}^n \left[\int_0^\tau W(t)\left\{\boldsymbol{Z}_i(t) - \hat{E}_Z(t)\right\} d\hat{M}_i(t) - \int_0^\tau \frac{W(t)\hat{R}(t)}{S_0(t;\hat{\boldsymbol{\gamma}}_T)}\,d\hat{M}_i^*(t)\right.$$
$$\left. - \hat{P}\,\hat{D}^{-1}\int_0^\tau \left\{\boldsymbol{Z}_i(t) - \bar{\boldsymbol{Z}}(t;\hat{\boldsymbol{\gamma}}_T)\right\} d\hat{M}_i^*(t)\right]^{\otimes 2}\,.$$

5.5.3 Determination of Estimators

This subsection discusses the determination of the estimators $\hat{\boldsymbol{\beta}}_T$ and $\hat{\mu}_0(t)$ described in the previous subsection. For the determination of $\hat{\boldsymbol{\gamma}}_T$ and $\hat{\tilde{\mu}}_0(t;\boldsymbol{\gamma})$, the readers are referred to Cook and Lawless (2007) among others. Let $s_1 < s_2 < \ldots < s_m$ denote the distinct ordered observation times of $\{t_{i,j}; j = 1, \ldots, m_i, i = 1, \ldots, n\}$. Then at time s_j, Eq. (5.18) can be rewritten as

$$\sum_{i=1}^{n}\sum_{l=1}^{m_i} N_i(t_{i,l})\, I(t_{i,l}=s_j) - \sum_{i=1}^{n} g\left\{\mu_0(s_j)\exp(\boldsymbol{\beta}^T \boldsymbol{Z}_i(s_j))\right\} Y_i(s_j)$$
$$\times \exp\left\{\boldsymbol{\gamma}^T \boldsymbol{Z}_i(s_j)\right\} d\mu_0(s_j) = 0,$$

$j = 1, \ldots, m$. Let $\hat{\mu}_0(t;\boldsymbol{\beta},\boldsymbol{\gamma})$ denote the solution to the equation above for given $\boldsymbol{\beta}$ and $\boldsymbol{\gamma}$. Then by replacing $\boldsymbol{\gamma}$ and $\mu_0(t)$ with the estimators $\hat{\boldsymbol{\gamma}}_T$ and $\hat{\mu}_0(t;\boldsymbol{\beta},\hat{\boldsymbol{\gamma}}_T)$, respectively, the estimating equation $U_T(\boldsymbol{\beta};\boldsymbol{\gamma}) = 0$ has the form

$$\sum_{i=1}^{n}\sum_{l=1}^{m_i} W(t_{i,l})\, \boldsymbol{Z}_i(t_{i,l})\, N_i(t_{i,l}) - \sum_{j=1}^{m} W(s_j) \sum_{i=1}^{n} \boldsymbol{Z}_i(s_j)$$
$$\times g\left\{\hat{\mu}_0(s_j;\boldsymbol{\beta},\hat{\boldsymbol{\gamma}}_T)\exp(\boldsymbol{\beta}^T \boldsymbol{Z}_i(s_j))\right\} Y_i(s_j) \exp\left\{\hat{\boldsymbol{\gamma}}_T^T \boldsymbol{Z}_i(s_j)\right\} d\hat{\mu}_0(s_j;\hat{\boldsymbol{\gamma}}_T) = 0.$$

It is apparent that once $\hat{\boldsymbol{\beta}}_T$ is obtained, we have $\hat{\mu}_0(t) = \hat{\mu}_0(t;\hat{\boldsymbol{\beta}}_T,\hat{\boldsymbol{\gamma}}_T)$. Note that for a given data set, the estimator $\hat{\mu}_0(t)$ obtained above may not be a non-decreasing function sometimes. In this case, one simple approach is to apply some justification such as defining the estimator at time t as $\max\{\hat{\mu}_0(s); 0 \leq s \leq t\}$.

In general, there are no closed forms for $\hat{\boldsymbol{\beta}}_T$ and $\hat{\mu}_0(t;\boldsymbol{\beta},\boldsymbol{\gamma})$ and some iterative algorithms have to be used to solve the equations above. Hence the computation for the determination of these estimators could be slow, especially in simulation. The same is true for the determination of the estimated covariance matrix due to its complexity although it does have a closed form.

On the other hand, for some special situations, the estimators $\hat{\boldsymbol{\beta}}_T$ and $\hat{\mu}_0(t;\boldsymbol{\beta},\boldsymbol{\gamma})$ do have closed forms and thus their determination is straightforward. For example, assume $g(t) = t^\eta$, where η is a positive constant. In this case, we have

$$g\{\hat{\mu}_0(t;\boldsymbol{\beta},\boldsymbol{\gamma})\} = \frac{\sum_{i=1}^{n} Y_i(t)\, N_i(t)\, dH_i(t)}{\sum_{i=1}^{n} g\{\exp(\boldsymbol{\beta}^T \boldsymbol{Z}_i(t))\} Y_i(t) \exp\{\boldsymbol{\gamma}^T \boldsymbol{Z}_i(t)\}\, d\tilde{\mu}_0(t)} \cdot \frac{1}{.}$$

That is, $\hat{\mu}_0(t;\boldsymbol{\beta},\boldsymbol{\gamma})$ has an explicit expression. Also in this situation, $U_T(\boldsymbol{\beta};\hat{\boldsymbol{\gamma}}_T) = 0$ becomes

$$\sum_{i=1}^{n}\int_0^\tau W(t)\left\{\boldsymbol{Z}_i(t) - \bar{\boldsymbol{Z}}(t;\boldsymbol{\beta},\hat{\boldsymbol{\gamma}}_T)\right\} Y_i(t)\, N_i(t)\, dH_i(t) = 0,$$

where

$$\bar{Z}(t;\boldsymbol{\beta},\hat{\boldsymbol{\gamma}}_T) = \frac{\sum_{i=1}^n \boldsymbol{Z}_i(t) g\{\exp(\boldsymbol{\beta}^T \boldsymbol{Z}_i(t))\} Y_i(t) \exp\{\hat{\boldsymbol{\gamma}}_T^T \boldsymbol{Z}_i(t)\}}{\sum_{i=1}^n g\{\exp(\boldsymbol{\beta}^T \boldsymbol{Z}_i(t))\} Y_i(t) \exp\{\hat{\boldsymbol{\gamma}}_T^T \boldsymbol{Z}_i(t)\}}.$$

Another special case where the determination of $\hat{\boldsymbol{\beta}}_T$ and $\hat{\mu}_0(t;\boldsymbol{\beta},\boldsymbol{\gamma})$ is straightforward is when $g(t) = \log(t)$. In this case, the estimator $\hat{\mu}_0(t;\boldsymbol{\beta},\boldsymbol{\gamma})$ also has a closed form that can be obtained by

$$g\{\hat{\mu}_0(t;\boldsymbol{\beta},\boldsymbol{\gamma})\} = \frac{\sum_{i=1}^n Y_i(t) N_i(t) dH_i(t)}{\sum_{i=1}^n Y_i(t) \exp\{\boldsymbol{\gamma}^T \boldsymbol{Z}_i(t)\}} \frac{1}{d\mu_0(t)}$$
$$- \frac{\sum_{i=1}^n g\{\exp(\boldsymbol{\beta}^T \boldsymbol{Z}_i(t))\} Y_i(t) \exp\{\boldsymbol{\gamma}^T \boldsymbol{Z}_i(t)\}}{\sum_{i=1}^n Y_i(t) \exp\{\boldsymbol{\gamma}^T \boldsymbol{Z}_i(t)\}}.$$

For $\hat{\boldsymbol{\beta}}_T$, we have

$$U_T(\boldsymbol{\beta};\hat{\boldsymbol{\gamma}}_T) = \sum_{i=1}^n \int_0^\tau W(t) \{\boldsymbol{Z}_i(t) - \bar{\boldsymbol{Z}}(t;\hat{\boldsymbol{\gamma}}_T)\} Y_i(t) \Big[N_i(t) dH_i(t)$$
$$- \boldsymbol{\beta}^T \boldsymbol{Z}_i(t) \exp\{\hat{\boldsymbol{\gamma}}_T^T \boldsymbol{Z}_i(t)\} d\hat{\mu}_0(t;\hat{\boldsymbol{\gamma}}_T) \Big],$$

where $\bar{\boldsymbol{Z}}(t;\boldsymbol{\gamma})$ is the same as defined in the previous subsection. This yields

$$\hat{\boldsymbol{\beta}}_T = \left[\sum_{i=1}^n \int_0^\tau W(t) \{\boldsymbol{Z}_i(t) - \bar{\boldsymbol{Z}}(t;\hat{\boldsymbol{\gamma}}_T)\} \boldsymbol{Z}_i^T(t) Y_i(t) e^{\hat{\boldsymbol{\gamma}}_T^T \boldsymbol{Z}_i(t)} d\hat{\mu}_0(t;\hat{\boldsymbol{\gamma}}_T) \right]^{-1}$$
$$\times \sum_{i=1}^n \int_0^\tau W(t) \{\boldsymbol{Z}_i(t) - \bar{\boldsymbol{Z}}(t;\hat{\boldsymbol{\gamma}}_T)\} Y_i(t) N_i(t) dH_i(t).$$

That is, $\hat{\boldsymbol{\beta}}_T$ has a closed form too.

For the determination of $\hat{\boldsymbol{\beta}}_T$ and $\hat{\mu}_0(t)$ for a given data set, another issue is to choose or specify the function g in model (5.15). As seen above, this can have large effects on the determination. As with the same topic in other fields such as longitudinal data analysis (Lin et al., 2001) and failure time data analysis (Zhang et al., 2005), the selection of an appropriate g is a very difficult issue in general. A common strategy is to try several choices and compare the obtained estimation results. Similarly as with the selection of g, one also needs to choose the weight function $W(t)$ and it does not seem to exist an established procedure in the literature for this. A practical approach again is to try different choices and compare the results.

5.5.4 A Goodness-of-Fit Test

As with model (1.4), a natural question about model (5.15) is to assess its adequacy with a given g. To address this, we now describe a goodness-of-fit test procedure. Note that of course, one could ask the same question about model (5.16) and for that, the readers are referred to Cook and Lawless (2007) and Lin et al. (2000).

To present the test procedure, let the $\hat{M}_i(t)$'s, $\hat{M}_i^*(t)$'s, $W(t)$, $\hat{E}_Z(t)$, $\hat{R}(t)$, $\hat{D}$, $\hat{P}$ and A_T be defined as in Sect. 5.5.2. Motivated by the idea used in Sun et al. (2007a), we consider the following cumulative sum of residuals process

$$\mathcal{F}(t, z) = n^{-1/2} \sum_{i=1}^{n} \int_0^t I\{\mathbf{Z}_i(u) \leq z\} d\hat{M}_i(u). \quad (5.22)$$

In the above, $I\{\mathbf{Z}_i(u) \leq z\}$ means that each component of $\mathbf{Z}_i$ is not larger than the corresponding component of z. Note that under model (5.15), the process $\mathcal{F}(t, z)$ is expected to fluctuate randomly around zero. Hence it is natural to construct a goodness-of-fit test based on the supremum statistic $\sup_{t,z} |\mathcal{F}(t, z)|$.

To employ the statistic $\sup_{t,z} |\mathcal{F}(t, z)|$, one needs to know its distribution, which is usually difficult to derive. For this, we use the following approximation for the determination of the p-value for the goodness-of-fit test. Define

$$\hat{\Psi}_i(t, z) = \int_0^t \left\{ I(\mathbf{Z}_i(u) \leq z) - \bar{\Phi}(u, z) \right\} d\hat{M}_i(u) - \int_0^t \frac{S(u, z)}{S_0(u; \hat{\gamma}_T)} d\hat{M}_i^*(u)$$

$$-\hat{\Upsilon}_1^T(t, z) A_T^{-1} \left[\int_0^\tau W(u) \{\mathbf{Z}_i(u) - \hat{E}_Z(u)\} d\hat{M}_i(u) - \int_0^\tau \frac{W(u) \hat{R}(u)}{S_0(u; \hat{\gamma}_T)} d\hat{M}_i^*(u) \right.$$

$$\left. - \hat{P}\hat{D}^{-1} \int_0^\tau \{\mathbf{Z}_i(u) - \bar{\mathbf{Z}}(u; \hat{\gamma}_T)\} d\hat{M}_i^*(u) \right]$$

$$- \hat{\Upsilon}_2^T(t, z) \hat{D}^{-1} \int_0^\tau \{\mathbf{Z}_i(u) - \bar{\mathbf{Z}}(u; \hat{\gamma}_T)\} d\hat{M}_i^*(u),$$

where

$$\bar{\Phi}(u, z) = \frac{\sum_{i=1}^n I(\mathbf{Z}_i(u) \leq z) Y_i(u) \dot{g}\{\hat{\mu}_0(u) e^{\hat{\beta}_T^T \mathbf{Z}_i(u)}\} e^{\hat{\beta}_T^T \mathbf{Z}_i(u) + \hat{\gamma}_T^T \mathbf{Z}_i(u)}}{\sum_{i=1}^n Y_i(u) \dot{g}\{\hat{\mu}_0(u) e^{\hat{\beta}_T^T \mathbf{Z}_i(u)}\} e^{\hat{\beta}_T^T \mathbf{Z}_i(u) + \hat{\gamma}_T^T \mathbf{Z}_i(u)}},$$

$$S(u, z) = \frac{1}{n} \sum_{i=1}^n I(\mathbf{Z}_i(u) \leq z) Y_i(u) g\{\hat{\mu}_0(u) \exp(\hat{\beta}_T^T \mathbf{Z}_i(u))\} \exp\{\hat{\gamma}_T^T \mathbf{Z}_i(u)\},$$

$$\hat{\Upsilon}_1(t, z) = \frac{1}{n} \sum_{i=1}^n \int_0^t I(\mathbf{Z}_i(u) \leq z) Y_i(u) g\left\{\hat{\mu}_0(u) \exp(\hat{\beta}_T^T \mathbf{Z}_i(u))\right\}$$

$$\times \left\{\mathbf{Z}_i(u) - \hat{E}_Z(u)\right\} \exp\left\{\hat{\beta}_T^T \mathbf{Z}_i(u) + \hat{\gamma}_T^T \mathbf{Z}_i(u)\right\} \hat{\mu}_0(u) d\hat{\tilde{\mu}}_0(u; \hat{\gamma}_T),$$

and

$$\hat{\varUpsilon}_2(t, z) = \frac{1}{n}\sum_{i=1}^{n}\int_0^t \left\{I(\boldsymbol{Z}_i(u) \leq z) - \bar{\varPhi}(u, z)\right\}Y_i(u)g\left\{\hat{\mu}_0(u)\exp(\hat{\boldsymbol{\beta}}_T^T\boldsymbol{Z}_i(u))\right\}$$
$$\times \exp\left\{\hat{\boldsymbol{\gamma}}_T^T\boldsymbol{Z}_i(u)\right\}\left\{\boldsymbol{Z}_i(u) - \bar{\boldsymbol{Z}}(u; \hat{\boldsymbol{\gamma}}_T)\right\}d\hat{\bar{\mu}}_0(u; \hat{\boldsymbol{\gamma}}_T).$$

Then by following the arguments similar to those used in Lin et al. (2000), one can show that the null distribution of $\mathcal{F}(t, z)$ can be approximated by the zero-mean Gaussian process

$$\tilde{F}(t, z) = n^{-1/2}\sum_{i=1}^{n}\hat{\varPsi}_i(t, z).$$

Furthermore, one can approximate the distribution of $\tilde{F}(t, z)$ by the zero-mean Gaussian process

$$\hat{\mathcal{F}}(t, z) = n^{-1/2}\sum_{i=1}^{n}\hat{\varPsi}_i(t, z)\, G_i,$$

where $(G_1, \ldots, G_n)$ are a simple random sample of size n from the standard normal distribution independent of the observed data. This suggests that the p-value can be obtained by comparing the observed value of $\sup_{0 \leq t \leq \tau, z}|\mathcal{F}(t, z)|$ to a large number of realizations of $\sup_{0 \leq t \leq \tau, z}|\hat{\mathcal{F}}(t, z)|$ given by repeatedly generating the standard normal random sample $(G_1, \ldots, G_n)$ while fixing the observation data. As a graphical tool, one could also plot $\mathcal{F}(t, z)$ along with a few realizations of $\hat{\mathcal{F}}(t, z)$, and an unusual pattern of $\mathcal{F}(t, z)$ would suggest a lack-of-fit of model (5.15).

5.6 Analysis of National Cooperative Gallstone Study

In this section, we illustrate the regression analysis procedures discussed in the previous sections by applying them to the gallstone data described in Sect. 1.2.2 and analyzed in Sect. 4.4.1. As discussed before, the study yielding the data concerns the effects of the use of the natural bile acid chenodeoxycholic acid, cheno, on the dissolution of cholesterol gallstones. The observed data include the incidences of digestive symptoms commonly associated with the gallstone disease and in particular, the incidence of nausea. More specifically, on the occurrences of nausea, the observed information is given by the form of panel count data. For the analysis, as before, we focus on the data given in the data set I of Chap. 9 from the 113 patients in the placebo and high dose groups during the first 52 weeks of the follow-up.

5.6 Analysis of National Cooperative Gallstone Study

To perform the regression analysis, let $N_i(t)$ denote the underlying recurrent event process controlling the occurrence of nausea for subject i, $i = 1, \ldots, 113$. Define $Z_i = 0$ if subject i was in the placebo group and 1 otherwise. To estimate the effect of treatment cheno on the occurrence of nausea, first we assume that the $N_i(t)$'s are non-homogeneous Poisson processes satisfying the proportional mean model (1.4). The application of the pseudo-likelihood estimation procedure described in Sect. 5.2 gives $\hat{\beta}_L = -0.533$ with the estimated standard error of 0.543 based on 200 bootstrap samples. This corresponds to the p-value of 0.326 for testing no treatment effect on the occurrence of nausea. The result suggests that the treatment cheno did not seem to have a significant effect in reducing the occurrence rate of nausea for the floating gallstone patients.

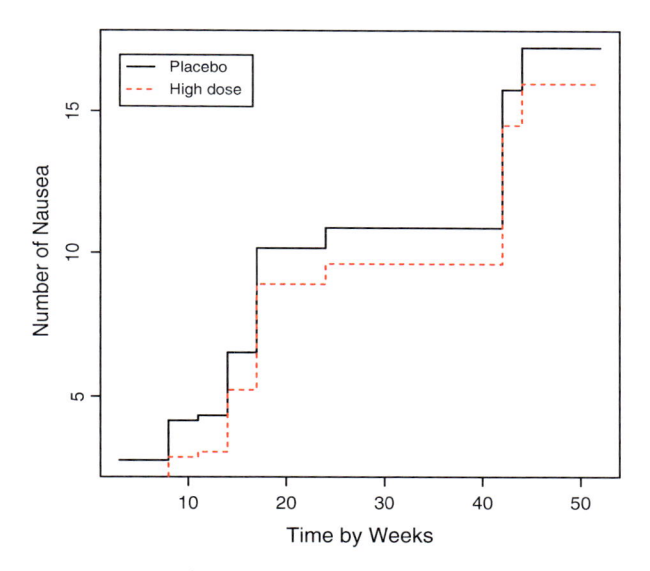

Fig. 5.1. Estimated mean functions of the occurrence processes of nausea under model (5.15) with $g(t) = \log(t)$

As discussed before, the pseudo-likelihood estimation procedure used above relies on the Poisson process assumption, which may not hold. To avoid this, consider the estimation procedures given in Sect. 5.4, which do not require the assumption but still assume that the $N_i(t)$'s follow the proportional mean model (1.4). First we apply the conditional estimation procedure and obtain $\hat{\beta}_{II}^C = -0.419$ with the estimated standard error being 0.537, yielding the p-value of 0.540 for testing no treatment effect. The application of the unconditional estimation procedure gives $\hat{\beta}_{II}^M = -0.527$ and the estimated standard error of 0.628. This result gives the same conclusion as the conditional estimation procedure as well as the pseudo-likelihood estimation procedure. Together with the result above, we also obtain $\hat{\gamma} = -0.024$ with the estimated standard error of 0.040 for model (5.12). This indicates that the treatment also did not seem to have any significant effect on the patient's visiting process.

Table 5.1. Estimated treatment effects and p-values

Link function	$\hat{\beta}_T$	SE($\hat{\beta}_T$)	p-value for $\beta = 0$	p-value for model-checking
$g(t) = t$	-0.527	0.533	0.323	0.445
$g(t) = t^2$	-0.263	0.266	0.323	0.077
$g(t) = \log(t)$	-1.276	1.419	0.368	0.572

Now we consider the application of the estimation procedure derived based on the semiparametric transformation model (5.15). For this, note that it is easy to see from Figs. 3.2 and 3.4 that the proportional mean model (1.4) could be questionable. Thus it is natural to consider model (5.15). Table 5.1 presents the results obtained on the estimator $\hat{\beta}_T$ based on three different link functions, $g(t) = t$, t^2 and $\log(t)$, respectively. In additional to $\hat{\beta}_T$, the table also gives the corresponding estimated standard errors (SE), the p-values for testing $\beta = 0$ in model (5.15), and the p-values given by the goodness-of-fit test described in Sect. 5.5.4 for testing the adequacy of model (5.15). One can see that overall the results are similar to those obtained above and indicate that there is no significant difference between the occurrence rates of nausea for the patients in the two treatment groups. It is interesting to note that the semiparametric transformation model (5.15) with either $g(t) = t$ or $g(t) = \log(t)$ seems to be a better or more appropriate choice than that with $g(t) = t^2$. To give a graphical idea about the estimated treatment effect, Fig. 5.1 presents the estimated mean functions of the occurrence processes of nausea for the two groups under model (5.15) with $g(t) = \log(t)$.

For the application of the estimation procedures given in Sect. 5.3, note that they require centered covariates. For this, we redefine $Z_i = -65/113$ for the patients in the placebo group and $48/113$ otherwise. For the analysis, we first consider the fitting of model (5.5) and it gives $\hat{\tau} = -0.161$ with the estimated standard error being 0.153. This suggests that one should employ the estimation procedure described in Sect. 5.3.3, which yields $\hat{\beta}_{I,1} = -0.409$ with the estimated standard error of 0.559. The result again indicates that the treatment cheno did not have significant effects on the occurrence process of nausea.

5.7 Bibliography, Discussion, and Remarks

As mentioned before, there exists a great deal of literature on regression analysis of simple count data and recurrent event data (Andersen et al. 1993; Cook and Lawless 2007; Lawless 1987a; Vermunt 1997). In comparison, only limited literature exists for regression analysis of panel count data, which can be regarded as dependent count data arising from point processes. For regression analysis of panel count data, the existing methods can be generally classified into two types. One is likelihood-based approaches such as those described in Chap. 2 and Sect. 5.2 and the other is estimating equation-based approaches such as those discussed in Sects. 5.3–5.5. For the former, some Poisson-type assumptions are usually needed although they may not be realistic sometimes. Note that as pointed out before, an alternative to these two types procedures is to regard panel count data as longitudinal data and apply the existing methods for regression analysis of longitudinal data (Diggle et al., 1994; Sun, 2010). However, it is easy to see that the use of these methods would not take into account the special structure of panel count data. More importantly, they may not provide direct answers to the questions that are only of interest for recurrent event processes.

In addition to those mentioned above, other authors who have investigated regression analysis of panel count data include Cheng and Wei (2000), Cheng et al. (2011), He (2007), Lawless and Zhan (1998), Lu et al. (2009), Nielsen and Dean (2008), Staniswalls et al. (1997), Sun and Matthews (1997), and Wellner et al. (2004). In particular, Sun and Matthews (1997) discussed a situation where the irregular and real observation process can be described by a constant or fixed process plus some random effects. Lawless and Zhan (1998) studied the proportional rate model and suggested to approximate the baseline rate function by a piecewise constant rate function. For estimation, they gave a Poisson-based likelihood procedure and a GEE-based robust procedure.

Also Cheng and Wei (2000) developed an estimator similar to the estimator $\hat{\boldsymbol{\beta}}_{II}^M$ for $\boldsymbol{\beta}$ in model (1.4) while assuming that $\boldsymbol{\gamma} = 0$ in model (5.12). More specifically, they defined their estimator using the estimating function

$$\sum_{i=1}^{n} \int_0^\tau w(t) \, I(C_i \geq t) \, \boldsymbol{Z}_i(t) \, d\left[\tilde{N}_i(t) - \int_0^t \exp\left\{ \boldsymbol{\beta}^T \boldsymbol{Z}_i(s) \right\} d\hat{\tilde{\mu}}_0^*(s; \boldsymbol{\beta}) \right]$$

with time-dependent covariates. In contrast to the methods described above, Lu et al. (2009), Nielsen and Dean (2008) and Staniswalls et al. (1997) gave some methods that employ some smoothing techniques along with Poisson process-related assumptions. In particular, Lu et al. (2009) used monotone B-splines to approximate the baseline mean function in the proportional mean model, while Nielsen and Dean (2008) modeled smooth intensity functions by penalized splines.

With respect to the comparison of Poisson or likelihood-based methods and estimating equation-based procedures, as discussed before, the former could be much more complicated than the latter. This is partly because the former involves estimation of an unknown baseline function. On the other hand, it is clear that the former could be more efficient than the latter if the Poisson process-related assumption is valid. Of course, in practice, it may be difficult to check or verify this assumption without prior information. Another advantage of the estimating equation-based procedures is that they give closed-form estimation of the variance.

An issue that is similar to the appropriateness of Poisson process-related assumptions is the adequacy of model (1.4) or (5.15). For this, one could apply the goodness-of-fit test given in Sect. 5.5. However, the selection of an appropriate or the optimal link function g in model (5.15) is generally difficult as commented above. Also one may ask the sensitivity of estimation results to the selection of the function g and in general, the estimated effects of covariates could be biased if there is model misspecification. For this, in addition to applying model checking procedures as mentioned above, another method is to develop robust estimation procedures. But of course, in general, the robust estimators could be less efficient.

6
Regression Analysis of Panel Count Data II

6.1 Introduction

This chapter discusses the same problem as in the previous chapter, but under different situations. A basic assumption behind the methods described in the last chapter is that the underlying recurrent event process of interest and the observation process are independent of each other conditional on covariates. As pointed out before, sometimes this assumption may not hold. In other words, the observation process may depend on or contain relevant information about the recurrent event process. In a study on the occurrence of asthma attacks, for example, the observations on or clinical visits of asthma patients may be related to or driven by the numbers of the asthma attacks before the visits. The same can occur for similar recurrent event studies such as these on some disease infections or tumor development. In these situations, it is clear that the methods given in Chap. 5 are not valid as they would lead to biased estimation or wrong conclusions. The data arising from these cases are often referred to as panel count data with informative or dependent observation processes.

For regression analysis of panel count data with dependent observation processes, in the following, we first describe a simple joint modeling procedure in Sect. 6.2. The method allows all three processes, the underlying recurrent event process of interest, the observation process and the follow-up process, to be correlated with each other even conditional on covariates. The assumption behind the approach is that their relationship can be characterized through some latent variables. A three-step procedure involving the use of the EM algorithm is given for estimation of all involved parameters. A drawback of the procedure is that it may not be robust to the specified relationship. To address this, Sect. 6.3 considers a class of much more general models for the relationship and gives a robust inference procedure for estimation of the effects of covariates.

In both Sects. 6.2 and 6.3, it is assumed that the effects of covariates on the underlying recurrent event process of interest can be described by the proportional mean model. As discussed in Sect. 5.5, the model could be restrictive in practice. Corresponding to this, Sect. 6.4 generalizes the semiparametric transformation model (5.15) to allow the dependence between the recurrent event process and the observation process. The new model is a conditional one and assumes that the occurrence rate of the recurrent events of interest may depend on the observation process. For estimation of regression parameters, an estimating equation approach is described.

In all of the previous discussions, it has been assumed that the censoring or follow-up time can be either independent of or related to the underlying recurrent event process of interest. For both cases, the implication is that the recurrent events of interest can continue to occur after the follow-up time although not observable. On the other hand, sometimes the follow-up may be determined by some event whose occurrence stops or terminates the occurrence of future recurrent events of interest. A simple example of such events is death and they are often referred to as terminal events. For example, tumors would not develop after death. In the presence of terminal events, an important issue arises if the terminal event is correlated with the recurrent events of interest as well as the observation process. Section 6.5 investigates this situation in more details and discusses how to conduct valid inference about covariate effects. Section 6.6 gives some bibliographical notes and discusses some issues not discussed in the previous sections.

6.2 Analysis by a Joint Modeling Procedure

As mentioned above, this section discusses a simple joint modeling approach for regression analysis of panel count data with dependent observation processes. The basic idea behind the approach, borrowed from longitudinal and failure time data analysis, is to employ some shared frailty models. In the following, we first discuss the assumptions and models needed for the approach. A three-step estimation procedure is then presented for estimation of all concerned parameters and followed by some remarks and discussion.

6.2.1 Assumptions and Models

Consider a recurrent event study that consists of n independent subjects and yields only panel count data. As in the previous chapters, let the $N_i(t)$'s and $\tilde{H}_i(t)$'s denote the underlying recurrent event processes of interest and observation processes, respectively. Specifically, $N_i(t)$ represents the number of occurrences of the recurrent event of interest up to time t for subject i, and $\tilde{H}_i(t)$ is a counting process with jumps at $t_{i,1} < t_{i,2} < \ldots$, the potential observation times on $N_i(t)$. Also as before, suppose that for subject i, there

6.2 Analysis by a Joint Modeling Procedure

exists a vector of covariates denoted by $\boldsymbol{Z}_i$, whose effects on the $N_i(t)$'s are of main interest.

Furthermore, assume that there exist two follow-up times C_i^* and τ_i and one only observes $C_i = \min(C_i^*, \tau_i)$ and $\delta_i = I(C_i = C_i^*)$. Here it is assumed that C_i^* may be related to $N_i(t)$ and $\tilde{H}_i(t)$, but τ_i is independent of them. Define $H_i(t) = \tilde{H}_i\{\min(t, C_i)\} = \sum_{j=1}^{m_i} I(t_{i,j} \leq t)$, representing the real observation process on subject i, where $m_i = \tilde{H}_i(C_i)$ as before, $i = 1, \ldots, n$. Then $N_i(t)$ is observed only at the time points where $H_i(t)$ jumps and the observed data consist of the independent and identically distributed

$$\{ H_i(t), N_i(t)\, dH_i(t), C_i, \delta_i, \boldsymbol{Z}_i\, ; t \geq 0\, , i = 1, \ldots, n \,\}. \tag{6.1}$$

To describe the possible effects of covariates on $N_i(t)$, $\tilde{H}_i(t)$ and C_i^* and the relationship among the three processes or variables, we assume that there exist two independent latent variables u_i and v_i and given $\boldsymbol{Z}_i$, u_i and v_i, $N_i(t)$, $\tilde{H}_i(t)$ and C_i^* are independent. Also it is assumed that given $\boldsymbol{Z}_i$, u_i and v_i, $N_i(t)$ follows the proportional mean model

$$E\{\, N_i(t) | \boldsymbol{Z}_i, u_i, v_i\, \} = \mu_0(t)\, \exp(\boldsymbol{\beta}_1^T \boldsymbol{Z}_i + \beta_2 u_i + \beta_3 v_i)\,. \tag{6.2}$$

Here as before, $\mu_0(t)$ is a completely unknown continuous baseline mean function and $\boldsymbol{\beta}_1$, β_2 and β_3 are unknown regression parameters. For $\tilde{H}_i(t)$ and C_i^*, it is supposed that given $\boldsymbol{Z}_i$, u_i and v_i, $\tilde{H}_i(t)$ is a non-homogeneous Poisson process with the intensity function

$$\lambda_{ih}(t) = \lambda_{0h}(t)\, \exp(\boldsymbol{\alpha}_1^T \boldsymbol{Z}_i + u_i)\,, \tag{6.3}$$

and the hazard function of C_i^* has the form

$$\lambda_{ic}(t) = \lambda_{0c}(t)\, \exp(\boldsymbol{\gamma}_1^T \boldsymbol{Z}_i + \gamma_2 u_i + v_i)\,. \tag{6.4}$$

In the above, $\lambda_{0h}(t)$ is a completely unknown continuous baseline intensity function, $\lambda_{0c}(t)$ denotes an unknown baseline hazard function, and $\boldsymbol{\alpha}_1$, $\boldsymbol{\gamma}_1$ and γ_2 are unknown regression parameters.

Under the models above, it is easy to see that the relationship between the recurrent event process of interest $N_i(t)$ and the observation process $\tilde{H}_i(t)$ is represented by the regression parameter β_2. A positive β_2 means that the two are positively correlated and they are negatively correlated if $\beta_2 < 0$. Similarly β_3 characterizes the relationship between $N_i(t)$ and the follow-up process defined by C_i^*, while the parameter γ_2 represents the relationship between the observation process and the follow-up process. If $\beta_2 = \beta_3 = \gamma_2 = 0$, the three processes are independent given covariates. The parameters $\boldsymbol{\beta}_1$, $\boldsymbol{\alpha}_1$ and $\boldsymbol{\gamma}_1$ represent the effects of covariates on each of the three processes, respectively, after adjusting for their correlation among the three processes.

As discussed before, there exists a great deal of research in the literature on the type of model (6.2) and the same is true on both models (6.3) and

(6.4) as well as their special cases. For example, Huang and Wang (2004) give a model similar to model (6.3) for regression analysis of recurrent event data, and model (6.3) reduces to model (1.8) if $u_i = 0$. Model (6.4) without the latent variables gives the PH model (5.5) and a number of methods have been developed for model (6.4) with $\gamma_2 = 0$. Also in the case of $u_i = v_i = 0$ for all i, models (6.2)–(6.4) reduce to models (1.4), (5.4) and (5.5), respectively. In other words, models (6.2)–(6.4) can be regarded as generalizations of the models discussed in Sect. 5.3 as well as Sect. 5.4.

In the following, we discuss joint analysis of all three models together with the focus on estimation of regression parameters $\boldsymbol{\beta}_1$, $\boldsymbol{\alpha}_1$ and $\boldsymbol{\gamma}_1$. Let $\Lambda_{0h}(t) = \int_0^t \lambda_{0h}(s)\,ds$. For the parameter identifiability, we assume that $\Lambda_{0h}(\tau) = 1$ and $E(u_i|\boldsymbol{Z}_i) = E(u_i)$, where τ denotes the length of study. Also for simplicity, we assume that $v_i \sim N(0, \sigma^2)$, where σ^2 is an unknown parameter. The procedure given below still applies for other distributional assumptions on the v_i's.

6.2.2 Estimation of Parameters

Now we consider estimation of regression parameters $\boldsymbol{\beta}_1$, $\boldsymbol{\alpha}_1$ and $\boldsymbol{\gamma}_1$ as well as other parameters. For this, we describe a three-step procedure, proposed by He et al. (2009), which is basically a combination of three existing estimation procedures for models (6.2)–(6.4), respectively. For $i = 1, \ldots, n$, let $\boldsymbol{Z}_{1i} = (\boldsymbol{Z}_i^T, u_i)^T$, $\boldsymbol{Z}_{2i} = (\boldsymbol{Z}_i^T, u_i, v_i)^T$, $\boldsymbol{\beta} = (\boldsymbol{\beta}_1^T, \beta_2, \beta_3)^T$, $\boldsymbol{\alpha} = (\boldsymbol{\alpha}_1^T, 1, 0)^T$, and $\boldsymbol{\gamma} = (\boldsymbol{\gamma}_1^T, \gamma_2)^T$. The estimation procedure consists of the following three steps.

6.2.2.1 Step 1: Estimation of the Parameters in Model (6.3)

First we consider estimation about model (6.3). As in the previous chapters, let the s_l's denote the ordered and distinct time points of all the observation times $\{t_{i,j}\}$, d_l the number of the observation times equal to s_l, and n_l the number of the observation times satisfying $t_{i,j} \le s_l \le C_i$ among all subjects. Define $\boldsymbol{Z}_{3i} = (\boldsymbol{Z}_i^T, 1)^T$, $\boldsymbol{\alpha}_* = (\boldsymbol{\alpha}_1^T, \alpha_2)^T = (\boldsymbol{\alpha}_1^T, E(u_i))^T$. To estimate the parameters in model (6.3), note that we have recurrent event data on the model and hence some estimation procedures for recurrent event data can be used. In particular, Huang and Wang (2004) suggest to estimate $\Lambda_{0h}(t)$ and $\boldsymbol{\alpha}_*$ by

$$\hat{\Lambda}_{0h}(t) = \prod_{s_l > t}\left(1 - \frac{d_l}{n_l}\right)$$

6.2 Analysis by a Joint Modeling Procedure

and the estimating equation

$$\sum_{i=1}^{n} w_i \, \mathbf{Z}_{3i} \left\{ m_i \, \hat{\Lambda}_{0h}^{-1}(C_i) - \exp(\boldsymbol{\alpha}_*^T \mathbf{Z}_{3i}) \right\} = 0, \qquad (6.5)$$

respectively. In the estimating equation above, the w_i's are some weights that could depend on $\mathbf{Z}_i$, C_i and Λ_{0h}.

A key fact used in deriving the estimating equation above is that conditional on $(\mathbf{Z}_i, C_i, u_i, m_i)$, the observation times $\{T_{i,1} = t_{i,1}, \ldots, T_{i,m_i} = t_{i,m_i}\}$ can be seen as the order statistics of a simple random sample of size m_i from the density function

$$\frac{\lambda_{0h}(t) \, \exp(\boldsymbol{\alpha}_1^T \mathbf{Z}_i + u_i)}{\Lambda_{0h}(C_i) \, \exp(\boldsymbol{\alpha}_1^T \mathbf{Z}_i + u_i)} I(0 \le t \le C_i) = \frac{\lambda_{0h}(t)}{\Lambda_{0h}(C_i)} I(0 \le t \le C_i).$$

Let $\hat{\boldsymbol{\alpha}}_* = (\hat{\boldsymbol{\alpha}}_1^T, \hat{\boldsymbol{\alpha}}_2)^T$ denote the estimator of $\boldsymbol{\alpha}_*$ given by Eq. (6.5). Given $\hat{\Lambda}_{0h}(t)$ and $\hat{\boldsymbol{\alpha}}_*$ and for the estimation of the unobserved u_i based on the observed data, note that conditional on $(\mathbf{Z}_i, C_i, u_i)$, the expected value of m_i is equal to $\Lambda_{0h}(C_i) \exp(\boldsymbol{\alpha}_1^T \mathbf{Z}_i + u_i)$. Thus it is natural to estimate u_i by

$$\hat{u}_i = \log \left\{ \frac{m_i}{\hat{\Lambda}_{0h}(C_i) \, \exp(\hat{\boldsymbol{\alpha}}_1^T \mathbf{Z}_i)} \right\}. \qquad (6.6)$$

6.2.2.2 Step 2: Estimation of the Parameters in Model (6.4)

Now we discuss the estimation of model (6.4). For this, let $O_i = (C_i, \delta_i, \mathbf{Z}_i, u_i)$, the observed data related to model (6.4) on subject i assuming that u_i is known, and $O = (O_1, \ldots, O_n)$. Also let $c_1 < \cdots < c_r$ denote the ordered observed C_i^*'s and assume that we can write $\Lambda_{0c}(t) = \int_0^t \lambda_{0c}(s) \, ds$ as

$$\Lambda_{0c}(t) = \sum_{j=1}^{r} a_j \, I(t \ge c_j),$$

where $\boldsymbol{a} = (a_1, \ldots, a_r)^T$ is a vector of unknown parameters. Define $\boldsymbol{\theta} = (\boldsymbol{a}^T, \boldsymbol{\gamma}^T, \sigma^2)^T$. Then the full likelihood function based on the pseudo complete data O and the v_i's has the form

$$L(\boldsymbol{\theta}) = \prod_{i=1}^{n} \left\{ \lambda_{0c}(C_i) e^{\boldsymbol{\gamma}^T \mathbf{Z}_{1i} + v_i} \right\}^{\delta_i} \exp \left\{ -\Lambda_{0c}(C_i) e^{\boldsymbol{\gamma}^T \mathbf{Z}_{1i} + v_i} \right\} \phi(v_i; \sigma),$$

where $\phi(\cdot; \sigma)$ denotes the density function of $N(0, \sigma^2)$.

To estimate $\boldsymbol{\theta}$, it is natural to maximize $L(\boldsymbol{\theta})$ with replacing the u_i's by their predicted values given by (6.6). Also it is natural to employ the EM algorithm since the maximization of $L(\boldsymbol{\theta})$ has no closed form. To implement the EM algorithm, we first consider the E-step, which computes the conditional expectation of the log likelihood function $l(\boldsymbol{\theta}) = \log L(\boldsymbol{\theta})$ given the current estimator of $\boldsymbol{\theta}$ and the observed data O. To this end, note that $l(\boldsymbol{\theta})$ can be written as

$$l(\boldsymbol{\theta}) = \sum_{i=1}^{n} \left[\delta_i \left\{ \log\{\lambda_{0c}(C_i)\} + \boldsymbol{\gamma}^T \boldsymbol{Z}_{1i} + v_i \right\} - \Lambda_{0c}(C_i) e^{\boldsymbol{\gamma}^T \boldsymbol{Z}_{1i} + v_i} + \log \phi(v_i; \sigma) \right]$$

$$= \sum_{i=1}^{n} \delta_i \left[\log\{\lambda_{0c}(C_i)\} + \boldsymbol{\gamma}^T \boldsymbol{Z}_{1i} \right] + \sum_{i=1}^{n} g(v_i; \boldsymbol{\theta}),$$

where

$$g(v_i; \boldsymbol{\theta}) = \delta_i v_i - \Lambda_{0c}(C_i) \exp\left\{\boldsymbol{\gamma}^T \boldsymbol{Z}_{1i} + v_i\right\} + \log \phi(v_i; \sigma).$$

To calculate $E\{l(\boldsymbol{\theta})|O, \boldsymbol{\theta}^{(k)}\}$ given the current estimator $\boldsymbol{\theta}^{(k)}$ of $\boldsymbol{\theta}$, one needs to calculate

$$E_i\left\{g(v_i; \boldsymbol{\theta})|O_i, \boldsymbol{\theta}^{(k)}\right\} = \int g(v_i; \boldsymbol{\theta}) f(v_i|O_i, \boldsymbol{\theta}^{(k)}) \, dv_i. \tag{6.7}$$

In the above,

$$f(v_i|O_i, \boldsymbol{\theta}) = \frac{\exp\{\delta_i v_i - \Lambda_{0c}(C_i) \exp(\boldsymbol{\gamma}^T \boldsymbol{Z}_{1i} + v_i)\} \phi(v_i; \sigma)}{\int \exp\{\delta_i v - \Lambda_{0c}(C_i) \exp(\boldsymbol{\gamma}^T \boldsymbol{Z}_{1i} + v)\} \phi(v; \sigma) \, dv}$$

is the conditional density of v_i given O_i and $\boldsymbol{\theta}$. It is apparent that the integration (6.7) has no closed form. For this, let $\{v_i^{(l)}; i = 1, \ldots, n, l = 1, \ldots, L\}$ be L independent and identically distributed samples from $N(0, \{\sigma^{(k)}\}^2)$ for sufficiently large L. Then one can approximate the integration (6.7) by

$$\hat{E}_i\left\{g(v_i; \boldsymbol{\theta})|O_i, \boldsymbol{\theta}^{(k)}\right\} = \frac{\sum_{l=1}^{L} b_l \, g(v_i^{(l)}; \boldsymbol{\theta})}{\sum_{l=1}^{L} b_l}, \tag{6.8}$$

where

$$b_l = \exp\left\{\delta_i v_i^{(l)} - \Lambda_{0c}^{(k)}(C_i) \exp(\boldsymbol{\gamma}^{(k)T} \boldsymbol{Z}_{1i} + v_i^{(l)})\right\}.$$

For the M-step of the EM algorithm, one needs to maximize $E\{l(\boldsymbol{\theta})|O, \boldsymbol{\theta}^{(k)}\}$ with respect to $\boldsymbol{\theta}$. For this, by taking its derivatives with respect to $\boldsymbol{\theta}$ and setting the derivatives equal to zero, we can obtain

$$a_j^{(k+1)} = \left[\sum_{i=1}^{n} E_i \left\{ \exp(\boldsymbol{\gamma}^T \boldsymbol{Z}_{1i} + v_i) \, I(C_i \geq c_j) \right\} \right]^{-1} \tag{6.9}$$

for $j = 1, \ldots, r$, $\sigma^{(k+1)} = \{n^{-1} \sum_{i=1}^{n} E_i(v_i^2)\}^{1/2}$, and

6.2 Analysis by a Joint Modeling Procedure

$$\sum_{i=1}^{n} E_i \left[\boldsymbol{Z}_{1i} \left\{ \delta_i - \Lambda_{0c}(C_i) \exp(\boldsymbol{\gamma}^T \boldsymbol{Z}_{1i} + v_i) \right\} \right] = 0 \quad (6.10)$$

for the updated estimator $\boldsymbol{\theta}^{(k+1)}$ of $\boldsymbol{\theta}$. Note that E_i above and $\hat{E}_i$ below are defined in (6.7) and (6.8), respectively. For the implementation, one can first obtain the $a_j^{(k+1)}$'s from (6.9) by letting $\boldsymbol{\theta} = \boldsymbol{\theta}^{(k)}$ and thus $\Lambda_{0c}^{(k+1)}$. Then by replacing Λ_{0c} with $\Lambda_{0c}^{(k+1)}$, one can obtain the updated estimators $\{\sigma^{(k+1)}\}^2$ and $\boldsymbol{\gamma}^{(k+1)}$ by solving equation (6.10). Let $\hat{\boldsymbol{\theta}}$ denote the estimator of $\boldsymbol{\theta}$ at the convergence. As with the u_i's, one may also want to estimate the v_i's and a natural one is clearly given by the conditional expectation of v_i

$$\hat{v}_i = \hat{E}_i(v_i | O_i, \hat{\boldsymbol{\theta}}), \quad (6.11)$$

which can be approximated by (6.8) again.

6.2.2.3 Step 3: Estimation of the Parameters in Model (6.2)

Now we are ready to estimate the parameters in model (6.2). For this, as before, define $Y_i(t) = I(t \leq C_i)$ and

$$S_j(t; \boldsymbol{\beta}) = \frac{1}{n} \sum_{i=1}^{n} Y_i(t) \exp\left\{ (\boldsymbol{\beta} + \boldsymbol{\alpha})^T \boldsymbol{Z}_{2i} \right\} \boldsymbol{Z}_{2i}^{\otimes j},$$

for $j = 0, 1, 2$. Note that if all the u_i's and v_i's were known and fixed, the problem considered here would reduce to the one discussed in Chap. 5 and thus one could employ the estimation procedures discussed there. Based on this fact and by following the estimating function $U_{II}^M(\tilde{\boldsymbol{\beta}}, w)$ defined in Sect. 5.4, it is natural to consider the following estimating function

$$U_J(\boldsymbol{\beta}) = \frac{1}{\sqrt{n}} \sum_{i=1}^{n} \int_0^\tau \left\{ \hat{\boldsymbol{Z}}_{2i} - \frac{\hat{S}_1(t; \boldsymbol{\beta})}{\hat{S}_0(t; \boldsymbol{\beta})} \right\} N_i(t) d H_i(t). \quad (6.12)$$

In the above, $\hat{\boldsymbol{Z}}_{2i} = (\boldsymbol{Z}_i^T, \hat{u}_i, \hat{v}_i)^T$ with $\hat{u}_i$ and $\hat{v}_i$ given by (6.6) and (6.11), and $\hat{S}_j(t; \boldsymbol{\beta})$ denotes $S_j(t; \boldsymbol{\beta})$ with the $\boldsymbol{Z}_{2i}$'s and $\boldsymbol{\alpha}$ replaced by the $\hat{\boldsymbol{Z}}_{2i}$'s and $\hat{\boldsymbol{\alpha}} = (\hat{\boldsymbol{\alpha}}_1^T, 1, 0)^T$, respectively.

Define the estimator $\hat{\boldsymbol{\beta}}_J$ of $\boldsymbol{\beta}$ as the solution to $U_J(\boldsymbol{\beta}) = 0$. Then it is easy to show that $\hat{\boldsymbol{\beta}}_J$ exists and is unique by noting that

$$\frac{\partial U_J(\boldsymbol{\beta})}{\partial \boldsymbol{\beta}} = -\frac{1}{\sqrt{n}} \sum_{i=1}^{n} \int_0^\tau \frac{\hat{S}_2(t; \boldsymbol{\beta}) \hat{S}_0(t; \boldsymbol{\beta}) - \hat{S}_1(t; \boldsymbol{\beta}) \hat{S}_1^T(t; \boldsymbol{\beta})}{\hat{S}_0^2(t; \boldsymbol{\beta})} N_i(t) \, dH_i(t)$$

is strictly negative. For inference, He et al. (2009) suggest that one can approximate the distribution of $\sqrt{n}\,(\hat{\boldsymbol{\beta}}_J - \boldsymbol{\beta}_0)$ by the multivariate normal distribution with mean zero, where $\boldsymbol{\beta}_0$ denotes the true value of $\boldsymbol{\beta}$ as before. Note that it is possible to derive a consistent estimator of the covariance matrix of $\hat{\boldsymbol{\beta}}_J$, but the estimator could be too complicated to be useful. Corresponding to this, He et al. (2009) suggest to apply the simple bootstrap procedure. Specifically, let B be a given integer and $\hat{\boldsymbol{\beta}}_J^{(1)}, \ldots, \hat{\boldsymbol{\beta}}_J^{(B)}$ denote the proposed estimators of $\boldsymbol{\beta}$ based on B bootstrap samples of sizes n drawn with replacement from the observed data. Then one can estimate the covariance matrix of $\hat{\boldsymbol{\beta}}_J$ by

$$\hat{\Sigma}_J = \frac{1}{B-1} \sum_{b=1}^{B} \left\{ \hat{\boldsymbol{\beta}}_J^{(b)} - \frac{1}{B} \sum_{b=1}^{B} \hat{\boldsymbol{\beta}}_J^{(b)} \right\}^{\otimes 2}.$$

To implement the estimation procedure above, one needs to choose constants L and B. In general, for a practical problem, one may start with some reasonable large values and then increase them until the resulting estimators are stable. For example, it is common to choose $L = 200$ and $B = 100$. On the other hand, to save computational effort in simulation studies, small values may be used as long as there is a large number of replications.

6.2.3 Discussion

A main feature of the approach described above is that it allows both observation process and follow-up process to be related with the underlying recurrent event process of interest. In the case where the follow-up process is independent of the other two processes given covariates, two approaches similar to the one given above have been proposed. In Huang et al. (2006), they assume that $N_i(t)$ is a non-homogeneous Poisson process whose intensity function has the form

$$u_i^* \, \lambda_0(t) \, \exp(\boldsymbol{\beta}^T \boldsymbol{Z}_i)$$

given $\boldsymbol{Z}_i$ and a nonnegative latent variable u_i^*. Furthermore, they assume that $N_i(t)$ and $\tilde{H}_i(t)$ are related only through $\boldsymbol{Z}_i$ and u_i^* but the dependence of the observation process on u_i^* is arbitrary. It is apparent that the model above and model (6.3) are equivalent.

The other similar approach is given by Sun et al. (2007b), who suggest to use the model

$$E\{N_i(t)|\boldsymbol{Z}_i, u_i^*\} = u_i^{*\phi} \, \mu_0(t) \, \exp(\boldsymbol{\beta}^T \boldsymbol{Z}_i) \qquad (6.13)$$

for the conditional mean of $N_i(t)$ instead of model (6.2). In the above, again u_i^* is a nonnegative latent variable and ϕ is an unknown scale parameter.

6.3 Analysis by a Robust Estimation Procedure

For the observation process, they assume that $\tilde{H}_i(t)$ is a non-homogeneous Poisson process with the intensity function

$$u_i^* \, \lambda_0(t) \, \exp(\boldsymbol{\alpha}^T \boldsymbol{Z}_i)$$

given $\boldsymbol{Z}_i$ and u_i^*. It is easy to see that the above two models can be actually seen as special cases of models (6.2) and (6.3), respectively.

Several remarks are needed for the approach described in this section. For parameter estimation, sometimes it may be reasonable to assume that $N_i(t)$ is also a non-homogeneous Poisson process as $\tilde{H}_i(t)$. In this case, instead of the three-step procedure given above, one could develop a full likelihood approach such as those discussed in Sect. 5.2 or a conditional likelihood approach like the one given in Huang et al. (2006). Furthermore, the EM algorithm and the approach given in Louis (1982) can be used for the determination of parameter estimators and variance estimation, respectively. Of course, this approach can be very computationally intensive. So far in this section, it has been assumed that covariates are time-independent. For the case with time-dependent covariates, one can still use model (6.2) and the estimating function given in (6.12) but may need different estimation procedures with respect to models (6.3) and (6.4).

With respect to the estimating function $U_J(\boldsymbol{\beta})$ given in (6.12), as with the estimating function given in (6.5), one could also add some weights in the front of the integration. However, as with (6.5), it may be difficult to establish some procedures for choosing appropriate or optimal weights. Lastly we remark that it is not hard to see that sometimes the assumptions and models described above may not be valid and also it may be difficult or impossible to verify or assess them. To address this, one way is to conduct some sensitivity analysis against possible assumption violation or model misspecification. Another, also more general, approach is to develop some robust estimation procedures as discussed in the next section.

6.3 Analysis by a Robust Estimation Procedure

For the regression procedure described in the previous section, a couple of the assumptions used there could be questionable in practice. One is the format of the latent variables in model (6.2) or (6.13) or the way by which the latent variables affect the recurrent event process of interest. The other is the Poisson process assumption on the observation processes $\tilde{H}_i(t)$'s. To address these, in this section, we first introduce some new models that include the models considered in the previous section as special cases. A robust estimation procedure is then presented along with a model checking procedure. The methodology is illustrated along with the method given in the previous section by the bladder tumor data discussed in Sect. 1.2.3.

6.3.1 Assumptions and Models

Consider a recurrent event study that consists of n independent subjects and gives panel count data as in the previous section. Also let the $N_i(t)$'s, $\tilde{H}_i(t)$'s, $H_i(t)$'s, $\boldsymbol{Z}_i$'s and $t_{i,j}$'s be defined and assume that $\{N_i(t), H_i(t), C_i, \boldsymbol{Z}_i, 0 \leq t \leq \tau\}_{i=1}^n$ are independent and identically distributed as in the previous section. In this section, for the simplicity, we assume that the follow-up time C_i is independent of $\{N_i(t), \tilde{H}_i(t), \boldsymbol{Z}_i\}$.

To describe the effect of covariates $\boldsymbol{Z}_i$ on the recurrent event process of interest $N_i(t)$, we assume that there exists a positive latent variable u_i and given $\boldsymbol{Z}_i$ and u_i, the mean function of $N_i(t)$ has the form

$$E\{N_i(t)|\boldsymbol{Z}_i, u_i\} = \mu_0(t) g(u_i) \exp(\boldsymbol{\beta}^T \boldsymbol{Z}_i). \qquad (6.14)$$

Here $\mu_0(t)$ and $\boldsymbol{\beta}$ are defined as in model (1.4) or (6.13) and g is a positive, completely unspecified link function. For the observation process, it is assumed that $\tilde{H}_i(t)$ satisfies the following proportional rate model

$$E\{d\tilde{H}_i(t)|\boldsymbol{Z}_i, u_i\} = u_i h(\boldsymbol{Z}_i) d\tilde{\mu}_0(t). \qquad (6.15)$$

In the above, as g in model (6.14), h is a positive, completely unspecified function and $\tilde{\mu}_0(t)$ is also a completely unspecified continuous function as in model (5.4).

It is easy to see that model (6.14) includes both models (6.2) and (6.13) as special cases and model (6.15) can be seen as a generalization of model (5.4) or (5.12). Also the assumption on $\tilde{H}_i(t)$ above is much less restrictive than that used in Sect. 6.2. Model (6.14) allows the latent variable u_i to affect the mean function of $N_i(t)$ in an arbitrary way. It is apparent that one can equivalently express model (6.15) in the same format as model (6.14) with respect to u_i because it is unobservable and can follow an arbitrary distribution. In the following, we assume that $N_i(t)$ and $\tilde{H}_i(t)$ are independent given $\boldsymbol{Z}_i$ and u_i and discuss a robust estimation procedure for the regression parameter $\boldsymbol{\beta}$ in model (6.14). Also a goodness-of-fit procedure is described for checking the adequacy of models (6.14) and (6.15).

6.3.2 Inference Procedure

Now we consider estimation of regression parameter $\boldsymbol{\beta}$ in model (6.14) and for this, we discuss an approach similar to those given in Sects. 5.3 and 5.4. Specifically, let $\tilde{N}_i(t)$ denote the process defined in Sect. 5.4, $i = 1, \ldots, n$. Then under models (6.14) and (6.15), we have

$$E\left\{\tilde{N}_i(\tau)|\boldsymbol{Z}_i\right\} = \exp(\boldsymbol{\beta}^T \boldsymbol{Z}_i) h(\boldsymbol{Z}_i) E\{u_i g(u_i)\} \int_0^\tau P(C_i \geq t) \mu_0(t) d\tilde{\mu}_0(t)$$

6.3 Analysis by a Robust Estimation Procedure

and
$$E(m_i|\mathbf{Z}_i) = E(u_i)\,E\{\tilde{\mu}_0(C_i)\}\,h(\mathbf{Z}_i).$$

These yield
$$E\left\{\tilde{N}_i(\tau)\,|\mathbf{Z}_i\right\} = E(m_i|\mathbf{Z}_i)\exp\left(\boldsymbol{\beta}^T\mathbf{Z}_i + \theta\right), \qquad (6.16)$$

where
$$\theta = \log\left[\frac{E\{u_i g(u_i)\}}{E(u_i)E\{\tilde{\mu}_0(C_i)\}}\int_0^\tau P(C_i \geq t)\,\mu_0(t)\,d\tilde{\mu}_0(t)\right],$$

an unknown parameter.

Define $\boldsymbol{\beta}_1 = (\boldsymbol{\beta}^T, \theta)^T$ and $\mathbf{Z}_{1i} = (\mathbf{Z}_i^T, 1)^T$. For estimation of regression parameter $\boldsymbol{\beta}$ or $\boldsymbol{\beta}_1$, motivated by Eq. (6.16) and the approaches discussed in Sects. 5.3 and 5.4, we can use the following estimating equation

$$U_R(\boldsymbol{\beta}_1) = \sum_{i=1}^n w_i\,\mathbf{Z}_{1i}\left\{\tilde{N}_i(\tau) - m_i\exp\left(\boldsymbol{\beta}_1^T\mathbf{Z}_{1i}\right)\right\} = 0. \qquad (6.17)$$

In the above, the w_i's are some weights that could depend on $\mathbf{Z}_i$ as before. Let $\hat{\boldsymbol{\beta}}_{1R} = (\hat{\boldsymbol{\beta}}_R^T, \hat{\theta}_R)^T$ denote the estimator of $\boldsymbol{\beta}_1$ given by the solution to the equation above and $\boldsymbol{\beta}_{10} = (\boldsymbol{\beta}_0^T, \theta_0)^T$ the true value of $\boldsymbol{\beta}_1$. Zhao et al. (2013) show that under some regularity conditions, $\hat{\boldsymbol{\beta}}_{1R}$ is consistent and $\sqrt{n}(\hat{\boldsymbol{\beta}}_{1R} - \boldsymbol{\beta}_{10})$ asymptotically follows a multivariate normal distribution with mean zero and the covariance matrix that can be consistently estimated by $\hat{\Sigma}_R = A_R^{-1} B_R A_R^{-1}$. Here

$$A_R = \frac{1}{n}\sum_{i=1}^n\left\{w_i\,m_i\,\mathbf{Z}_{1i}\mathbf{Z}_{1i}^T\exp\left(\hat{\boldsymbol{\beta}}_1^T\mathbf{Z}_{1i}\right)\right\}$$

and $B_R = n^{-1}\sum_{i=1}^n \hat{\phi}_i\,\hat{\phi}_i'$, where

$$\hat{\phi}_i = w_i\,\mathbf{Z}_{1i}\left\{\tilde{N}_i(\tau) - m_i\exp\left(\hat{\boldsymbol{\beta}}_1^T\mathbf{Z}_{1i}\right)\right\}.$$

As discussed above, sometimes one may question the appropriateness of postulated regression models in practice. To assess the adequacy of models (6.14) and (6.15) for a given set of panel count data, we now present a goodness-of-fit test procedure similar to the one given in Sect. 5.5.4. Define

$$\mathcal{A}(t) = \frac{E\{u_i\,g(u_i)\}}{E(u_i)\,E\{\tilde{\mu}_0(C_i)\}}\int_0^t P(C_i \geq u)\,\mu_0(u)\,d\tilde{\mu}_0(u).$$

Then under models (6.14) and (6.15), we have

$$E\left\{\tilde{N}_i(t)|\mathbf{Z}_i\right\} = E(m_i|\mathbf{Z}_i)\exp\left(\boldsymbol{\beta}^T\mathbf{Z}_i\right)\mathcal{A}(t).$$

It follows that a natural estimator of $\mathcal{A}(t)$ is given by

$$\hat{\mathcal{A}}(t) = \sum_{i=1}^{n}\int_0^t \frac{N_i(u)\,dH_i(u)}{\sum_{i=1}^{n} m_i \exp(\hat{\boldsymbol{\beta}}_R^T\mathbf{Z}_i)}$$

and one can define the residual process as

$$\hat{R}_i(t) = \int_0^t N_i(u)\,dH_i(u) - m_i\exp\left(\hat{\boldsymbol{\beta}}_R^T\mathbf{Z}_i\right)\hat{\mathcal{A}}(t).$$

For the assessment of models (6.14) and (6.15), as the statistic $\mathcal{F}(t,\mathbf{z})$ given in (5.22), it is natural to define a goodness-of-fit test statistic as

$$\Phi(t,\mathbf{z}) = n^{-1/2}\sum_{i=1}^{n} I(\mathbf{Z}_i \leq \mathbf{z})\hat{R}_i(t).$$

In the above, as before, the event $I(\mathbf{Z}_i \leq \mathbf{z})$ means that each of the components of $\mathbf{Z}_i$ is not larger than the corresponding component of $\mathbf{z}$. It is easy to see that $\Phi(t,\mathbf{z})$ is the cumulative sum of $\hat{R}_i(t)$ over the values of the $\mathbf{Z}_i$'s. To describe the asymptotic behavior of $\Phi(t,\mathbf{z})$, define

$$S_0 = \frac{1}{n}\sum_{i=1}^{n} m_i \exp\left(\hat{\boldsymbol{\beta}}_R^T\mathbf{Z}_i\right),$$

$$S(\mathbf{z}) = \frac{1}{n}\sum_{i=1}^{n} I(\mathbf{Z}_i \leq \mathbf{z})m_i \exp\left(\hat{\boldsymbol{\beta}}_R^T\mathbf{Z}_i\right),$$

and

$$B(t,\mathbf{z}) = \frac{1}{n}\sum_{i=1}^{n}\left\{I(\mathbf{Z}_i \leq \mathbf{z}) - \frac{S(\mathbf{z})}{S_0}\right\}m_i\,\mathbf{Z}_i^T \exp\left(\hat{\boldsymbol{\beta}}_R^T\mathbf{Z}_i\right)\hat{\mathcal{A}}(t).$$

Zhao et al. (2013) show that the null distribution of $\Phi(t,\mathbf{z})$ can be approximated by the zero-mean Gaussian process

$$\hat{\Phi}(t,\mathbf{z}) = \frac{1}{\sqrt{n}}\sum_{i=1}^{n}\left\{I(\mathbf{Z}_i \leq \mathbf{z}) - \frac{S(\mathbf{z})}{S_0}\right\}\hat{R}_i(t)G_i - B^T(t,\mathbf{z})\frac{1}{\sqrt{n}}\sum_{i=1}^{n}\hat{d}_iG_i.$$

In the above, $\hat{d}_i$ is the vector $A_R^{-1}\hat{\phi}_i$ without the last entry and $(G_1,\ldots,G_n)$ are a simple random sample from the standard normal distribution independent of the data.

The results above suggest that for the distribution of $\Phi(t,\mathbf{z})$, we can first obtain a large number of realizations of $\hat{\Phi}(t,\mathbf{z})$ by repeatedly generating the

6.3 Analysis by a Robust Estimation Procedure 133

standard normal random sample $(G_1, \ldots, G_n)$ given the observed data. Then it can be approximated by the empirical distribution of the realizations. For the assessment of the overall fit of models (6.14) and (6.15) based on $\varPhi(t, z)$, one can obtain the p-value by comparing the observed value of $\sup_{t,z} |\varPhi(t, z)|$ to the corresponding realizations of $\sup_{t,z} |\hat{\varPhi}(t, z)|$.

6.3.3 Analysis of Bladder Cancer Study

In this subsection, we illustrate the two estimation procedures described in the previous and this sections using the bladder tumor data discussed in Sects. 1.2.3, 2.4.3 and 4.5.2 and given in the data set II of Chap. 9. For the data set, as mentioned before, the observed information includes discrete clinical visit or observation times and the numbers of bladder tumors that occurred between the observation times. Also it involves two treatment groups, placebo group (47 patients) and thiotepa treatment group (38 patients), and two covariates, the number of initial bladder tumors and the size of the largest initial bladder tumor. The main goal here is to determine the treatment effect on the tumor recurrence as well as the covariate effects.

Before the formal analysis, some preliminary analysis of the data is needed to investigate the relationship between the underlying tumor recurrence process and the observation process. For the patients in the placebo and treatment groups, the average numbers of bladder tumor recurrences are 39.81 and 17.03, while the average numbers of clinical visits or observations are 8.66 and 13.50, respectively. They suggest that the patients in the placebo group seem to have smaller numbers of observations but larger numbers of tumor recurrences than those in the treatment group. Note that the difference between the observation processes in the two groups was also discussed in Sect. 4.5.1 and shown in Fig. 4.1. To further see the relationship between the tumor recurrence process and the observation process, we divide the patients into two groups, the rare visit group with at most nine visits and the frequent visit group with more than nine visits. Figure 6.1 displays the separate IRE of the cumulative mean functions of the tumor recurrence processes for the two groups. Plot (a) is for all patients, while the other is for the patients in the placebo group only. They suggest that the patients in the frequent visit group seem to have a higher tumor recurrence rate than those in the rare visit group. That is, the underlying tumor recurrence process and the observation process seem to be positively correlated.

Now we apply the two estimation procedures discussed above to the data. For this, define $\boldsymbol{Z}_i = (Z_{i1}, Z_{i2}, Z_{i3})^T$ with $Z_{i1} = 1$ if subject i is in the thiotepa treatment group and 0 otherwise and Z_{i2} and Z_{i3} denoting the number of initial tumors and the size of the largest initial tumor of the ith patient, respectively, $i = 1, \ldots, 85$. First assume that the recurrence process of the bladder tumors, the clinical visit process and the follow-up process can be described by models (6.2)–(6.4), respectively. The application of

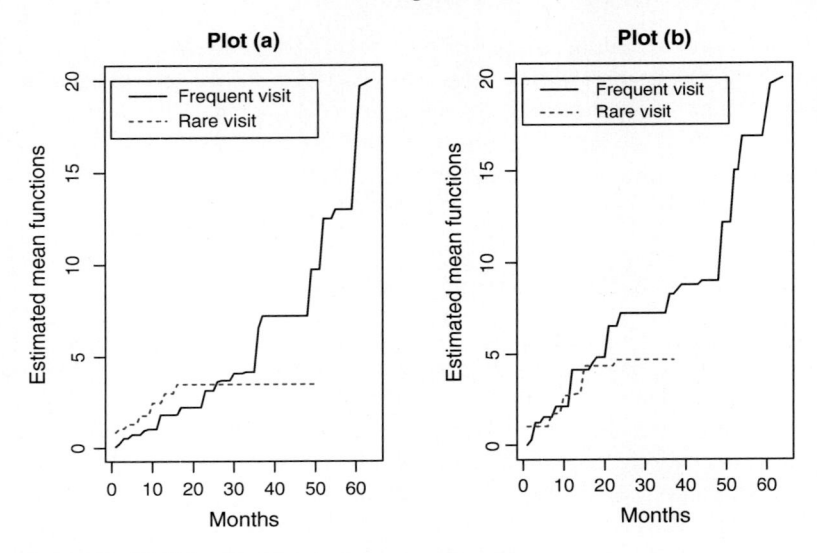

Fig. 6.1. The IRE for bladder tumor recurrence processes

the estimation procedure given in the previous section with $L = 200$ and $B = 100$ yields $\hat{\boldsymbol{\beta}}_J = (-1.8483, 0.1996, 0.0015)^T$ with the estimated standard errors of $(0.6879, 0.3181, 0.3562)^T$. The use of large values for both L and B gives similar results. By assuming that the tumor process and the observation process follow models (6.14) and (6.15), one can obtain $\hat{\boldsymbol{\beta}}_R = (-1.3862, 0.3282, 0.0000)^T$ with the estimated standard errors of $(0.3282, 0.0668, 0.0956)^T$.

The results above all suggest that the thiotepa treatment significantly reduced the recurrence rate of the bladder tumors. Also the recurrence rate did not seem to be significantly related with the size of the largest initial tumor. With respect to the number of initial tumors, the estimator $\hat{\boldsymbol{\beta}}_J$ suggests that it did not have significant effect on the tumor recurrence rate, but the estimator $\hat{\boldsymbol{\beta}}_R$ tells a different story. For comparison, the application of the estimation approach discussed in Sect. 5.3 gives $\hat{\boldsymbol{\beta}}_I = (-2.0249, 0.6620, -0.1229)^T$ with the estimated standard errors of $(0.4500, 0.2133, 0.2035)^T$. One can see that although the results from all three methods are similar, the approach that does not take into account the correlation between the recurrence and observation processes overestimates the treatment effect. One possible reason for this is that the part of the estimated effects given by the latter may be due to the correlation of the two processes.

Note that the approach discussed in the previous section requires the Poisson process assumption for the observation process. To assess this, Fig. 6.2 gives the residual plot obtained after fitting the data on the observation process to model (6.3). Also the use of a simple Kolomogorov-Smirnov test statistic procedure (Gibbons and Chakraborti, 2011) gives the p-value of

6.3 Analysis by a Robust Estimation Procedure

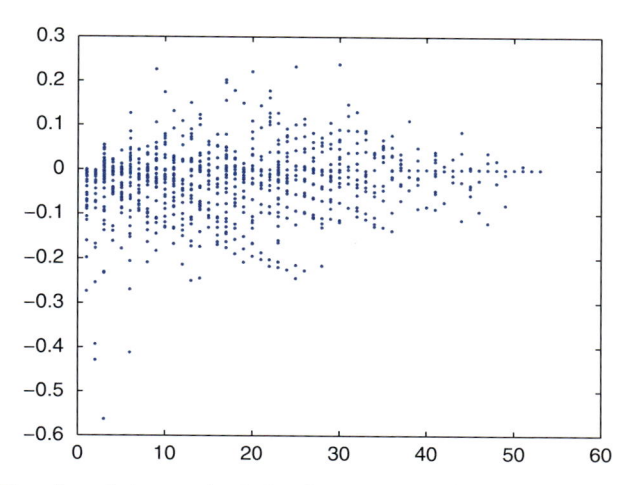

Fig. 6.2. The plot of the residuals for fitting model (6.3) to bladder tumor data

0.07 for testing the Poisson process assumption. Both the figure and the test suggest that the Poisson process assumption with model (6.3) may be questionable although not significant. For the appropriateness of models (6.14) and (6.15), one can apply the goodness-of-fit test procedure in the previous subsection, which gives the p-value of 0.768. This suggests that these models seem to be appropriate for the bladder cancer data considered here.

6.3.4 Discussion

Compared to the approaches discussed in the previous section, a key advantage of the inference procedure described in this section is that it allows the correlation between the recurrent event process of interest and the observation process in a much more general format. In other words, the latter is robust. This could be very important in practice since the format of the relationship between the two processes is generally unknown and could be very complicated. Thus some flexible models and robust procedures may be more appropriate or preferred unless there exists some prior information. Another advantage of the approach described in this section is that it does not require the Poisson assumption, which can be questionable in reality as discussed in the previous subsection. Also it is apparent that the new methodology is much easier in its implementation.

For the preceding discussion, we have assumed that the follow-up time C_i is independent of $\{N_i(t), \tilde{H}_i(t), Z_i\}$. Of course this may not be true and in this case, models such as the one given in (6.4) can be used to model the relationship between them and an estimation procedure similar to that given above can be easily developed. Another generalization of the approach given above is to replace models (6.14) and (6.15) by

$$E\{\, N_i(t)|\bm{Z}_i, u_i \,\} \;=\; \mu_0(t)\, g_1(u_{1i}) \exp(\bm{\beta}^T \bm{Z}_i)$$

and

$$E\{\, d\tilde{H}_i(t)|\bm{Z}_i, u_i \,\} \;=\; g_2(u_{2i})\, h(\bm{Z}_i)\, d\tilde{\mu}_0(t)\,,$$

respectively. In the above, as g in model (6.14), g_1 and g_2 are positive, completely unspecified link functions and u_{1i} and u_{2i} are two correlated latent variables. For estimation of the regression parameter $\bm{\beta}$ in the model above, an estimating function similar to $U_R(\bm{\beta}_1)$ given in (6.17) can be derived.

As one can easily see and also pointed out above, the methods discussed in both the previous and this sections are joint modeling procedures. In some situations, conditional modeling approaches may be preferred depending on the problems of interest. In the next section, we generalize the conditional method discussed in Sect. 5.5 to the situation where the recurrent event process of interest and the observation process are correlated.

6.4 Analysis with Semiparametric Transformation Models

In this section, we introduce some generalizations of the models and estimation procedure discussed in Sect. 5.5 for the situation with dependent observation processes. As in the previous section, we begin with describing the assumptions and models used in this section. An estimation procedure, a simple generalization of the one discussed in Sect. 5.5, is then presented. Both the assumed models and the inference procedure reduce to those given in Sect. 5.5 if the recurrent event process of interest and the observation process are independent conditional on covariates. The approach is illustrated again by the panel count data arising from the bladder tumor study, which is followed by some discussion on the comparison of the inference procedures discussed in the previous sections and this section.

6.4.1 Assumptions and Models

Consider a recurrent event study that consists of n independent subjects and gives panel count data as in the previous section. Also we employ the same notation and suppose that $\{\, N_i(t), H_i(t), C_i, \bm{Z}_i(t); 0 \le t \le \tau \,\}_{i=1}^n$ are independent and identically distributed as in the previous section. Note that here we assume that the covariates $\bm{Z}_i(t)$'s may be time-dependent as in Sect. 5.5. Furthermore, as in Sect. 5.5, we assume that the observation process $\tilde{H}_i(t)$ is a non-homogeneous Poisson process satisfying the proportional rate model (5.16).

6.4 Analysis with Semiparametric Transformation Models

To describe the relationship between the recurrent event process of interest $N_i(t)$ and the observation process $\tilde{H}_i(t)$ as well as the covariate process $\mathbf{Z}_i(t)$, for subject i, define $\mathcal{F}_{it} = \{\tilde{H}_i(s); 0 \le s < t\}$, the history or filtration of the observation process up to time $t-$, $i = 1, \ldots, n$. In the following, we assume that given $\mathbf{Z}_i(t)$ and $\mathcal{F}_{it}$, the conditional mean function of $N_i(t)$ is specified by the following semiparametric transformation model

$$E\{N_i(t)|\mathbf{Z}_i(t), \mathcal{F}_{it}\} = g\left\{\mu_0(t)\exp\left(\boldsymbol{\beta}^T\mathbf{Z}_i(t) + \boldsymbol{\alpha}^T\mathbf{Q}(\mathcal{F}_{it})\right)\right\}. \quad (6.18)$$

Here $g(t)$, $\mu_0(t)$ and $\boldsymbol{\beta}$ are defined as in model (5.15), $\boldsymbol{\alpha}$ is a vector of unknown regression parameters, and $\mathbf{Q}$ is a vector of known functions of $\mathcal{F}_{it}$. Model (6.18) supposes that the observation process $\tilde{H}_i(t)$ may be informative about or affect the underlying recurrent event process $N_i(t)$ through its mean process, and $N_i(t)$ depends on $\mathcal{F}_{it}$ through $\boldsymbol{\alpha}$. If $\boldsymbol{\alpha} = 0$, model (6.18) reduces to model (5.15). Also in the following, it is assumed that given $\mathbf{Z}_i(t)$, C_i is independent of both $N_i(t)$ and $\tilde{H}_i(t)$ and given $\mathbf{Z}_i(t)$ and $\mathcal{F}_{it}$, $N_i(t)$ and $\tilde{H}_i(t)$ are independent.

The semiparametric transformation model (6.18) is motivated by the models used in Lin et al. (2001) and Sun et al. (2005). The former considers a similar model for point processes with an independent observation process, while the latter discusses the situation where $N_i(t)$ is a general longitudinal process whose mean function is given by

$$E\{N_i(t)|\mathbf{Z}_i(t), \mathcal{F}_{it}\} = \mu_0(t) + \boldsymbol{\beta}^T\mathbf{Z}_i(t) + \boldsymbol{\alpha}^T\mathbf{Q}(\mathcal{F}_{it}).$$

As with model (5.15), model (6.18) allows various types of dependence of the mean function of $N_i(t)$ on $\mathbf{Z}_i(t)$ and $\tilde{H}_i(t)$. By taking g to be the commonly referred Box-Cox transformation, one obtains

$$E\{N_i(t)|\mathbf{Z}_i(t), \mathcal{F}_{it}\} = \frac{[\mu_0(t)\exp\{\boldsymbol{\beta}^T\mathbf{Z}_i(t) + \boldsymbol{\alpha}^T\mathbf{Q}(\mathcal{F}_{it})\} + 1]^\rho - 1}{\rho}$$

for $\rho > 0$ and

$$E\{N_i(t)|\mathbf{Z}_i(t), \mathcal{F}_{it}\} = \log\left\{\mu_0(t)\exp\left(\boldsymbol{\beta}^T\mathbf{Z}_i(t) + \boldsymbol{\alpha}^T\mathbf{Q}(\mathcal{F}_{it})\right) + 1\right\}$$

with $\rho = 0$ in the above.

With respect to the function vector $\mathbf{Q}$ in model (6.18), it can have different forms depending on the dependence of $N_i(t)$ on $\tilde{H}_i(t)$. For example, one may take $\mathbf{Q}(\mathcal{F}_{it}) = \tilde{H}_i(t-)$ if it is believed that $N_i(t)$ may depend on the total number of the observations before time t. This could be the case in a medical study in which patients may pay more visits to clinics or their doctors because they feel worse than usual either with or without treatments. A similar choice is to let $\mathbf{Q}(\mathcal{F}_{it}) = \tilde{H}_i(t-) - \tilde{H}_i(t-a)$, meaning that $N_i(t)$ may depend on the number of the observations over the period $[t-a, t)$, where a is a constant. That is, instead of the total number of observations, $N_i(t)$ may depend only on the number of observations over a certain time period right before the current time. Of course, $N_i(t)$ could depend on both $\tilde{H}_i(t-)$ and $\tilde{H}_i(t-) - \tilde{H}_i(t-a)$. More discussion on this is given below.

6.4.2 Inference Procedure

For estimation of regression parameters $\boldsymbol{\beta}$, $\boldsymbol{\alpha}$ and $\boldsymbol{\gamma}$ (in model (5.16)) as well as other parameters, it is straightforward to generalize the estimation procedure given in Sect. 5.5 to the current situation. Specifically, define

$$\boldsymbol{X}_i(t) = (\boldsymbol{Z}_i^T(t), \boldsymbol{Q}^T(\mathcal{F}_{it}))^T \,,\; \boldsymbol{\theta} = (\boldsymbol{\beta}^T, \boldsymbol{\alpha}^T)^T \,,$$

and

$$M_i^*(t;\boldsymbol{\theta},\boldsymbol{\gamma}) = \int_0^t Y_i(u)\, N_i(u)\, dH_i(u) - \int_0^t g\left\{\mu_0(u)\, e^{\boldsymbol{\beta}^T \boldsymbol{Z}_i(u) + \boldsymbol{\alpha}^T \boldsymbol{Q}(\mathcal{F}_{iu})}\right\} \\ \times Y_i(u)\, \exp\left\{\boldsymbol{\gamma}^T \boldsymbol{Z}_i(u)\right\}\, d\tilde{\mu}_0(u)\,. \tag{6.19}$$

In the above, $Y_i(t) = I(C_i \geq t)$ as before, $i = 1, \ldots, n$.

Note that the process $M_i^*(t;\boldsymbol{\theta},\boldsymbol{\gamma})$ is $M_i(t;\boldsymbol{\beta},\boldsymbol{\gamma})$ defined in (5.17) with $\boldsymbol{\beta}^T \boldsymbol{Z}_i(u)$ replaced by $\boldsymbol{\theta}^T \boldsymbol{X}_i(u)$. Under models (5.16) and (6.18), we have that

$$E\left\{Y_i(t) N_i(t) d\tilde{H}_i(t)\right\} = E\left[E\{Y_i(t) N_i(t) d\tilde{H}_i(t) | \boldsymbol{Z}_i(t), \mathcal{F}_{it}\}\right]$$
$$= E\left[E\{Y_i(t)|\boldsymbol{Z}_i(t)\}\, E\{N_i(t)|\boldsymbol{Z}_i(t), \mathcal{F}_{it}\}\, E\left\{d\tilde{H}_i(t)|\boldsymbol{Z}_i(t)\right\}\right]$$
$$= E\left\{E\left[Y_i(t)g\{\mu_0(t)e^{\boldsymbol{\beta}^T \boldsymbol{Z}_i(t) + \boldsymbol{\alpha}^T \boldsymbol{Q}(\mathcal{F}_{it})}\}e^{\boldsymbol{\gamma}^T \boldsymbol{Z}_i(t)} d\tilde{\mu}_0(t)|\boldsymbol{Z}_i(t), \mathcal{F}_{it}\right]\right\}$$
$$= E\left[Y_i(t)g\left\{\mu_0(t)\exp\{\boldsymbol{\beta}^T \boldsymbol{Z}_i(t) + \boldsymbol{\alpha}^T \boldsymbol{Q}(\mathcal{F}_{it})\}\right\} e^{\boldsymbol{\gamma}^T \boldsymbol{Z}_i(t)} d\tilde{\mu}_0(t)\right] \,.$$

$i = 1, \ldots, n$. So as the $M_i(t;\boldsymbol{\beta},\boldsymbol{\gamma})$'s, the $M_i^*(t;\boldsymbol{\theta},\boldsymbol{\gamma})$'s are also zero-mean stochastic processes and can be used to construct the needed estimating functions as before.

Let $\hat{\boldsymbol{\gamma}}_T$ and $\hat{\tilde{\mu}}_0(t;\hat{\boldsymbol{\gamma}}_T)$ denote the estimators of $\boldsymbol{\gamma}$ and $\tilde{\mu}_0(t)$ defined in Sect. 5.5 or given by Eqs. (5.20) and (5.21), respectively. Also let $U_T^*(\boldsymbol{\theta},\boldsymbol{\gamma})$ denote the estimating function $U_T(\boldsymbol{\beta},\boldsymbol{\gamma})$ given in (5.19) with replacing $\exp\{\boldsymbol{\beta}^T \boldsymbol{Z}_i(t)\}$ by $\exp\{\boldsymbol{\theta}^T \boldsymbol{X}_i(t)\}$ or $M_i(t;\boldsymbol{\beta},\boldsymbol{\gamma})$ by $M_i^*(t;\boldsymbol{\theta},\boldsymbol{\gamma})$, $i = 1, \ldots, n$. For estimation of $\boldsymbol{\beta}$ and $\boldsymbol{\alpha}$ or $\boldsymbol{\theta}$ along with $\mu_0(t)$, similarly as in Sect. 5.5, we can first estimate $\mu_0(t)$ by the solution to

$$\sum_{i=1}^n dM_i^*(t;\boldsymbol{\theta},\boldsymbol{\gamma}) = \sum_{i=1}^n \left[Y_i(t) N_i(t) dH_i(t)\right.$$
$$\left. - Y_i(t)\, g\left\{\mu_0(t)\exp\{\boldsymbol{\beta}^T \boldsymbol{Z}_i(t) + \boldsymbol{\alpha}^T \boldsymbol{Q}(\mathcal{F}_{it})\}\right\} \exp\left\{\hat{\boldsymbol{\gamma}}_T^T \boldsymbol{Z}_i(t)\right\} d\hat{\tilde{\mu}}_0(t;\hat{\boldsymbol{\gamma}}_T)\right] = 0\,.$$

6.4 Analysis with Semiparametric Transformation Models

Then $\boldsymbol{\theta}$ can be estimated by the solution, denoted by $\hat{\boldsymbol{\theta}}_{DT} = (\hat{\boldsymbol{\beta}}_{DT}^T, \hat{\boldsymbol{\alpha}}_{DT}^T)^T$, to the estimating equation $U_T^*(\boldsymbol{\theta}, \boldsymbol{\gamma}) = 0$ with all other unknowns replaced by their estimators. Li et al. (2010) show that as with $\hat{\boldsymbol{\beta}}_T$, $\hat{\boldsymbol{\theta}}_{DT}$ is consistent. Also for large n, one can approximate the distribution of $n^{1/2}(\hat{\boldsymbol{\theta}}_{DT} - \boldsymbol{\theta}_0)$ by the multivariate normal distribution with mean zero and the covariance matrix $\hat{\Sigma}_{DT} = A_{DT}^{-1} B_{DT} A_{DT}^{-1}$. Here $\boldsymbol{\theta}_0 = (\boldsymbol{\beta}_0^T, \boldsymbol{\alpha}_0^T)^T$ denotes the true value of $\boldsymbol{\theta}$, and A_{DT} and B_{DT} are A_T and B_T defined in Sect. 5.5.2 with $\exp\{\boldsymbol{\beta}^T \boldsymbol{Z}_i(t)\}$ replaced by $\exp\{\boldsymbol{\theta}^T \boldsymbol{X}_i(t)\}$, respectively.

As with the estimation procedure, it is also straightforward to generalize the goodness-of-fit test procedure discussed in Sect. 5.5.4 to the current situation. Specifically, one needs to replace $\boldsymbol{Z}_i(t)$, $\boldsymbol{\beta}^T \boldsymbol{Z}_i(t)$, $\hat{\boldsymbol{\beta}}_T^T \boldsymbol{Z}_i(t)$ and $\boldsymbol{z}$ by $\boldsymbol{X}_i(t)$, $\boldsymbol{\theta}^T \boldsymbol{X}_i(t)$, $\hat{\boldsymbol{\theta}}_{DT}^T \boldsymbol{X}_i(t)$ and $\boldsymbol{x}$, respectively, in all concerned quantities or processes, where $\boldsymbol{x}$ is a vector of the same dimension as $\boldsymbol{X}_i$. For example, corresponding to the cumulative sum of residuals process $\mathcal{F}(t, \boldsymbol{z})$ defined in (5.22), we now have

$$\mathcal{F}^*(t, \boldsymbol{x}) = \frac{1}{\sqrt{n}} \sum_{i=1}^n \int_0^t I\{\boldsymbol{X}_i(u) \leq \boldsymbol{x}\} d\hat{M}_i^{**}(u).$$

In the above, $\hat{M}_i^{**}(u)$ denotes $M_i^*(u; \boldsymbol{\theta}, \boldsymbol{\gamma})$ with all unknowns replaced by their estimators defined above. Let $\hat{\mathcal{F}}^*(t, \boldsymbol{x})$ denote the new process corresponding to $\hat{\mathcal{F}}(t, \boldsymbol{z})$ defined in Sect. 5.5.4. Then for testing the goodness-of-fit of model (6.18), we first obtain a large number of realizations of $\hat{\mathcal{F}}^*(t, \boldsymbol{x})$ by repeatedly generating the standard normal random sample while fixing the observation data. The p-value can then be determined by comparing the observed value of $\sup_{0 \leq t \leq \tau, \boldsymbol{x}} |\mathcal{F}^*(t, \boldsymbol{x})|$ to all the realizations of $\sup_{0 \leq t \leq \tau, \boldsymbol{x}} |\hat{\mathcal{F}}^*(t, \boldsymbol{x})|$.

6.4.3 An Illustration

To illustrate the methodology discussed above, we apply it to the bladder cancer panel count data analyzed in Sect. 6.3.3. As discussed before, the data include the clinical visit or observation times (in months) and the numbers of bladder tumors that occurred between clinical visits. There are 85 patients with bladder tumors, 47 in the placebo group and 38 in the thiotepa treatment group. For the patients in these two groups, the number of observations ranges from 1 to 38 and the number of new tumors found ranges from 0 to 9. Also the average numbers of observations and new tumors found are 8.66 and 0.70, respectively, for the patients in the placebo group, while the corresponding numbers for the patients in the thiotepa group are 13.50 and 0.23, respectively. Again as pointed out in Sect. 6.3.3, these numbers suggest that there seems to exist some correlation between the underlying tumor recurrence process and the observation process. In addition to the treatment,

Table 6.1. Estimated regression parameters with $Q(\mathcal{F}_{it}) = \tilde{H}_i(t-)$

Function $g(t)$	$\hat{\beta}_{DT,1}$ SE($\hat{\beta}_{DT,1}$) 95% CI for β_1	$\hat{\beta}_{DT,2}$ SE($\hat{\beta}_{DT,2}$) 95% CI for β_2	$\hat{\alpha}_{DT}$ SE($\hat{\alpha}_{DT}$) 95% CI for α
$g(t) = t$	-2.2165 0.4532 $(-3.1047, -1.3282)$	0.2563 0.0780 $(0.1034, 0.4092)$	0.1095 0.0225 $(0.0653, 0.1537)$
$g(t) = t^2$	-1.1082 0.2266 $(-1.5524, -0.6641)$	0.1281 0.0390 $(0.0517, 0.2046)$	0.0547 0.0113 $(0.0327, 0.0768)$
$g(t) = \log(t)$	-0.9579 0.1797 $(-1.3101, -0.6057)$	0.1832 0.0485 $(0.0882, 0.2781)$	0.0646 0.0284 $(0.0090, 0.1203)$

there exist two baseline covariates, the number of initial tumors and the size of the largest initial tumor. In the following, for the simplicity, we consider only the number of initial tumors since the other baseline covariate has been shown to have no effect on both the underlying tumor recurrence and the observation processes. We are interested in assessing the effects of thiotepa treatment (β_1) and the number of initial tumors (β_2) on the recurrence process of bladder tumors as well as the effect of the observation history (α) on the recurrence process.

For the analysis, define $\boldsymbol{Z}_i = (Z_{i1}, Z_{i2})^T$ with $Z_{i1} = 0$ for the patients in the placebo group and $Z_{i1} = 1$ otherwise and Z_{i2} denoting the number of initial tumors, $i = 1, \ldots, 85$. We assume that the visiting or observation process and the recurrence process of the bladder tumors follow models (5.16) and (6.18), respectively. Note that to apply the approach discussed above, we need to select the link functions g and $\boldsymbol{Q}(\mathcal{F}_{it})$ in model (6.18). For the former, we consider three choices: $g(t) = t$, $g(t) = t^2$ and $g(t) = \log(t)$. For the latter, two choices are considered and they are $Q(\mathcal{F}_{it}) = \tilde{H}_i(t-)$ and $Q(\mathcal{F}_{it}) = \tilde{H}_i(t-) - \tilde{H}_i(t-6)$. The former assumes that the recurrence rate of bladder tumors may depend on the total number of patient's visits, while the latter supposes that the recurrence rate may depend only on the number of patient's visits during the 6-month period before. The latter choice is motivated by the fact that sometimes it is the most recent visits that may carry information about the response variable. Also note that for the third choice of the function g above, we define $N_i(t)$ to be the natural logarithm of the cumulative number of the observed bladder tumors up to time t plus 1 to avoid 0. In contrast, for the other two choices, $N_i(t)$ is defined to be just the cumulative number of the observed bladder tumors up to time t.

Table 6.1 gives the results obtained on estimation of the three regression parameters β_1, β_2 and α for the case of $Q(\mathcal{F}_{it}) = \tilde{H}_i(t-)$, and the results based on $Q(\mathcal{F}_{it}) = \tilde{H}_i(t-) - \tilde{H}_i(t-6)$ are presented in Table 6.2. For both cases, we use $W(t) = 1$. The results include the point estimates $\hat{\boldsymbol{\beta}}_{DT}$ and $\hat{\alpha}_{DT}$, their estimated standard errors (SE) and the estimated 95% confidence intervals (CI). They all suggest that the thiotepa treatment significantly re-

6.4 Analysis with Semiparametric Transformation Models

Table 6.2. Estimated regression parameters with $Q(\mathcal{F}_{it}) = \tilde{H}_i(t-) - \tilde{H}_i(t-6)$

Function $g(t)$	$\hat{\beta}_{DT,1}$ SE($\hat{\beta}_{DT,1}$) 95% CI for β_1	$\hat{\beta}_{DT,2}$ SE($\hat{\beta}_{DT,2}$) 95% CI for β_2	$\hat{\alpha}_{DT}$ SE($\hat{\alpha}_{DT}$) 95% CI for α
$g(t) = t$	−1.7864 0.3756 (−2.5226, −1.0502)	0.2501 0.0682 (0.1163, 0.3838)	0.3846 0.0898 (0.2086, 0.5606)
$g(t) = t^2$	−0.8932 0.1878 (−1.2613, −0.5251)	0.1250 0.0341 (0.0582, 0.1919)	0.1923 0.0449 (0.1043, 0.2803)
$g(t) = \log(t)$	−0.9013 0.1811 (−1.2562, −0.5464)	0.1791 0.0465 (0.0881, 0.2702)	0.1959 0.0720 (0.0548, 0.3370)

duced the recurrence rate of the bladder tumor after adjusting for the dependent visiting process. Also the recurrence rate was positively significantly related to the initial number of bladder tumors, and these conclusions are similar to those given in Sect. 6.3.3. It is interesting to note that the results on estimation of the effects of the treatment and the initial tumors seem to be consistent with respect to the function g and $Q(\mathcal{F}_{it})$ although the magnitudes differ. Note that the magnitudes are expected to be different due to the scale difference under different g.

In terms of the relationship between the recurrence process of bladder tumors and the visiting process, it seems that the recurrence rate significantly depended on both the total number of visits and the number of visits during the last 6 months. In particular, the results indicate that a higher number of visits would mean a higher tumor recurrence rate. Also the effect of the number of visits over the last 6 months on the recurrence rate seems to be greater than that of the total number of visits. Note that the estimated effects here are after adjusting for other factors.

To finish the analysis, the goodness-of-fit test procedure described at the end of Sect. 6.4.2 is applied. It gives the p-values of 0.546, 0.550 and 0.161 for the cases of $Q(\mathcal{F}_{it}) = \tilde{H}_i(t-)$ with the three g functions considered above, respectively, based on 1,000 realizations of $\sup_{0 \le t \le \tau, \boldsymbol{x}} |\hat{\mathcal{F}}^*(t, \boldsymbol{x})|$. These results suggest that all three functions and their specified relationships seem to be reasonable for the observed data. The procedure with the use of $Q(\mathcal{F}_{it}) = \tilde{H}_i(t-) - \tilde{H}_i(t-6)$ gives similar p-values.

6.4.4 Discussion

There exist several differences among the inference procedures discussed in the previous two sections and this section. A basic one is that the procedures given in Sects. 6.2 and 6.3 are joint modeling approaches and allow one to directly describe or estimate the relationship between $N_i(t)$ and $\tilde{H}_i(t)$, the underlying recurrent event process of interest and the observation process. In contrast, the procedure given in this section is a conditional approach with respect to the relationship between the two processes and does not allow one to estimate the relationship quantitatively. Another difference of the three procedures is that it is easy to see that the one given in Sect. 6.2 could be more efficient than the other two if the assumed models are appropriate. On the other hand, it could yield biased results or suffer model misspecification-related problems more often than the other two. This is because the latter two employ much more flexible or general models.

In comparison to the robust procedure described in Sect. 6.3, as the procedure given in Sect. 6.2, a limitation of the procedure discussed in this section is that it requires the observation process $\tilde{H}_i(t)$ to be a Poisson process. As discussed above, this could be questionable in practice. On the other hand, as mentioned before, we have recurrent event data on the $\tilde{H}_i(t)$'s, and thus the assessment of this assumption is relatively easy as discussed in Sect. 6.3.3.

To implement the method described in this section, one needs to choose the link function g. It is apparent that it would be helpful to develop some procedures for selecting or estimating it. However, this is generally quite difficult as in all other similar situations as discussed before. Also as discussed before, one may ask the sensitivity of the results to the misspecification of g and the same can be asked about the robust inference procedure discussed in Sect. 6.3 too. In practice, it may be difficult or impossible to determine the exact relationship between the recurrent event process and the observation process. As discussed in the previous subsection, a simple and natural way is to try different choices for the link function g and see how the resulting estimators change.

A major motivation behind model (6.18) is to extract or take into account the relevant information about the underlying recurrent event process of interest that may exist in or be carried by the observation process. As mentioned above, the model and the associated inference procedure should not be used if the goal is to characterize or estimate the relationship between the two processes. A related and reverse situation that may occur in practice is that one may be more interested in the observation process than the recurrent event process. This corresponds to the situation where one faces regression analysis of recurrent event data with the covariate process suffering incompleteness or missingness. Of course, here the covariate process could be a general longitudinal process rather than just a recurrent event process.

6.5 Analysis with Dependent Terminal Events

In recurrent event studies, as discussed above, sometimes there may exist some terminal events. In this case, there are two possibilities with respect

6.5 Analysis with Dependent Terminal Events

to the relationship between the recurrent event of interest and the terminal event. One is that their occurrences are independent of each other and in this situation, one can simply treat the censoring caused by terminal events as the ordinary censoring such as in the previous section. The other is that the events are related and their correlation needs to be taken into account for the inference about the recurrent event process of interest. An example of such related situations is that a higher rate of the recurrent events caused by a disease may be associated with an increased rate of the death, the terminal event, from the disease. In the literature, such terminal events are often referred to as dependent terminal events or simply terminal events. It is apparent that for this latter situation, the inference procedures different from those discussed above are needed.

There exists considerable work on regression analysis of recurrent event data with dependent terminal events. For inference in this situation, most of the existing procedures adopt one of the following two approaches. One is the marginal model approach that models the marginal occurrences of both recurrent and terminal events and leaves their correlation arbitrary (Cook and Lawless, 2007; Ghosh and Lin, 2002; Zhao et al., 2011b; Zhu et al., 2010, 2011a). The other, similar to those discussed in Sects. 6.2 and 6.3, is the frailty model approach that employs some latent variables to account for the correlation. In this case, the two event processes are usually assumed to be independent given the frailty (Huang and Wang, 2004; Liu et al., 2004; Wang et al., 2001; Ye et al., 2007; Zeng and Cai, 2010).

For regression analysis of panel count data in the presence of dependent terminal events, the literature is relatively much limited. In this section, we describe a marginal modeling approach that can be regarded as a generalization of the approach described in the previous section. Specifically, as before, we first introduce the notation and the assumed models, which have great flexibility and allow for a variety of patterns for the underlying recurrent event process. For estimation of regression parameters, the estimating equation approach is adopted. The methodology leaves the correlation between the recurrent event and the terminal event unspecified. Also it makes use of the inverse probability weighting technique to take into account the fact that the subjects who are terminated cannot experience further occurrence of the events of interest. Then we revisit the bladder tumor panel count data discussed in Sects. 6.3.3 and 6.4.3 assuming that the recurrence process of bladder tumors and the death of the patients may be related. It is followed by some discussion and remarks.

6.5.1 Assumptions and Models

Consider a recurrent event study with the same set-up and the same problem of interest as in the previous section. Let the $N_i(t)$'s and $\tilde{H}_i(t)$'s along with all other notation used below be defined too as in the previous section. In addition, assume that there exists a terminal event denoted by D_i for subject i that may be related to $N_i(t)$, $i = 1, \ldots, n$. Define $N_{di}^*(t) = N_i(t \wedge D_i)$ and $H_{di}^*(t) = \tilde{H}_i(t \wedge D_i)$, which are the terminal event-adjusted recurrent event process of interest and observation process and shall stay constant after D_i. Of course, the observed recurrent event process and the actual observation process are $N_{di}(t) = N_{di}^*(t \wedge C_i)$ and $H_{di}(t) = H_{di}^*(t \wedge C_i)$, respectively. Define $T_{di} = C_i \wedge D_i$ and $\delta_{di} = I(D_i \leq C_i)$, $i = 1, \ldots, n$. Then the observed data have the form

$$\{\, H_{di}(t), N_{di}(t)\, dH_{di}(t), T_{di}, \delta_{di}, \boldsymbol{Z}_i(t)\,;\, t \geq 0\,,\, i = 1, \ldots, n\,\}.$$

To describe the covariate effects on the recurrent event process, define $\mathcal{Z}_i(t) = \{\, \boldsymbol{Z}_i(s);\, 0 \leq s \leq t\,\}$, the history of the covariate process. In the following, we assume that given $\mathcal{Z}_i(t)$, $\mathcal{F}_{it}$ and $D_i \geq t$, the conditional mean function of the adjusted recurrent event process $N_{di}^*(t)$ has the form

$$E\{\, N_{di}^*(t) \mid \mathcal{Z}_i(t), \mathcal{F}_{it}, D_i \geq t\,\} = g\left\{\, \mu_0(t)\, \exp\{\boldsymbol{\beta}^T \boldsymbol{Z}_i(t) + \boldsymbol{\alpha}^T \boldsymbol{Q}(\mathcal{F}_{it})\}\,\right\}. \qquad (6.20)$$

In the above, all $g(\cdot)$, $\mu_0(t)$, $\boldsymbol{Q}$, $\boldsymbol{\beta}$ and $\boldsymbol{\alpha}$ are defined as with model (6.18). As discussed before, the link function $g(\cdot)$ can take many forms to account for various types of dependence of $N_{di}^*(t)$ on $\mathcal{Z}_i(t)$ and $\mathcal{F}_{it}$. For example, $g(x) = x$ and $g(x) = \log x$ give the proportional mean model and the additive mean model, respectively. Also one can let $g(\cdot)$ to be the Box-Cox transformation $g(x) = \{(x + 1)^a - 1\}/a$ for a positive constant a and $g(x) = \log(x + 1)$. The discussion in the previous section on the link function vector $\boldsymbol{Q}$ applies here too.

Note that here we focus on the adjusted mean function and the same idea can be found in the analysis of recurrent event data (Cook and Lawless, 2007; Ghosh and Lin, 2002). Assume that the terminal event is death for the time being. Among others, one advantage for the approach here is that no assumption is needed for the recurrent event process after the death (Luo and Huang, 2010). In contrast, if one simply treats the death as a censoring variable as with the methods described in the previous sections, the estimation of the mean function could be biased. In addition, the analysis would not be able to take into account the fact that the subjects who die can not experience any further recurrent events. It is obvious that if there does not exist death or $D_i = \infty$, $E\{\, N_{di}^*(t) \mid \mathcal{Z}_i(t), \mathcal{F}_{it}, D_i \geq t\,\}$ reduces to $E\{\, N_{di}^*(t) \mid \mathcal{Z}_i(t), \mathcal{F}_{it}\,\}$. In the presence of death, one can show that

$$E\{\, N_{di}^*(t) \mid \mathcal{Z}_i(t), \mathcal{F}_{it}\,\} = \int_0^t S(u|\boldsymbol{Z}_i)\, E\{\, dN_{di}^*(u) \mid \mathcal{Z}_i(u), \mathcal{F}_{iu}, D_i \geq u\,\}$$

given $\mathcal{Z}_i(t)$ and $\mathcal{F}_{it}$ and after adjusting for the fact that the death precludes further recurrent events, where $S(t|\boldsymbol{Z}_i) = P\{\, D_i \geq t|\mathcal{Z}_i(t)\,\}$. It then follows

6.5 Analysis with Dependent Terminal Events

that
$$E\{\,N_{di}^*(t)\,|\,\mathcal{Z}_i(t), \mathcal{F}_{it}, D_i \geq t\,\} \;>\; E\{N_{di}^*(t)\,|\,\mathcal{Z}_i(t), \mathcal{F}_{it}\,\}$$
for t greater than the first observed death time.

In reality, as discussed above, both the adjusted observation process $H_{di}^*(t)$ and the terminal event time D_i may also depend on the covariate process $\mathcal{Z}_i(t)$. With respect to the former, we assume that given $\mathcal{Z}_i(t)$, $H_{di}^*(t)$ follows the proportional rate model

$$E\{\,dH_{di}^*(t)\,|\,\mathcal{Z}_i(t)\,\} \;=\; \exp\{\boldsymbol{\gamma}^T \boldsymbol{Z}_i(t)\}\, d\tilde{\mu}_0(t)\,. \tag{6.21}$$

Here $\boldsymbol{\gamma}$ and $\tilde{\mu}_0(t)$ are defined as in model (5.16). For the terminal event time D_i, it is assumed that it follows the proportional hazards model given by

$$\lambda_d(t|\boldsymbol{Z}_i(t)) \;=\; \lambda_{d0}(t)\,\exp\{\boldsymbol{\tau}^T \boldsymbol{Z}_i(t)\}\,. \tag{6.22}$$

In the above, as with model (5.5), $\lambda_{d0}(t)$ is an unspecified baseline hazard function and $\boldsymbol{\tau}$ is a vector of unknown regression parameters. Under the model above, we have

$$S(t|\boldsymbol{Z}_i) \;=\; \exp\left\{-\int_0^t \lambda_{d0}(s)\,\exp\{\boldsymbol{\tau}^T \boldsymbol{Z}_i(s)\}\,ds\right\}\,.$$

It is easy to see that models (5.16) and (6.21) are the same if the covariates $\boldsymbol{Z}_i(t)$'s are time-independent. Also note that model (6.21) is the same as model (2) of Ghosh and Lin (2002) and it is a marginal model. As an alternative, instead of $E\{\,dH_{di}^*(t)\,|\,\mathcal{Z}_i(t)\,\}$, one may naturally choose to model $E\{\,dH_{di}^*(t)\,|\,\mathcal{Z}_i(t), D_i \geq t\,\}$, which would be a conditional model. A main advantage of model (6.21) is that it allows one to focus on the marginal mean of the cumulative number of observations over time and Ghosh and Lin (2002) give more comments on this. Some discussion on this can also be found in Luo and Huang (2010). In the following, it is assumed that $N_{di}^*(t)$ and $H_{di}^*(t)$ are independent given $\mathcal{Z}_i(t)$, $D_i \geq t$ and $\mathcal{F}_{it}$. Also we assume that C_i is independent of $\{\,N_{di}^*(t), H_{di}^*(t), D_i\,\}$ conditional on $\mathcal{Z}_i(t)$.

6.5.2 Estimation of Regression Parameters

Now we discuss estimation of regression parameters defined in the previous subsection along with other parameters. Let $\boldsymbol{X}_i(t)$, $\boldsymbol{\theta}$ and $Y_i(t)$ be defined as in Sect. 6.4.2 and define

$$\begin{aligned}dM_{di}^*(t;\boldsymbol{\theta},\boldsymbol{\gamma}) \;=\;& N_{di}(t)\,dH_{di}(t) - Y_i(t)\,g\{\mu_0(t)\,\exp\{\boldsymbol{\theta}^T \boldsymbol{X}_i(t)\}\}\\&\times \exp\{\boldsymbol{\gamma}^T \boldsymbol{Z}_i(t)\}\,d\tilde{\mu}_0(t)\,,\end{aligned}$$

$i = 1, \ldots, n$. Note that under models (6.20) and (6.21) and given the conditional independent assumption for $N_{di}^*(t)$, $H_{di}^*(t)$ and C_i, one can show that

$$\begin{aligned} E\{ N_{di}(t)\, dH_{di}(t) \} &= E\Big[E\{ Y_i(t)\, N_{di}^*(t)\, dH_{di}^*(t) \mid \mathcal{Z}_i(t), \mathcal{F}_{it} \} \Big] \\ &= E\Big[E\{ Y_i(t) \mid \mathcal{Z}_i(t) \}\, E\{ N_{di}^*(t)\, dH_{di}^*(t) \mid \mathcal{Z}_i(t), \mathcal{F}_{it} \} \Big] \\ &= E\Big[E\{ Y_i(t) \mid \mathcal{Z}_i(t) \}\, E\{ N_{di}^*(t) \mid \mathcal{Z}_i(t), \mathcal{F}_{it}, D_i \geq t \}\, E\{ dH_{di}^*(t) \mid \mathcal{Z}_i(t) \} \Big] \\ &= E\Big[E\big\{ Y_i(t) g\big\{ \mu_0(t) \exp\{\boldsymbol{\theta}^T \boldsymbol{X}_i(t)\} \big\} \exp\{\boldsymbol{\gamma}^T \boldsymbol{Z}_i(t)\}\, d\tilde{\mu}_0(t) \big| \mathcal{Z}_i(t), \mathcal{F}_{it} \big\} \Big] \\ &= E\Big[Y_i(t)\, g\big\{ \mu_0(t) \exp\{\boldsymbol{\theta}^T \boldsymbol{X}_i(t)\} \big\} \exp\{\boldsymbol{\gamma}^T \boldsymbol{Z}_i(t)\}\, d\tilde{\mu}_0(t) \Big]. \end{aligned}$$

It follows that the $dM_{di}^*(t; \boldsymbol{\theta}, \boldsymbol{\gamma})$'s are zero-mean stochastic processes and hence can be used to construct some estimating equations.

On the other hand, note that in practice, C_i is unobservable when $D_i \leq C_i$ and thus one cannot directly use $dM_{di}^*(t; \boldsymbol{\theta}, \boldsymbol{\gamma})$. To overcome this, one way is to employ the inverse probability weighting technique to replace $Y_i(t)$. Specifically, define $\omega_i(t) = I(T_{di} \geq t)/S(t|\boldsymbol{Z}_i)$ and note that $E\{I(T_{di} \geq t)|\mathcal{Z}_i(t)\} = E\{ I(C_i \geq t)|\mathcal{Z}_i(t) \} S(t|\boldsymbol{Z}_i)$ based on the independence between C_i and D_i given $\boldsymbol{Z}_i(\cdot)$. It follows that

$$E\{ \omega_i(t) \mid \mathcal{Z}_i(t) \} = E\{ I(C_i \geq t) \mid \mathcal{Z}_i(t) \}.$$

This motivates us to consider

$$\begin{aligned} dM_{di}(t; \boldsymbol{\theta}, \boldsymbol{\gamma}) = N_{di}(t)\, dH_{di}(t) &- \omega_i(t)\, g\big\{ \mu_0(t) \exp\{\boldsymbol{\theta}^T \boldsymbol{X}_i(t)\} \big\} \\ &\times \exp\{\boldsymbol{\gamma}^T \boldsymbol{Z}_i(t)\}\, d\tilde{\mu}_0(t), \end{aligned}$$

$i = 1, \ldots, n$, and it can be easily shown that the $dM_{di}(t; \boldsymbol{\theta}, \boldsymbol{\gamma})$'s are also zero-mean stochastic processes. Note that here $\omega_i(t)$ is still unobservable, but it can be easily estimated by, for example, $\hat{\omega}_i(t) = I(T_{di} \geq t)/\hat{S}(t|\boldsymbol{Z}_i)$. Here

$$\hat{S}(t|\boldsymbol{Z}_i) = \exp\left[-\int_0^t \exp\{\hat{\boldsymbol{\tau}}^T \boldsymbol{Z}_i(s)\}\, d\hat{\Lambda}_{d0}(s) \right],$$

where $\hat{\boldsymbol{\tau}}$ and $\hat{\Lambda}_{d0}(t)$ denote the maximum partial likelihood estimator of $\boldsymbol{\tau}$ and the Breslow estimator of $\Lambda_{d0}(t) = \int_0^t \lambda_{d0}(s)ds$, respectively, based on model (6.22). By following the arguments similar to those in Lin et al. (2001), one can show that for large n, the estimator $\hat{\omega}_i(t)$ always exists and is unique and consistent.

As in the previous section, let $\hat{\boldsymbol{\gamma}}_T$ and $\hat{\tilde{\mu}}_0(t; \hat{\boldsymbol{\gamma}}_T)$ denote the estimators of $\boldsymbol{\gamma}$ and $\tilde{\mu}_0(t)$ defined by Eqs. (5.20) and (5.21), respectively. For estimation of $\boldsymbol{\theta}$ and $\mu_0(t)$ in model (6.20), as discussed before, it is natural to employ the following estimating equations

6.5 Analysis with Dependent Terminal Events

$$\sum_{i=1}^{n}\left[N_{di}(t)\,dH_{di}(t)-\hat{\omega}_i(t)g\left\{\mu_0(t)\exp\{\boldsymbol{\theta}^T\boldsymbol{X}_i(t)\}\right\}\exp\left\{\boldsymbol{\gamma}^T\boldsymbol{Z}_i(t)\right\}d\tilde{\mu}_0(t)\right]=0 \tag{6.23}$$

for $0 \leq t \leq \tau$, and

$$U_D(\boldsymbol{\theta},\boldsymbol{\gamma}) = \sum_{i=1}^{n}\int_0^{\tau} W(t)\,\boldsymbol{X}_i(t)\left[N_{di}(t)\,dH_{di}(t) - \hat{\omega}_i(t)\right.$$
$$\left.\times g\left\{\mu_0(t)\exp\{\boldsymbol{\theta}^T\boldsymbol{X}_i(t)\}\right\}\exp\left\{\boldsymbol{\gamma}^T\boldsymbol{Z}_i(t)\right\}d\tilde{\mu}_0(t)\right] = 0 \tag{6.24}$$

with replacing $\boldsymbol{\gamma}$ and $\tilde{\mu}_0(t)$ by $\hat{\boldsymbol{\gamma}}_T$ and $\hat{\tilde{\mu}}_0(t;\hat{\boldsymbol{\gamma}}_T)$, respectively. In the above, as before, $W(t)$ denotes a possibly data-dependent weight function.

Let $\hat{\boldsymbol{\theta}}_D$ and $\hat{\mu}_D(t;\hat{\boldsymbol{\theta}}_D,\hat{\boldsymbol{\gamma}}_T)$ denote the estimators of $\boldsymbol{\theta}$ and $\mu_0(t)$ given by the solutions to Eqs. (6.23) and (6.24). For their determination, one can develop a procedure similar to the one discussed in Sect. 5.5.3 and the comments given there also apply here. In particular, in general, these estimators have no closed forms except in some special cases. One such case is when $g(t) = t^m$, where m is a positive number, and in this situation, $\hat{\mu}_D(t;\boldsymbol{\theta},\boldsymbol{\gamma})$ has an explicit expression. Another special case is when $g(t) = \log t$ and for this situation, one can easily derive

$$\hat{\boldsymbol{\theta}}_D = \left[\sum_{i=1}^{n}\int_0^{\tau} W(t)\{\boldsymbol{X}_i(t) - \bar{\boldsymbol{X}}(t;\hat{\boldsymbol{\gamma}}_T)\}\boldsymbol{X}_i^T(t)\hat{\omega}_i(t)\,e^{\hat{\boldsymbol{\gamma}}_T^T\boldsymbol{Z}_i(t)}\,d\hat{\tilde{\mu}}_0(t;\hat{\boldsymbol{\gamma}}_T)\right]^{-1}$$
$$\times \sum_{i=1}^{n}\int_0^{\tau} W(t)\{\boldsymbol{X}_i(t) - \bar{\boldsymbol{X}}(t;\hat{\boldsymbol{\gamma}}_T)\}N_{di}(t)\,dH_{di}(t),$$

and

$$\hat{\mu}_D(t;\boldsymbol{\theta},\boldsymbol{\gamma}) = \exp\left\{\frac{\sum_{i=1}^{n} N_{di}(t)\,dH_{di}(t)}{\sum_{i=1}^{n}\hat{\omega}_i(t)\exp\{\boldsymbol{\gamma}^T\boldsymbol{Z}_i(t)\}\,d\hat{\tilde{\mu}}_0(t;\boldsymbol{\gamma})} - \boldsymbol{\theta}^T\bar{\boldsymbol{X}}(t;\boldsymbol{\gamma})\right\},$$

where

$$\bar{\boldsymbol{X}}(t;\boldsymbol{\gamma}) = \frac{\sum_{i=1}^{n}\boldsymbol{X}_i(t)\,\hat{\omega}_i(t)\,\exp\{\boldsymbol{\gamma}^T\boldsymbol{Z}_i(t)\}}{\sum_{i=1}^{n}\hat{\omega}_i(t)\,\exp\{\boldsymbol{\gamma}^T\boldsymbol{Z}_i(t)\}}.$$

With respect to the asymptotic properties of $\hat{\boldsymbol{\theta}}_D$, Zhao et al. (2013a) show that under some regularity conditions, it is consistent. To describe its asymptotic distribution, let $\boldsymbol{\theta}_0$ denote the true value of $\boldsymbol{\theta}$ and $\hat{M}_{di}^{(1)}(t)$ be $M_{di}(t;\boldsymbol{\theta},\boldsymbol{\gamma})$ with all unknowns replaced by their estimates. Define

$$\hat{M}_{di}^{(2)}(t) = H_{di}(t) - \int_0^t \hat{\omega}_i(s)\,\exp\left\{\hat{\boldsymbol{\gamma}}_T^T\boldsymbol{Z}_i(s)\right\}d\hat{\tilde{\mu}}_0(s;\hat{\boldsymbol{\gamma}}_T),$$

$$\hat{M}_{di}^{(3)}(t) = I(T_{di} \leq t, \delta_{di} = 1) - \int_0^t Y_i(s)\exp\left\{\hat{\boldsymbol{\tau}}^T\boldsymbol{Z}_i(s)\right\}d\hat{\Lambda}_{d0}(s),$$

$$\hat{E}_X(t;\boldsymbol{\theta},\boldsymbol{\gamma}) = \frac{\sum_{i=1}^n \boldsymbol{X}_i(t)\,\hat{\omega}_i(t)\,\dot{g}\{\hat{\mu}_D(t;\boldsymbol{\theta},\boldsymbol{\gamma})e^{\boldsymbol{\theta}^T\boldsymbol{X}_i(t)}\}e^{\boldsymbol{\theta}^T\boldsymbol{X}_i(t)+\boldsymbol{\gamma}^T\boldsymbol{Z}_i(t)}}{\sum_{i=1}^n \hat{\omega}_i(t)\dot{g}\{\hat{\mu}_D(t;\boldsymbol{\theta},\boldsymbol{\gamma})e^{\boldsymbol{\theta}^T\boldsymbol{X}_i(t)}\}e^{\boldsymbol{\theta}^T\boldsymbol{X}_i(t)+\boldsymbol{\gamma}^T\boldsymbol{Z}_i(t)}},$$

$$\hat{\Upsilon}(t;\boldsymbol{\theta},\boldsymbol{\gamma})=\frac{1}{n}\sum_{i=1}^n \{\boldsymbol{X}_i(t)-\hat{E}_X(t;\boldsymbol{\theta},\boldsymbol{\gamma})\}\hat{\omega}_i(t)g\{\hat{\mu}_D(t;\boldsymbol{\theta},\boldsymbol{\gamma})e^{\boldsymbol{\theta}^T\boldsymbol{X}_i(t)}\}e^{\boldsymbol{\gamma}^T\boldsymbol{Z}_i(t)},$$

$$R^{(k)}(t;\boldsymbol{\tau}) = \frac{1}{n}\sum_{i=1}^n I(T_{di}\geq t)\exp\{\boldsymbol{\tau}^T\boldsymbol{Z}_i(t)\}\,\boldsymbol{Z}_i(t)^{\otimes k},\ k=0,1,2,$$

$$\hat{A}(\boldsymbol{\theta},\boldsymbol{\gamma}) = \frac{1}{n}\sum_{i=1}^n \int_0^\tau W(t)\hat{\omega}_i(t)g\left\{\hat{\mu}_D(t;\boldsymbol{\theta},\boldsymbol{\gamma})\exp\{\boldsymbol{\theta}^T\boldsymbol{X}_i(t)\}\right\}\exp\{\boldsymbol{\gamma}^T\boldsymbol{Z}_i(t)\}$$
$$\times\left\{\boldsymbol{X}_i(t)-\hat{E}_X(t;\boldsymbol{\theta},\boldsymbol{\gamma})\right\}\left\{\boldsymbol{Z}_i(t)-\hat{\boldsymbol{Z}}(t;\boldsymbol{\gamma})\right\}^T d\hat{\tilde{\mu}}_0(t;\boldsymbol{\gamma}),$$

and

$$\hat{\Omega}(\boldsymbol{\gamma}) = \frac{1}{n}\sum_{i=1}^n\int_0^\tau \left\{\boldsymbol{Z}_i(t)-\hat{\boldsymbol{Z}}(t;\boldsymbol{\gamma})\right\}^{\otimes 2}\hat{\omega}_i(t)\exp\{\boldsymbol{\gamma}^T\boldsymbol{Z}_i(t)\}\,d\hat{\tilde{\mu}}_0(t;\boldsymbol{\gamma}),$$

where $\dot{g} = dg(t)/dt$ and $\hat{\boldsymbol{Z}}(t;\boldsymbol{\gamma}) = S^{(1)}(t;\boldsymbol{\gamma})/S^{(0)}(t;\boldsymbol{\gamma})$ with

$$S^{(k)}(t;\boldsymbol{\gamma}) = \frac{1}{n}\sum_{i=1}^n \hat{\omega}_i(t)\boldsymbol{Z}_i(t)^k\exp\{\boldsymbol{\gamma}^T\boldsymbol{Z}_i(t)\},\ k=0,1.$$

Also define

$$\hat{B}_1(t) = \frac{1}{n}\sum_{i=1}^n e^{\hat{\boldsymbol{\tau}}^T\boldsymbol{Z}_i(t)}\int_0^\tau I(t<s)\,\hat{B}_i^*(s)\,d\hat{\tilde{\mu}}_0(s;\hat{\boldsymbol{\gamma}}),$$

$$\hat{B}_2 = \frac{1}{n}\sum_{i=1}^n \int_0^\tau \hat{B}_i^*(t)\,\hat{H}(t;\boldsymbol{Z}_i)^T\hat{\Omega}_\tau^{-1}\,d\hat{\tilde{\mu}}_0(t;\hat{\boldsymbol{\gamma}}),$$

$$\hat{Q}_1 = \frac{1}{n}\sum_{i=1}^n \int_0^\tau \{\boldsymbol{Z}_i(t)-\hat{\boldsymbol{Z}}(t;\hat{\boldsymbol{\gamma}}_T)\}\hat{Q}_3(t;\boldsymbol{Z}_i)^T\hat{\Omega}_\tau^{-1}\,d\hat{M}_{di}^{(2)}(t),$$

and

$$\hat{Q}_2(t) = \frac{1}{n}\sum_{i=1}^n \exp\{\hat{\boldsymbol{\tau}}^T\boldsymbol{Z}_i(t)\}\int_0^\tau \{\boldsymbol{Z}_i(u)-\hat{\boldsymbol{Z}}(u;\hat{\boldsymbol{\gamma}}_T)\}I(u\geq t)\,d\hat{M}_{di}^{(2)}(u),$$

where

$$\hat{B}_i^*(t) = W(t)\hat{\omega}_i(t)\exp\{\hat{\boldsymbol{\gamma}}^T\boldsymbol{Z}_i(t)\}\left[\{\boldsymbol{X}_i(t)-\hat{E}_X(t;\hat{\boldsymbol{\theta}}_D,\hat{\boldsymbol{\gamma}}_T)\}\right.$$

6.5 Analysis with Dependent Terminal Events

$$\times g\left\{\hat{\mu}_D(t;\hat{\boldsymbol{\theta}}_D,\hat{\boldsymbol{\gamma}}_T)\exp\{\hat{\boldsymbol{\theta}}_D^T\boldsymbol{X}_i(t)\}\right\} - \frac{\hat{\Upsilon}(t;\hat{\boldsymbol{\theta}}_D,\hat{\boldsymbol{\gamma}}_T)}{S^{(0)}(t;\hat{\boldsymbol{\gamma}}_T)}\right],$$

$$\hat{H}(t;\boldsymbol{Z}_i) = \int_0^t \exp\left\{\hat{\boldsymbol{\tau}}^T\boldsymbol{Z}_i(u)\right\}\left\{\boldsymbol{Z}_i(u) - \frac{R^{(1)}(u;\hat{\boldsymbol{\tau}})}{R^{(0)}(u;\hat{\boldsymbol{\tau}})}\right\}d\hat{\Lambda}_{d0}(u),$$

$$\hat{\Omega}_\tau = \frac{1}{n}\sum_{i=1}^n \int_0^\tau \left[\frac{R^{(2)}(t;\hat{\boldsymbol{\tau}})}{R^{(0)}(t;\hat{\boldsymbol{\tau}})} - \left\{\frac{R^{(1)}(t;\hat{\boldsymbol{\tau}})}{R^{(0)}(t;\hat{\boldsymbol{\tau}})}\right\}^{\otimes 2}\right]d\hat{M}_{di}^{(3)}(t),$$

and

$$\hat{Q}_3(t;\boldsymbol{Z}_i) = \int_0^t \left\{\boldsymbol{Z}_i(u) - \hat{\boldsymbol{Z}}(u;\hat{\boldsymbol{\gamma}}_T)\right\}\exp\left\{\hat{\boldsymbol{\tau}}^T\boldsymbol{Z}_i(u)\right\}d\hat{\Lambda}_{d0}(u).$$

Under the same regularity conditions mentioned above, Zhao et al. (2013a) show that the distribution of $n^{1/2}(\hat{\boldsymbol{\theta}}_D - \boldsymbol{\theta}_0)$ can be asymptotically approximated by the normal distribution with mean zero and the covariance matrix $\hat{A}^{-1}(\hat{\boldsymbol{\theta}}_D,\hat{\boldsymbol{\gamma}}_T)\hat{\Sigma}_D\hat{A}^{-1}(\hat{\boldsymbol{\theta}}_D,\hat{\boldsymbol{\gamma}}_T)$. Here $\hat{\Sigma}_D = n^{-1}\sum_{i=1}^n (\hat{\xi}_{1i} - \hat{\xi}_{2i} - \hat{\xi}_{3i})^{\otimes 2}$ with

$$\hat{\xi}_{1i} = \int_0^\tau W(t)\left\{\boldsymbol{X}_i(t) - \hat{E}_X(t;\hat{\boldsymbol{\theta}}_D,\hat{\boldsymbol{\gamma}}_T)\right\}d\hat{M}_{di}^{(1)}(t),$$

$$\hat{\xi}_{2i} = \int_0^\tau \left[\frac{W(t)\hat{\Upsilon}(t;\hat{\boldsymbol{\theta}}_D,\hat{\boldsymbol{\gamma}}_T)}{S^{(0)}(t;\hat{\boldsymbol{\gamma}}_T)} + \hat{A}(\hat{\boldsymbol{\theta}}_D,\hat{\boldsymbol{\gamma}}_T)\hat{\Omega}^{-1}(\hat{\boldsymbol{\gamma}}_T)\left\{\boldsymbol{Z}_i(t) - \hat{\boldsymbol{Z}}(t;\hat{\boldsymbol{\gamma}}_T)\right\}\right]$$
$$d\hat{M}_{di}^{(2)}(t),$$

and

$$\hat{\xi}_{3i} = \int_0^\tau \left[\hat{A}(\hat{\boldsymbol{\theta}}_D,\hat{\boldsymbol{\gamma}}_T)\hat{\Omega}^{-1}(\hat{\boldsymbol{\gamma}}_T)\hat{Q}_1\left\{\boldsymbol{Z}_i(t) - \frac{R^{(1)}(t;\hat{\boldsymbol{\tau}})}{R^{(0)}(t;\hat{\boldsymbol{\tau}})}\right\} + \hat{A}(\hat{\boldsymbol{\theta}}_D,\hat{\boldsymbol{\gamma}}_T)\hat{\Omega}^{-1}(\hat{\boldsymbol{\gamma}}_T)\right.$$
$$\left.\times\frac{\hat{Q}_2(t)}{R^{(0)}(t;\hat{\boldsymbol{\tau}})} + \frac{\hat{B}_1(t)}{R^{(0)}(t;\hat{\boldsymbol{\tau}})} + \hat{B}_2\left\{\boldsymbol{Z}_i(t) - \frac{R^{(1)}(t;\hat{\boldsymbol{\tau}})}{R^{(0)}(t;\hat{\boldsymbol{\tau}})}\right\}\right]d\hat{M}_{di}^{(3)}(t).$$

6.5.3 Reanalysis of Bladder Cancer Study

Now we reanalyze the bladder cancer panel count data discussed in Sects. 6.3.3 and 6.4.3 assuming the existence of a dependent terminal event, death. For the analysis, as in Sect. 6.4.3, we confine ourselves to the data from the 85 bladder cancer patients in thiotepa (38) and placebo (47) groups. Also we consider only the effects of treatment and the number of initial tumors. As mentioned before, all patients had superficial bladder tumors when they entered the study and all these tumors were removed at the beginning. During the follow-up, the bladder tumors that were detected at each clinical

Table 6.3. Estimated regression parameters with $Q(\mathcal{F}_{it}) = \tilde{H}_i(t-)$

Function $g(t)$	$\hat{\beta}_{D,1}$ 95% CI for β_1 p-value for $\beta_1 = 0$	$\hat{\beta}_{D,2}$ 95% CI for β_2 p-value for $\beta_2 = 0$	$\hat{\alpha}_D$ 95% CI for α p-value for $\alpha = 0$
$g(t) = t$	-1.8955 $(-2.6442, -1.1467)$ < 0.001	0.2961 $(0.1487, 0.4436)$ < 0.001	0.0398 $(-0.0086, 0.0883)$ 0.1074
$g(t) = t^2$	-0.9474 $(-1.3217, -0.5731)$ < 0.001	0.1481 $(0.0743, 0.2218)$ < 0.001	0.0199 $(-0.0043, 0.0441)$ 0.1075
$g(t) = \log t$	-4.0501 $(-5.9544, -2.1459)$ < 0.001	0.8464 $(0.2636, 1.4292)$ 0.0044	0.0352 $(-0.1260, 0.1964)$ 0.6683

visit were also removed. Of the 85 study subjects, there are 22 patients died before the end of the follow-up. Here we assume that the death rate may be related to both the underlying recurrence process of bladder tumors and the visiting or observation process.

To apply the methodology described above, let $\mathbf{Z}_i$ be defined as in Sect. 6.4.3. In this case, unlike before, β_1 and β_2 denote the effects of the thiotepa treatment and the number of initial tumors on the terminal event-adjusted recurrence process of bladder tumors, respectively. Similarly α represents the effect of the visiting or observation process also on the terminal event-adjusted recurrent event process. Table 6.3 presents the results obtained with the use of the same three link functions g considered before, $Q(\mathcal{F}_{i,t}) = \tilde{H}_i(t-)$ and $W(t) = 1$. They include the estimated effects $\hat{\boldsymbol{\beta}}_D$ and $\hat{\boldsymbol{\alpha}}_D$, the 95% confidence intervals and the p-values for testing the corresponding effect being zero. The results with $Q(\mathcal{F}_{i,t}) = \tilde{H}_i(t-) - \tilde{H}_i(t-6)$ are given in Table 6.4 with all other set-ups being the same as in Table 6.3. One can easily see from the tables that as before, all results again suggest that both the thiotepa treatment and the initial number of tumors had significant effects on the recurrence rate of the bladder tumor. In particular, the thiotepa treatment seems to significantly reduce the recurrence of bladder tumors.

With respect to the relationship between the recurrence process of bladder tumors and the visit process, we now have different results compared with those obtained in Sect. 6.4.3. More specifically, the results here indicate that both the total number of visits and the number of visits during the last 6 months seem to have no significant effect on the recurrence rate of bladder tumors. One possible explanation for the difference is that the significant relationship detected in Sect. 6.4.3 may be due to the correlation between the bladder tumor occurrence process and the terminal event, death, which was assumed to be none. Note that in addition to the two choices considered above, sometimes one may argue that the recurrence process of bladder tumors could depend on the duration since the last visit. This corresponds to

6.5 Analysis with Dependent Terminal Events

Table 6.4. Estimated regression parameters with $Q(\mathcal{F}_{it}) = \tilde{H}_i(t-) - \tilde{H}_i(t-6)$

Function $g(t)$	$\hat{\beta}_{D,1}$ 95% CI for β_1 p-value for $\beta_1 = 0$	$\hat{\beta}_{D,2}$ 95% CI for β_2 p-value for $\beta_2 = 0$	$\hat{\alpha}_D$ 95% CI for α p-value for $\alpha = 0$
$g(t) = t$	-1.6750 $(-2.3786, -0.9713)$ < 0.001	0.2901 $(0.1483, 0.4318)$ < 0.001	0.0764 $(-0.0639, 0.2165)$ 0.2858
$g(t) = t^2$	-0.8373 $(-1.1890, -0.4854)$ < 0.001	0.1450 $(0.0742, 0.2159)$ < 0.001	0.0382 $(-0.0319, 0.1083)$ 0.2861
$g(t) = \log t$	-4.1338 $(-6.2092, -2.0584)$ < 0.001	0.8492 $(0.2780, 1.4205)$ 0.0036	0.2189 $(-0.0703, 0.5080)$ 0.1379

$Q(\mathcal{F}_{it}) = t - t_{i,j-1}$ with $t_{i,j-1} < t \leq t_{i,j}$, and the analysis with the use of this function actually gives similar results here.

Note that as for model (6.18), a procedure can be derived in the same way to assess the goodness-of-fit of model (6.20) and more discussion on this is given in the next subsection. The application of such procedure based on 1,000 realizations yields the p-values of 0.866, 0.857 and 0.594 for the situations with $Q(\mathcal{F}_{it}) = \tilde{H}_i(t-)$ and the three link functions $g(t) = t$, $g(t) = t^2$, and $g(t) = \log t$, respectively. The use of $Q(\mathcal{F}_{it}) = \tilde{H}_i(t-) - \tilde{H}_i(t-6)$ gives similar p-values and they all indicate that model (6.20) seems to be reasonable for the data.

6.5.4 Discussion

The focus of this section has been to take into account the dependent terminal event in regression analysis of panel count data. As discussed above, the analysis could give misleading or wrong results or conclusions if one treats the event as a simple censoring event. For the task, a key issue is how to model the relationship between the underlying recurrent event process of interest and the terminal event. It is easy to see that model (6.20) is a generalization of and reduces to model (6.18) if $D_i = \infty$ or there does not exist the terminal event. Model (6.20) should be of more clinical interest to some extent because it directly accounts for the covariate effects on the frequency of the recurrent events of interest among survivors. In other words, it does not model the recurrent event process after the terminal events or the correlation between the rates of recurrent and terminal events.

Instead of model (6.20), one could directly model the marginal mean function of the unadjusted recurrent event process of interest. An advantage of this approach is that the interpretation of the results may be easier than the model discussed above. Under the models considered above, if a treatment reduces the disease-related event recurrence and death rate simultaneously, it is clearly preferred. The same is true if the treatment reduces the disease-related event recurrence but has no significant impact on survival. However, if the treatment reduces the disease-related event recurrence but increases mortality, then it is more subtle to make a judgment on the treatment and one may need to do further analysis. In the context of recurrent event data, many authors have investigated the differences in terms of the uses of different types of models (Ghosh and Lin, 2000, 2003; Luo and Huang 2010).

As for model (6.18) discussed in Sect. 6.4, one can similarly develop an omnibus goodness-of-fit test procedure for model (6.20). For the current situation, the cumulative sum of residuals process corresponding to $\mathcal{F}^*(t, \boldsymbol{x})$ for model (6.18) has the form

$$\mathcal{F}_d^*(t, \boldsymbol{x}) = \frac{1}{\sqrt{n}} \sum_{i=1}^n \int_0^t I(\boldsymbol{X}_i(u) \leq \boldsymbol{x}) \, d\hat{M}_{di}^{(1)}(u),$$

and one can base the test on the statistic $\sup_{0 \leq t \leq \tau, \boldsymbol{x}} |\mathcal{F}_d^*(t, \boldsymbol{x})|$. To implement this, again as before, we can apply the approximation technique to obtain the p-value instead of deriving and using the exact distribution of the test statistic. More specifically, one can first construct a zero-mean Gaussian process $\hat{\mathcal{F}}_d^*(t, \boldsymbol{x})$ that is a function of a simple random sample of size n from the standard normal distribution independent of the observed data. The p-value can then be determined by comparing the observed value of $\sup_{0 \leq t \leq \tau, \boldsymbol{x}} |\mathcal{F}_d^*(t, \boldsymbol{x})|$ to a large number of realizations from $\sup_{0 \leq t \leq \tau, \boldsymbol{x}} |\hat{\mathcal{F}}_d^*(t, \boldsymbol{x})|$, which can be obtained by repeatedly generating the standard normal random samples given the observed data.

Of course one can ask the same model checking question about models (6.21) and (6.22). As pointed out before in other similar situations, for both models, complete data are available and so are some existing procedures in the literature (Lin et al., 2000, 1993; Schoenfeld, 1982). Also there exist many other models in the literature that one could apply for $H_{di}^*(t)$ and D_i instead of these two models. For modeling the terminal event, for example, some alternative models include the additive hazards model, the accelerated failure time model, and the linear transformation model (Kalbfleisch and Prentice, 2002).

6.6 Bibliography, Discussion, and Remarks

As mentioned before, the literature on regression analysis of panel count data with dependent observation processes is relatively new and limited. The authors who started the detailed investigation of this area include Huang et al. (2006), Kim (2006) and Sun et al. (2007b), and they gave some joint modeling

6.6 Bibliography, Discussion, and Remarks

inference procedures similar to those discussed in Sect. 6.2. Following them, He et al. (2009), Zhao and Tong (2011) and Zhao et al. (2013) also provided some joint modeling approaches for the problem. Other references on the topic include Buzkova (2010), Li (2011), Li et al. (2010), Li et al. (2013) and Zhao et al. (2013a) and the latter four developed some marginal approaches by employing semiparametric transformation models.

Also as mentioned before, panel count data can be regarded as a special type of longitudinal data. Although there exists a great deal of work on regression analysis of longitudinal data, the literature on longitudinal data with dependent observation processes is also limited (Liang et al., 2009; Lin et al., 2004; Liu et al., 2008; Sun et al., 2005, 2007a, 2012; Sun and Tong, 2009; Zhu et al., 2011b). Here by the dependent observation process, we mean that the longitudinal process of interest and the process that generates observation times are correlated. On the other hand, many authors have investigated the situation where there exists a terminal event such as a survival event that is related to the longitudinal process of interest. For the situation, most of the developed approaches assume that the longitudinal process and the observation process are independent of each other completely or given covariates. Furthermore, they are joint procedures aiming at the joint analysis of longitudinal and time-to-event data (DeGruttola and Tu, 1994; Elashoff et al., 2008; Jin et al., 2006; Liu and Ying, 2007; Roy and Lin, 2002; Song et al., 2002, 2012; Sun et al., 2007a, 2012; Tsiatis and Davidian, 2004).

Given the approaches discussed in the previous sections, a question of practical interest may be how to choose an appropriate procedure for a given set of panel count data. It is apparent that this will partly depend on the questions of interest. The methods described in Sects. 6.2 and 6.3 allow one to investigate the effects of covariates on all concerned processes, while the procedures given in Sects. 6.4 and 6.5 focus only on the effects of covariates on the recurrent event process of interest. A similar question is the selection of the link functions g and Q in models (6.18) and (6.20). They determine the patterns of the underlying recurrent event process or the relationship among the recurrent event process, the observation process and the covariate process. Both questions are clearly quite difficult in general. On the other hand, for a given specific model or set of models, as commented above, one could apply some goodness-of-fit test or model checking procedures.

Finally note that to model two related variables or processes, one can either model them jointly as in Sects. 6.2 and 6.3, or model one marginally and the other conditional on the first one. The models discussed in Sects. 6.4 and 6.5 assume that the observation process carries some relevant information about the recurrent event process of interest and specify how the information affects the recurrent event process. Sometimes it could be more natural to ask or model how the observation process depends on the history information of the recurrent event process. In other words, how the recurrent event process affects the observation process. To address this, we may want to develop some models on $\tilde{H}_i(t)$ conditional on $\{N_i(s)\,;\, 0 \leq s < t\}$.

7
Analysis of Multivariate Panel Count Data

7.1 Introduction

This chapter discusses statistical analysis of multivariate panel count data, which arise when there exist several related types of recurrent events and study subjects are observed only at discrete time points. As remarked before, in this case, an issue that does not exist for univariate panel count data is the correlation between different types of events. To deal with it, two approaches are commonly used as with multivariate failure time data (Hougaard, 2000). One is the marginal model approach that leaves the correlation arbitrary, and the other is the joint model approach that characterizes the correlation through the use of some latent or random variables. In this chapter, we mainly adopt the marginal model approach and consider two problems, nonparametric comparison of treatments in terms of mean functions and regression analysis.

As discussed before, for nonparametric or semiparametric analysis of univariate panel count data, it is usually convenient to focus on or model the rate or mean functions of the underlying recurrent event processes. This is the same for the analysis of multivariate panel count data. In the following, we first consider in Sect. 7.2 the nonparametric treatment comparison problem with the hypothesis formulated by the mean functions of the processes of interest as in Chap. 4. To conduct the hypothesis test, a class of test statistics based on the comparison of the estimated mean functions is presented.

Sections 7.3–7.5 discuss regression analysis of multivariate panel count data. First we consider in Sect. 7.3 the situation where the recurrent event processes of interest and the observation process can be assumed to be independent given covariates. For the problem, a marginal model approach is described under some general regression models for the mean functions of both the recurrent event processes and the observation process. The models can be regarded as generalizations of the proportional mean models (1.4) and (5.4). Some estimating equations are introduced for estimation of regression parameters.

Sections 7.4 and 7.5 investigate the regression problem about multivariate panel count data when the recurrent event processes of interest and the observation process may be related as in Chap. 6. For this, we first describe a marginal model approach that is a generalization of the approach discussed in Sect. 6.3. Specifically, we consider the situation where the marginal mean functions of each individual recurrent event process of interest and the observation process can be characterized by models (6.14) and (6.15), respectively. In Sect. 7.5, we discuss situations that are similar to those considered in Sect. 6.4. More specifically, it is assumed that the conditional marginal mean function of each individual recurrent event process given the observation process can be described by model (6.18). For both cases, the estimating equation approach is employed for estimation of regression parameters of interest. Finally Sect. 7.6 gives some bibliographical notes and discusses some issues not touched in the previous sections.

7.2 Nonparametric Comparison of Cumulative Mean Functions

Consider a recurrent event study that involves n independent subjects and in which each subject may experience K different types of recurrent events. Suppose that only panel count data are available for the underlying recurrent event processes of interest. In this section, we consider the nonparametric treatment comparison problem with the focus on the two-sample situation. The idea described can be easily generalized to general cases and some discussion on it is given below. In the following, it is assumed that the underlying recurrent event process and the observation process are independent.

For each i and k, let $N_{ik}(t)$ denote the recurrence event process given by subject i with respect to the kth type recurrent event, $i = 1,\ldots,n$, $k = 1,\ldots,K$. In other word, $N_{ik}(t)$ represents the cumulative number of the occurrences of the kth type recurrent event of interest that subject i has experienced up to time t. For simplicity, suppose that the first n_1 subjects are in the control group and the remaining n_2 are in the treatment group, where $n_1 + n_2 = n$. Furthermore, define $\mu_{k1}(t) = \mathrm{E}\{N_{ik}(t)\}$ for $i = 1,\ldots,n_1$ and $\mu_{k2}(t) = \mathrm{E}\{N_{ik}(t)\}$ for $i = n_1 + 1,\ldots,n$. That is, $\mu_{k1}(t)$ and $\mu_{k2}(t)$ are the mean functions of $N_{ik}(t)$ for subjects in the control and treatment groups, respectively. Suppose that the goal is to test the null hypothesis

$$H_0^K : \mu_{11}(t) = \mu_{12}(t)\,,\,\ldots\,,\,\mu_{K1}(t) = \mu_{K2}(t)\,.$$

Note that if $K = 1$, the test problem above reduces the one discussed in Chap. 4 and thus one can readily employ the approaches discussed there. The same methods can also be used if one is interested in the treatment effect

7.2 Nonparametric Comparison of Cumulative Mean Functions

only on one particular type of recurrent events. Otherwise it is apparent that one needs different procedures as the one described below for an efficient test.

7.2.1 Two-Sample Nonparametric Test Procedures

In this subsection, we describe a class of test statistics for testing the hypothesis H_0^K. For this, let $0 < t_{i,1} < \cdots < t_{i,m_i}$ denote the observation times on $N_{ik}(t)$ or subject i and $n_{i,k,j} = N_{ik}(t_{i,j})$, the observed value of $N_{ik}(t)$ at $t_{i,j}$, $i = 1, \ldots, n$, $k = 1, \ldots, K$, $j = 1, \cdots, m_i$. Then the observed data are

$$\{\, t_{i,j}, n_{i,k,j} \,;\, j = 1, \ldots, m_i,\, i = 1, \ldots, n,\, k = 1, \ldots, K \,\}.$$

Note that here for simplicity, we assume that the observation times for different types of recurrent events from the same subject are the same. The approach given below can be easily generalized to the situation where the observation times for different types of recurrent events are different.

To present the test statistics, let $\hat{\mu}_{I,k1}(t)$ and $\hat{\mu}_{I,k2}(t)$ denote the IRE of $\mu_{k1}(t)$ and $\mu_{k2}(t)$ based on the data on type k recurrent events and from the subjects in the control and treatment groups, respectively, $k = 1, \ldots, K$. Then by following the idea used in Sect. 4.2.2 and also commonly employed in failure time data analysis (Kalbfleisch and Prentice, 2002; Pepe and Fleming, 1989), one can consider the statistic

$$U_{ZVS} = \sqrt{\frac{n_1 n_2}{n}} \sum_{k=1}^{K} \int_0^{\tau} W_{n,k}(t) \{\hat{\mu}_{I,k1}(t) - \hat{\mu}_{I,k2}(t)\} dG_n(t), \quad (7.1)$$

first proposed in Zhao et al. (2013c). In the above, as before, τ denotes the largest observation time, $W_{n,k}(t)$ is a bounded weight process, and

$$G_n(t) = \frac{1}{n} \sum_{i=1}^{n} \sum_{j=1}^{m_i} I(t_{i,j} \leq t),$$

the empirical observation process. It is apparent that if $K = 1$, U_{ZVS} reduces to the test statistic U_{PSZ} discussed in Sect. 4.2.2 for univariate panel count data.

One can easily see that as U_{PSZ}, the statistic U_{ZVS} compares the estimators of individual mean functions directly and represents the integrated weighted differences between the estimated mean functions. As mentioned above, similar test statistics are commonly used in failure time data analysis for the comparison of survival functions as well as in other fields. Instead of using the statistic U_{ZVS}, one could construct test statistics that compare the estimators of individual mean functions to the estimator of the overall mean function under the hypothesis as the statistic U_{SF} discussed in Sect. 4.2.1.

In general, as commented before, it is natural to expect that the statistic U_{ZVS} has better power although the two should be asymptotically equivalent.

The statistic U_{ZVS} can be rewritten as

$$U_{ZVS} = \sqrt{\frac{n_1 n_2}{n^3}} \sum_{i=1}^{n} \sum_{k=1}^{K} \sum_{j=1}^{m_i} W_{n,k}(t_{i,j}) \{\hat{\mu}_{I,k1}(t_{i,j}) - \hat{\mu}_{I,k2}(t_{i,j})\}.$$

Under H_0^K and some regular condition, Zhao et al. (2013c) show that for large n, one can approximate the distribution of U_{ZVS} by the normal distribution with mean zero and the variance that can be consistently estimated by

$$\hat{\sigma}_{ZVS}^2 = \frac{n_2}{n\,n_1} \sum_{i=1}^{n_1} \left[\sum_{k=1}^{K} \sum_{j=1}^{m_i} W_{n,k}(t_{i,j}) \{N_{ik}(t_{i,j}) - \hat{\mu}_{I,k1}(t_{i,j})\} \right]^2$$

$$+ \frac{n_1}{n\,n_2} \sum_{i=n_1+1}^{n} \left[\sum_{k=1}^{K} \sum_{j=1}^{m_i} W_{n,k}(t_{i,j}) \{N_{ik}(t_{i,j}) - \hat{\mu}_{I,k2}(t_{i,j})\} \right]^2.$$

Hence one can perform the test of the null hypothesis H_0^K by using the statistic $U_{ZVS}^* = U_{ZVS}/\hat{\sigma}_{ZVS}$ based on the standard normal distribution.

In the above, it is assumed that $\hat{\mu}_{I,k1}(t)$ and $\hat{\mu}_{I,k2}(t)$ denote the isotonic regression estimators. Actually one can employ any consistent estimators of $\mu_{k1}(t)$ and $\mu_{k2}(t)$ such as the maximum likelihood estimators discussed in Chap. 3 and the results given above still hold (Zhao et al., 2013c). To apply the test procedure above, one needs to choose the weight process $W_{n,k}(t)$. It is clear that a simple and natural choice is to set all $W_{n,k}(t)$ to be the same such as $W_{n,k}(t) = 1$. Another natural choice is to take $W_{n,k}(t) = \sum_{i=1}^{n} I(t \leq t_{i,m_i})/n$. If observation times for different types of events are different, instead of the latter choice, one could also set $W_{n,k}(t)$ to be proportional to the number of subjects under observation at time t for type k recurrent events. It is apparent that the general comments given in Chap. 4 on the selection of weight processes apply here.

7.2.2 An Application

Now we illustrate the nonparametric comparison procedure described above by using the data arising from the skin cancer chemoprevention trial discussed in Sect. 1.2.4 and given in data set III of Chap. 9. As mentioned before, the data consist of 290 patients with a history of non-melanoma skin cancers and they were supposed to be assessed or observed every 6 months. However, as expected, the real observation and follow-up times differ from patient to patient. The patients were randomized to either a placebo group (147) or the DFMO group (143). In addition to the observation times, the observed data

7.2 Nonparametric Comparison of Cumulative Mean Functions

include the numbers of occurrences of two types of recurrent events, basal cell carcinoma and squamous cell carcinoma. One of the goals of the trial is to evaluate the overall effectiveness of DFMO in reducing the recurrence rates of both types of new skin cancers in these patients.

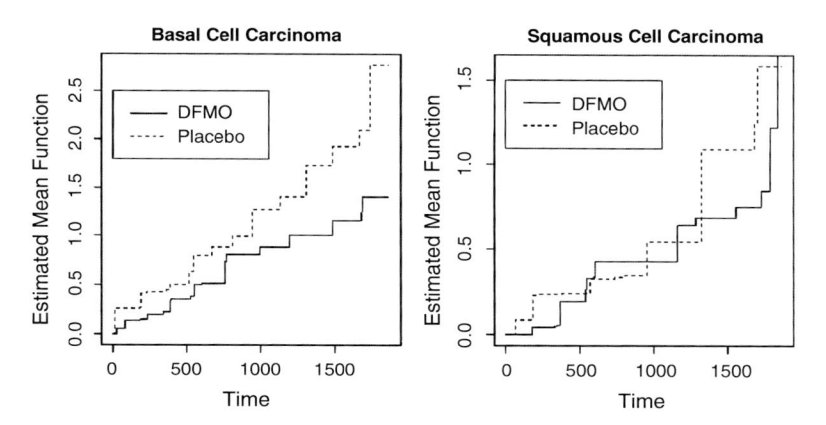

Fig. 7.1. Estimated mean functions of the recurrences of the new skin cancers

To apply the test procedure discussed in the previous subsection, for subject i, define $N_{i1}(t)$ and $N_{i2}(t)$ to be the processes representing the cumulative numbers of the occurrences of basal cell carcinoma and quamous cell carcinoma, respectively, up to time t, $i = 1, \ldots, 290$. Let $\mu_{11}(t)$ and $\mu_{21}(t)$ represent the cumulative mean functions of the occurrences of basal cell carcinoma and squamous cell carcinoma, respectively, for the patients in the DFMO treatment group. The functions $\mu_{12}(t)$ and $\mu_{22}(t)$ have the same meaning but for the patients in the placebo treatment group. The application of the test procedure with $W_{n,k}(t) = 1$ gives $U^*_{ZVS} = -1.748$. With the use of $W_{n,k}(t) = \sum_{i=1}^{n} I(t \leq t_{i,m_i})/n$, we have $U^*_{ZVS} = -1.660$. Both results indicate that overall the DFMO treatment seems to have some mild effects in reducing the recurrence rates of basal cell carcinoma and quamous cell carcinoma.

To give a graphical comparison of the two groups, Fig. 7.1 presents the IRE of the four mean functions $\mu_{11}(t)$, $\mu_{12}(t)$, $\mu_{21}(t)$ and $\mu_{22}(t)$ with the time scale being days. It suggests that the DFMO treatment seems to have some effects in reducing the recurrence rate of basal cell carcinoma but does not seem to have any effect on the recurrence rate of squamous cell carcinoma.

7.2.3 Discussion

As discussed in Chap. 4, the nonparametric treatment comparison based on univariate panel count data is needed or occurs in many fields including clinical trials, medical follow-up studies and tumorigenicity experiments. This is the same for multivariate panel count data. Also as pointed out before, the test procedure described above is a generalization of that given in Sect. 4.2.2 for univariate panel count data. Actually one could follow the same idea to generalize other test procedures discussed in Chap. 4. Note that the method adopted here is essentially a marginal approach in that it leaves the relationship between different types of recurrent events completely unspecified. Of course, one could develop some semiparametric or joint model approaches that involve modeling the correlation between different types of recurrent events. It is easy to see that the former is usually simpler and preferred in practice.

The test procedure described above can be easily generalized to general p-sample situations. To be specific, let $\mu_{kl}(t)$ denote the mean function of the recurrent event process for the kth type recurrent event corresponding to treatment l, $l = 1, \ldots, p$, $k = 1, \ldots, K$. Suppose that one is interested in testing the null hypothesis

$$H_0^{K*} : \mu_{k1}(t) = \ldots = \mu_{kp}(t) \text{ for all } k.$$

Let $\hat{\mu}_{I,kl}(t)$ denote the IRE of $\mu_{kl}(t)$ based on the lth sample on the kth type recurrent event, $l = 1, \ldots, p$, $k = 1, \ldots, K$. To test the hypothesis H_0^{K*}, similar to the statistic given in (7.1), one can consider the test statistic $U = (U_2, \ldots, U_p)^T$ with

$$U_l = \sqrt{\frac{n_1 n_l}{n}} \sum_{k=1}^{K} \int_0^{\tau} W_{n,kl}(t) \{ \hat{\mu}_{I,k1}(t) - \hat{\mu}_{I,kl}(t) \} \, dG_n(t),$$

$l = 2, \ldots, p$. In the above, n_l denotes the number of study subjects in the lth sample and the $W_{n,kl}(t)$'s are some bounded weight processes as the $W_{n,k}(t)$'s. The asymptotic normality of U under H_0^{K*} can be developed by following the argument similar to that used in Zhao et al. (2013c).

Note that for the test procedure given in the previous subsection, it has been assumed that the observation times or processes for different types of recurrent events are the same for simplicity. Although this is usually true for many recurrent event studies such as the skin cancer trial discussed above, sometimes different observation times may be used for different types of recurrent events. For this latter situation, the approach given above is actually still valid except that one needs to redefine the empirical observation process $G_n(t)$ used in (7.1).

Another assumption behind the test procedure above is that all observation times follow the same distribution for all subjects in different treatment groups. We remark that this assumption is generally reasonable for most of medical studies with periodic follow-ups such as clinical trials. In this situation, subjects are usually scheduled to be observed at prespecified observation time points. Although actual observation times may vary from these prespecified time points and from subject to subject, the variation can often be regarded as being independent of treatments. On the other hand, sometimes this may not be true as discussed in Chaps. 4 and 6 and in these situations, some new test procedures are needed. Also as discussed before, of course, the distributions of the observation times cannot be completely different among treatment groups as otherwise, it may not be possible for nonparametric comparison.

In the next section, we discuss methods for regression analysis of multivariate panel count data. For treatment comparison, as with univariate panel count data, one could also define some treatment indicators and employ the regression procedures discussed below.

7.3 Regression Analysis with Independent Observation Processes

This section discusses regression analysis of multivariate panel count data. For the discussion, we assume that the underlying recurrent event process of interest and the observation process are independent given covariates. The problem to be investigated is the same as that considered in Chap. 5 except that now there exist several related types of recurrent events rather than only one type of recurrent events as before. For the analysis, we first describe two marginal mean models for the recurrent event processes of interest and the observation process, respectively, along with some assumptions. Similar to the semiparametric transformation model (5.15), the models are quite general and include the proportional mean models (1.4) and (5.4) as special cases. Some estimating equations are then presented for estimation of regression parameters, and the estimation of the underlying mean functions is also discussed. The approach is illustrated by using a set of bivariate panel count data on psoriatic arthritis, collected from the University of Toronto Psoriatic Arthritis Clinic. It is followed by some discussion on the generalizations of the presented inference procedure among other issues.

7.3.1 Assumptions and Models

As in the previous section, consider a recurrent event study that involves n independent subjects and in which each subject may experience K different types of recurrent events. Also as before, suppose that only panel count data are available and let $N_{ik}(t)$'s be defined as in the previous section for $0 \leq t \leq \tau$, where τ is a known constant representing the study length, $i = 1, \ldots, n$, $k = 1, \ldots, K$. Furthermore, suppose that for each subject, there exist a positive random variable C_i representing the censoring or follow-up time on the subject and a $p \times 1$ vector of covariates denoted by $\boldsymbol{Z}_i$, $i = 1, \ldots, n$.

Note that here for the simplicity of presentation, we assume that the follow-up time or observation period and the covariates are the same for different types of recurrent events. Some comments on them are given below. Also we assume that the covariates are time-independent and the main goal of the study is to estimate the effects of $\mathbf{Z}_i$ on $N_{ik}(t)$.

To describe the observed panel count data, let $0 < t_{ik,1} < \ldots < t_{ik,m_{ik}}$ denote the observation times on $N_{ik}(t)$, where m_{ik} is the potential or scheduled number of observations on the kth type of recurrent events for subject i, $i = 1, \ldots, n$, $k = 1, \ldots, K$. For each i and k, define $H_{ik}(t) = \tilde{H}_{ik}\{\min(t, C_i)\}$, where $\tilde{H}_{ik}(t) = \sum_{j=1}^{m_{ik}} I(t_{ik,j} \leq t)$. It is easy to see that $H_{ik}(t)$ is a point process characterizing the observation process on subject i with respect to the kth type recurrent event, and it jumps by one only at the observation times on $N_{ik}(t)$. Then the observed data have the form

$$\{\, t_{ik,j}, N_{ik}(t_{ik,j}), C_i, \mathbf{Z}_i \,;\, j = 1, \ldots, m_{ik}, i = 1, \ldots, n, k = 1, \ldots, K \,\} \tag{7.2}$$

or

$$\{\, H_{ik}(t), N_{ik}(t)\, dH_{ik}(t), C_i, \mathbf{Z}_i \,;\, t \leq C_i, i = 1, \ldots, n, k = 1, \ldots, K \,\}. \tag{7.3}$$

For the effects of covariates on $N_{ik}(t)$, we assume that given $\mathbf{Z}_i$, the marginal mean function of $N_{ik}(t)$ has the form

$$E\{\, N_{ik}(t)\,|\,\mathbf{Z}_i \,\} = \mu_k(t)\, g_N(\mathbf{Z}_i^T \boldsymbol{\beta}). \tag{7.4}$$

Here $\mu_k(t)$ is an unknown, positive, strictly increasing and continuous baseline mean function, $\boldsymbol{\beta}$ a $p \times 1$ vector of regression parameters representing the effects of $\mathbf{Z}_i$ on $N_{ik}(t)$, and $g_N(\cdot)$ a known, positive function assumed to be strictly increasing and twice differentiable. With respect to the effects of covariates on the observation process, it is assumed that $\tilde{H}_{ik}(t)$ is a counting process with the marginal mean function

$$E\{\tilde{H}_{ik}(t)\,|\,\mathbf{Z}_i\} = \tilde{\mu}_k(t)\, g_H(\mathbf{Z}_i^T \boldsymbol{\gamma}) \tag{7.5}$$

given $\mathbf{Z}_i$. In the above, as with model (7.4), $\tilde{\mu}_k(t)$ is also a completely unknown, positive, strictly increasing and continuous baseline mean function, $\boldsymbol{\gamma}$ denotes the effects of covariates on $\tilde{H}_{ik}(t)$, and $g_H(\cdot)$ is a known, positive function also assumed to be strictly increasing and twice differentiable.

It is apparent that models (7.4) and (7.5) with $K = 1$ include models (1.4) and (5.4) as special cases, respectively, and different link functions $g_N(\cdot)$ and $g_H(\cdot)$ give different models. Model (7.4) assumes that baseline mean functions can be different for different types of recurrent events, but the effects of covariates on different types of recurrent events are identical. The same is true for model (7.5) with respect to the observation process. Some comments are given below for the situation where the covariate effects may be different for different types of recurrent events. With respect to the choice of the

7.3 Regression Analysis with Independent Observation Processes

link functions $g_N(\cdot)$ and $g_H(\cdot)$, a commonly used one is $g_N(x) = g_H(x) = \exp(x)$, which gives the proportional mean models. Some other choices include $g_N(x) = g_H(x) = 1 + x$ and $g_N(x) = g_H(x) = \log(1 + e^x)$. Of course, for a given problem, $g_N(\cdot)$ and $g_H(\cdot)$ do not have to be identical.

In the next subsection, we describe some estimating equations for estimation of regression parameters $\boldsymbol{\beta}$ as well as $\boldsymbol{\gamma}$. In this chapter, we assume that the C_i's follow the same distribution function.

7.3.2 Estimation Procedure

To derive the estimating equations for estimation of regression parameters, for each i and k, define

$$\bar{N}_{ik} = \sum_{j=1}^{m_{ik}} N_{ik}(t_{ik,j}) I(t_{ik,j} \leq C_i) = \int_0^T N_{ik}(t) \, dH_{ik}(t),$$

$i = 1, \ldots, n$, $k = 1, \ldots, K$. Note that conditional on $\boldsymbol{Z}_i$ and under models (7.4) and (7.5), we have

$$E\{\bar{N}_{ik} \mid \boldsymbol{Z}_i\} = \alpha_k \, g_N(\boldsymbol{Z}_i^T \boldsymbol{\beta}) \, g_H(\boldsymbol{Z}_i^T \boldsymbol{\gamma}),$$

where $\alpha_k = \int_0^T \mu_k(t) \, P(C_i \geq t) \, d\tilde{\mu}_k(t)$. Suppose that the covariates $\boldsymbol{Z}_i$'s are centered. Then by following the idea used in Sect. 5.3.2, a natural estimating function is given by

$$U_{MI}(\boldsymbol{\beta}, \boldsymbol{\gamma}) = \frac{1}{\sqrt{n}} \sum_{k=1}^K \sum_{i=1}^n \boldsymbol{Z}_i \, \bar{N}_{ik} \left\{ g_N(\boldsymbol{Z}_i^T \boldsymbol{\beta}) \right\}^{-1} \left\{ g_H(\boldsymbol{Z}_i^T \boldsymbol{\gamma}) \right\}^{-1} \quad (7.6)$$

assuming that $\boldsymbol{\gamma}$ is known.

Of course, the parameter $\boldsymbol{\gamma}$ is unknown in reality. For its estimation or the estimation of model (7.5), note that we have recurrent event data. Define $Y_i(t) = I(t \leq C_i)$, indicating if subject i is at risk of experiencing recurrent events at time t, $i = 1, \ldots, n$. Also define

$$S_k^{(d)}(t; \boldsymbol{\gamma}) = \frac{1}{n} \sum_{i=1}^n Y_i(t) \, \boldsymbol{Z}_i^{\otimes d} \, g_H^{(d)}(\boldsymbol{Z}_i^T \boldsymbol{\gamma}),$$

and

$$E_k(t; \boldsymbol{\gamma}) = \frac{S_k^{(1)}(t; \boldsymbol{\gamma})}{S_k^{(0)}(t; \boldsymbol{\gamma})},$$

$d = 0, 1, 2$, $k = 1, \ldots, K$. Suppose that the limits of $S_k^{(d)}(t; \boldsymbol{\gamma})$ and $E_k(t; \boldsymbol{\gamma})$ exist. Cai and Schaubel (2004) suggest to estimate $\boldsymbol{\gamma}$ by the following estimating equation

$$H_M(\boldsymbol{\gamma}) = \frac{1}{\sqrt{n}} \sum_{i=1}^{n} \sum_{k=1}^{K} \int_0^\tau \left\{ \boldsymbol{Z}_i \frac{g_H^{(1)}(\boldsymbol{Z}_i^T \boldsymbol{\gamma})}{g_H(\boldsymbol{Z}_i^T \boldsymbol{\gamma})} - E_k(s; \boldsymbol{\gamma}) \right\} dH_{ik}(s) = 0,$$

where $g_H^{(1)}(\cdot)$ denotes the derivative of $g_H(\cdot)$. It should be noted that the estimating equation above only makes use of the observed information on the observation processes $H_{ik}(t)$'s. Let $\hat{\boldsymbol{\gamma}}_M$ denote the solution to the equation above. Then it is natural to estimate $\boldsymbol{\beta}$ by the solution to $U_{MI}(\boldsymbol{\beta}, \hat{\boldsymbol{\gamma}}_M) = 0$.

Let $\hat{\boldsymbol{\beta}}_{MI}$ denote the estimator of $\boldsymbol{\beta}$ defined above and $\boldsymbol{\beta}_0$ and $\boldsymbol{\gamma}_0$ the true values of $\boldsymbol{\beta}$ and $\boldsymbol{\gamma}$, respectively. To describe the asymptotic properties of $\hat{\boldsymbol{\beta}}_{MI}$ as well as $\hat{\boldsymbol{\gamma}}_M$, for $k = 1, \ldots, K$, define

$$S_k^{(3)}(t; \boldsymbol{\gamma}) = \frac{1}{n} \sum_{i=1}^{n} Y_i(t) \boldsymbol{Z}_i^{\otimes 2} \left\{ g_H^{(1)}(\boldsymbol{Z}_i^T \boldsymbol{\gamma}) \right\}^2 \left\{ g_H(\boldsymbol{Z}_i^T \boldsymbol{\gamma}) \right\}^{-1},$$

$$V_k(t; \boldsymbol{\gamma}) = \frac{S_k^{(3)}(t; \boldsymbol{\gamma})}{S_k^{(0)}(t; \boldsymbol{\gamma})} - E_k(t; \boldsymbol{\gamma})^{\otimes 2},$$

and $H_{\cdot k}(t) = \sum_{i=1}^{n} H_{ik}(t)$. Assume that the limit of $V_k(t; \boldsymbol{\gamma})$ exists. He et al. (2008) show that under some mild regularity conditions, $\hat{\boldsymbol{\beta}}_{MI}$ is unique and consistent. Furthermore, they show that the distribution of $\sqrt{n}(\hat{\boldsymbol{\beta}}_{MI} - \boldsymbol{\beta}_0)$ can be asymptotically approximated by the multivariate normal distribution with mean zero and the covariance matrix

$$\hat{\Sigma}_{MI}(\hat{\boldsymbol{\beta}}_{MI}) = \hat{F}^{-1} \hat{G} \hat{\Gamma} \hat{G}^T \{\hat{F}^T\}^{-1}.$$

In the above, $\hat{G} = (I_p, -\hat{D}\hat{A}^{-1}(\hat{\boldsymbol{\gamma}}_M))$,

$$\hat{F} = -\frac{1}{n} \sum_{i=1}^{n} \sum_{k=1}^{K} \left\{ g_N(\boldsymbol{Z}_i^T \hat{\boldsymbol{\beta}}_{MI}) \right\}^{-2} g_N^{(1)}(\boldsymbol{Z}_i^T \hat{\boldsymbol{\beta}}_{MI}) \left\{ g_H(\boldsymbol{Z}_i^T \hat{\boldsymbol{\gamma}}_M) \right\}^{-1} \bar{N}_{ik} \boldsymbol{Z}_i \boldsymbol{Z}_i^T,$$

and

$$\hat{\Gamma} = \begin{pmatrix} \hat{\Sigma}_U & \hat{\Sigma}_{UH} \\ \hat{\Sigma}_{UH}^T & \hat{\Sigma}_H \end{pmatrix},$$

where I_p denotes the $p \times p$ identity matrix,

$$\hat{D} = -\frac{1}{n} \sum_{i=1}^{n} \sum_{k=1}^{K} \left\{ g_N(\boldsymbol{Z}_i^T \hat{\boldsymbol{\beta}}_{MI}) \right\}^{-1} g_H^{(1)}(\boldsymbol{Z}_i^T \hat{\boldsymbol{\gamma}}_M) \left\{ g_H(\boldsymbol{Z}_i^T \hat{\boldsymbol{\gamma}}_M) \right\}^{-2} \bar{N}_{ik} \boldsymbol{Z}_i \boldsymbol{Z}_i^T,$$

$$\hat{A}(\boldsymbol{\gamma}) = -\frac{1}{n} \sum_{k=1}^{K} \int_0^\tau V_k(t; \boldsymbol{\gamma}) \, dH_{\cdot k}(t),$$

7.3 Regression Analysis with Independent Observation Processes

$$\hat{\Sigma}_U = \frac{1}{n} \sum_{i=1}^{n} \left[\sum_{k=1}^{K} \mathbf{Z}_i \bar{N}_{ik} \left\{ g_N(\mathbf{Z}_i^T \hat{\boldsymbol{\beta}}_{MI}) \right\}^{-1} \left\{ g_H(\mathbf{Z}_i^T \hat{\boldsymbol{\gamma}}_M) \right\}^{-1} \right]^{\otimes 2},$$

$$\hat{\Sigma}_H = \frac{1}{n} \sum_{i=1}^{n} \left[\sum_{k=1}^{K} \int_0^\tau \left\{ \mathbf{Z}_i \frac{g_H^{(1)}(\mathbf{Z}_i^T \hat{\boldsymbol{\gamma}}_M)}{g_H(\mathbf{Z}_i^T \hat{\boldsymbol{\gamma}}_M)} - E_k(t; \hat{\boldsymbol{\gamma}}_M) \right\} d\hat{M}_{ik}(t; \hat{\boldsymbol{\gamma}}_M) \right]^{\otimes 2},$$

and

$$\hat{\Sigma}_{UH} = \frac{1}{n} \sum_{i=1}^{n} \left[\sum_{k=1}^{K} \mathbf{Z}_i \bar{N}_{ik} \left\{ g_N(\mathbf{Z}_i^T \hat{\boldsymbol{\beta}}_{MI}) \right\}^{-1} \left\{ g_H(\mathbf{Z}_i^T \hat{\boldsymbol{\gamma}}_M) \right\}^{-1} \right]$$

$$\times \left[\sum_{k=1}^{K} \int_0^\tau \left\{ \mathbf{Z}_i \frac{g_H^{(1)}(\mathbf{Z}_i^T \hat{\boldsymbol{\gamma}}_M)}{g_H(\mathbf{Z}_i^T \hat{\boldsymbol{\gamma}}_M)} - E_k(t; \hat{\boldsymbol{\gamma}}_M) \right\} d\hat{M}_{ik}(t; \hat{\boldsymbol{\gamma}}_M) \right]^T$$

with

$$d\hat{M}_{ik}(t; \boldsymbol{\gamma}) = dH_{ik}(t) - Y_i(t) g_H(\mathbf{Z}_i^T \boldsymbol{\gamma}) d\hat{\tilde{\mu}}_k(t; \boldsymbol{\gamma})$$

and

$$\hat{\tilde{\mu}}_k(t; \boldsymbol{\gamma}) = \int_0^t \frac{dH_{\cdot k}(s)}{n\, S_k^{(0)}(s; \boldsymbol{\gamma})}.$$

Note that the last quantity $\hat{\tilde{\mu}}_k(t; \boldsymbol{\gamma})$ is a generalization of the estimator (1.10) for the baseline mean function $\tilde{\mu}_k(t)$ given $\boldsymbol{\gamma}$, $i = 1, \ldots, n$, $k = 1, \ldots, K$.

In addition the distribution of $\hat{\boldsymbol{\beta}}_{MI}$, in practice, one may also be interested in or need the distribution of $\hat{\boldsymbol{\gamma}}_M$ or the joint distribution of $\hat{\boldsymbol{\beta}}_{MI}$ and $\hat{\boldsymbol{\gamma}}_M$ as well as the estimation of the baseline mean functions $\mu_k(t)$, $k = 1, \ldots, K$. For the former, He et al. (2008) prove that one can asymptotically approximate the joint distribution of $\sqrt{n}\,(\hat{\boldsymbol{\beta}}_{MI} - \boldsymbol{\beta}_0)$ and $\sqrt{n}\,(\hat{\boldsymbol{\gamma}}_M - \boldsymbol{\gamma}_0)$ by the multivariate normal distribution with mean zero and the covariance matrix

$$\hat{\Sigma}_{MI}(\hat{\boldsymbol{\beta}}_{MI}, \hat{\boldsymbol{\gamma}}_M) = -\hat{F}^{-1} \hat{G}\, \hat{\varGamma}\, \hat{G}_0^T.$$

Here $\hat{G}_0 = (0_p, -\hat{A}^{-1}(\hat{\boldsymbol{\gamma}}))$ with 0_p denoting the $p \times p$ zero matrix. For estimation of $\mu_k(t)$, one way is to apply the isotonic regression approach discussed in Sect. 3.3. A simpler method is to estimate $d\mu_k(t)$ first by the estimator similar to that given in (3.9) and then $\mu_k(t)$ by the integration of the estimated $d\mu_k(t)$. Specifically, given $\mathbf{Z}_i$ and $\boldsymbol{\beta}$ and under model (7.4), a natural estimator of the rate function $d\mu_k(t)$ based on subject i is given by the empirical estimator

$$d\hat{\mu}_{ik}(t; \boldsymbol{\beta}) = \sum_{j=1}^{m_{ik}} \frac{N_{ik}(t_{ik,j}) - N_{ik}(t_{ik,j-1})}{t_{ik,j} - t_{ik,j-1}} \left\{ g_N(\mathbf{Z}_i^T \boldsymbol{\beta}) \right\}^{-1} I(t_{ik,j-1} < t \le t_{ik,j}),$$

where $t_{ik,0} = 0$, $i = 1, \ldots, n$, $k = 1, \ldots, K$. This gives the empirical estimator

$$\hat{\mu}_k(t; \hat{\boldsymbol{\beta}}_{MI}) = \int_0^t \frac{\sum_{i=1}^n d\hat{\mu}_{ik}(s; \hat{\boldsymbol{\beta}}_{MI})}{\sum_{i=1}^n I(s \leq t_{ik,m_{ik}})} \qquad (7.7)$$

for $\mu_k(t)$, $0 \leq t \leq \max\{t_{ik,m_{ik}}\}$, $k = 1, \ldots, K$.

7.3.3 Analysis of Psoriatic Arthritis Data

In this subsection, we illustrate the methodology described above by using a set of bivariate panel count data collected from the University of Toronto Psoriatic Arthritis Clinic on the patients with psoriatic arthritis (Gladman et al., 1995). During the collection, the patients were examined or assessed from time to time, and at each assessment time, the number of the joints that were found to be damaged since the previous assessment time is recorded. In other words, the event of interest is if a joint is damaged. There exist two different methods for the assessment of patient's joints, which lead to or define two types of recurrent events. One is the functional assessment, which was scheduled annually and means that the patients undergo a detailed physical examination including a careful assessment of each joint. During the examination, a joint is classified as damaged if there is evidence of deformity or ankylosis, if it flails, or if it becomes damaged to the point that surgery is required. The other assessment method is the radiological assessment, which was scheduled to be performed on the patients at 2 year intervals. Based on the obtained films, a joint is classified as damaged if there is evidence of surface erosions of the bone in the joint, joint space narrowing, disorganization of the joint, or surgery being required.

For the panel count data above, it is apparent that the observation times are different for the two underlying point processes representing the occurrence processes of two types of damaged joints. Actually although each of the two types of assessments is scheduled at regular times, as expected, the actual assessment times and frequency of both types of assessments varied considerably from patient to patient. Also there exist some long periods during which no any assessment was made, and occasionally the two types of assessments did occur at the same time. In addition to the assessment times and the recorded numbers of damaged joints, the observed data also include information on three baseline covariates. They are the presence of a family history of psoriasis (yes/no), arthritis duration (years), and the number of active (defined as tender or swollen) joints at clinic entry. Our interest here is to evaluate the effects of the three baseline covariates on the occurrence rates of damaged joints. Also it is of interest to estimate and compare the occurrence rates between the two types of damaged joints. The analysis below is based on the 177 female patients who had baseline and at least one follow-up assessment with complete covariate data.

For the analysis of multivariate panel count data, as discussed above, one could equivalently conduct univariate analysis if different types of recurrent

7.3 Regression Analysis with Independent Observation Processes

events are not related. For the two types of damaged joints considered here, it is not hard to see that they are expected to be correlated. To further see this, we calculate the empirical or sample event rates defined as the total numbers of the detected damaged joints divided by the last assessment time for all patients and present them in Fig. 7.2. In the plot, the horizontal direction represents the sample rates for the functionally damaged joints, while the vertical direction is for the radiologically damaged joints corresponding to each subject. To give a reference, a dashed line with slope one is included in the figure. It suggests that as expected, the two types of recurrent events considered here are closely correlated. Furthermore, it seems that the rates of the radiologically damaged joints are higher than these of the functionally damaged joints although the difference may not be significant.

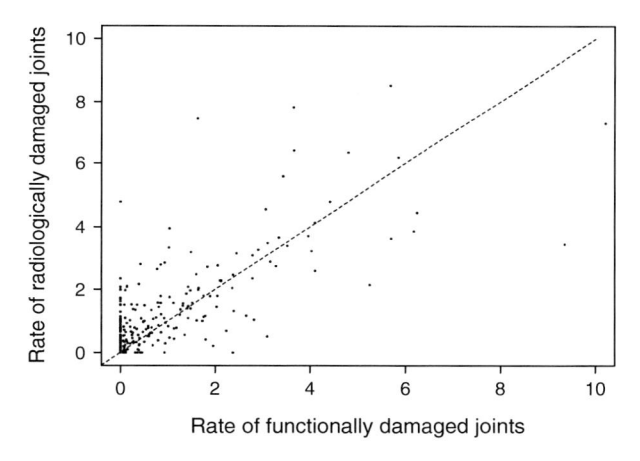

Fig. 7.2. Empirical rate functions of two types of damaged joints

To conduct the formal regression analysis, for patient i, define $N_{i1}(t)$ and $N_{i2}(t)$ to represent the cumulative numbers of radiologically and functionally damaged joints up to time t, respectively, $i = 1, \ldots, 177$. Also for patient i, define $Z_{i1} = 1$ if the patient had a family history of psoriasis and 0 otherwise, and Z_{i2} and Z_{i3} to be the arthritis duration and the number of active joints at clinic entry, respectively. The application of the methodology described above with $g_N(x) = g_H(x) = \exp(x)$ gives the results presented in Table 7.1. It includes $\hat{\gamma}_M$ and $\hat{\boldsymbol{\beta}}_{MI}$, the estimated effects of the baseline covariates on both the assessment time processes and the occurrence processes of damaged joints. For the estimated regression parameters, the table also gives their estimated standard errors (SE) and the p-values for testing each of the components equal to zero. For comparison, the univariate analysis, based on the same method but with setting $K = 1$, is also performed on the two types of damaged joints separately and the results are included in Table 7.1.

Table 7.1. Estimated effects of covariates on the assessment time processes and the occurrence processes of the two types of damaged joints

Covariate	$\hat{\gamma}_M$	SE($\hat{\gamma}_M$)	p-value	$\hat{\boldsymbol{\beta}}_{MI}$	SE($\hat{\boldsymbol{\beta}}_{MI}$)	p-value
Multivariate analysis						
Family history of psoriasis	0.1689	0.1165	0.1470	−1.4111	0.3913	0.0003
Duration of PsA in years	−0.0015	0.0057	0.7936	0.0587	0.0197	0.0029
Number of active joints	0.0030	0.0060	0.6106	0.0669	0.0194	0.0006
Univariate analysis of radiologically damaged joints						
Family history of psoriasis	0.1375	0.1403	0.3271	−0.9376	0.3653	0.0103
Duration of PsA in years	−0.0043	0.0063	0.4940	0.0340	0.0210	0.1057
Number of active joints	−0.0079	0.0075	0.2957	0.0751	0.0182	<0.0001
Univariate analysis of functionally damaged joints						
Family history of psoriasis	0.1609	0.1200	0.1799	−1.5467	0.4397	0.0004
Duration of PsA in years	−0.0007	0.0058	0.9024	0.0646	0.0206	0.0017
Number of active joints	0.0048	0.0059	0.4154	0.0662	0.0211	0.0017

The multivariate analysis results above indicate that all three baseline covariates had significant effects on the occurrence rates of the two types of damaged joints. In particular, it seems that the patients with a family history of psoriasis tend to have lower occurrence rates of damaged joints, and the rates are positively related to the duration of psoriatic arthritis and the initial number of active joints. In contrast, all covariates seem to have no significant effects on the assessment time processes. With respect to the two univariate analyses, one can see that the estimated effects across the two are actually quite close. This indicates that it is reasonable to assume that they are the same on the two types of damaged joints as implied in the multivariate analysis. Also the univariate analyses seem to give similar conclusions on all effects except on the effect of the arthritis duration on the occurrence rate of radiologically damaged joints. A possible explanation for this is the relatively higher efficiency of the multivariate analysis than the univariate analysis.

To give a graphical idea about the occurrence rates of the two types of damaged joints, Fig. 7.3 presents the estimated baseline cumulative mean functions $\hat{\mu}_k(t; \hat{\boldsymbol{\beta}}_{MI})$ given in (7.7). For comparison, the estimators of the same mean functions based on the univariate analysis are also obtained and included in Fig. 7.3. One can see that for both types of damaged joints, the estimators given by the multivariate and univariate analyses are close to each other, which again supports the same covariate effect assumption used in the multivariate analysis. Also it is worth noting that the occurrence rate of radiologically damaged joints is higher than that of functionally damaged joints. In other words, a joint is more likely to be identified to be damaged by the radiological assessment or criteria than by the functional assessment or criteria. Furthermore, Fig. 7.3 shows that the multivariate analysis suggests a larger difference between the two assessments than the univariate analysis,

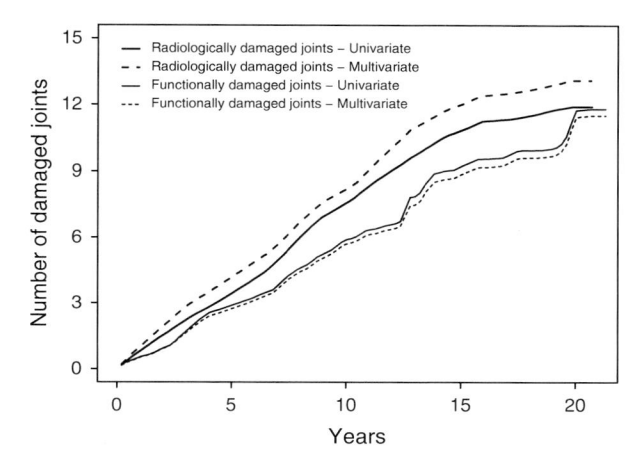

7.3 Regression Analysis with Independent Observation Processes

Fig. 7.3. Estimated baseline mean functions for two types of damaged joints

another indication that the former should be preferred in such situations rather than the latter.

7.3.4 Discussion

It is easy to see that the method described above is similar to those given in Sects. 5.3–5.5. As an alternative and similar to that discussed in Sect. 5.2, one could develop a likelihood-based approach if one is willing to make some Poisson process-related assumptions on the underlying recurrent event processes. For this, of course, some assumptions or models about the relationship between different types of recurrent event processes are needed. Actually the idea has been considered in Chen et al. (2005) under a mixed Poisson model with piecewise constant baseline intensities. For inference, they give both a likelihood-based approach, which characterizes the relationship through some log-normal random effects, and a marginal model-based procedure. It should be noted that the approaches given in Chen et al. (2005) are essentially parametric approaches. In contrast, the method described above is semiparametric and does not rely on the Poisson process and piecewise constant assumptions.

In the method described above, it has been assumed that the covariates that may affect the recurrent event processes of interest are same for different types of recurrent events. However, in practice, there may exist type-specific covariates. Another assumption that is used above and may not be true in reality is that the covariate effects in models (7.4) and (7.5) on different types of recurrent events are identical. To address these issues, one could generalize models (7.4) and (7.5) to

$$E\{N_{ik}(t) \mid \boldsymbol{Z}_{ik}\} = \mu_k(t) \, g_N(\boldsymbol{Z}_{ik}^T \boldsymbol{\beta}_k)$$

and
$$E\{\tilde{H}_{ik}(t) \,|\, \boldsymbol{Z}_{ik}\} \,=\, \tilde{\mu}_k(t)\, g_H(\boldsymbol{Z}_{ik}^T \boldsymbol{\gamma}_k)\,,$$

respectively, where $\boldsymbol{Z}_{ik}$, $\boldsymbol{\beta}_k$ and $\boldsymbol{\gamma}_k$ are type-specific covariates and regression parameters. Note that by redefining new and larger vectors of covariates, say $\boldsymbol{Z}_{ik}^*$, and regression parameters, say $\boldsymbol{\beta}^*$ and $\boldsymbol{\gamma}^*$, one could equivalently rewrite the two models above as

$$E\{\,N_{ik}(t)\,|\,\boldsymbol{Z}_{ik}^*\} \,=\, \mu_k(t)\, g_N(\boldsymbol{Z}_{ik}^{*T}\boldsymbol{\beta}^*)$$

and
$$E\{\tilde{H}_{ik}(t)\,|\,\boldsymbol{Z}_{ik}^*\} \,=\, \tilde{\mu}_k(t)\, g_H(\boldsymbol{Z}_{ik}^{*T}\boldsymbol{\gamma}^*)\,,$$

respectively. For these two latter models, an estimation procedure similar to that given in Sect. 7.3.2 can be easily developed. In addition, sometimes one may face situations where unlike required above, the distribution of the follow-up time C_i could depend on covariates. In this case, one way is to specify a model such as model (5.5) and develop some joint estimation procedures as in Sect. 5.3.2.

We conclude this section with some more comments on the differences between multivariate and univariate analyses of multivariate panel count data. One difference that has not been mentioned before is the fact that the former is usually used when the main interest is to provide a global assessment of covariate effects. In other words, the interest is to obtain the common estimators of covariate effects across several recurrent event processes. It is obvious that the univariate analysis cannot be used for this purpose. Among others, Wei et al. (1989) give some discussion on this in the context of regression analysis of multivariate failure time data. Also it is easy to see that unlike multivariate analysis, univariate analysis cannot estimate the correlations between different types of recurrent event processes. For a set of given multivariate data, it is apparent that the main advantage of conducting univariate analyses is its simplicity. Actually this is also true for the multivariate analysis based on the model with common covariate effects from the points of interpretation and discussion. In addition, the common effects can be estimated uniformly and more precisely as discussed before.

7.4 Joint Regression Analysis with Dependent Observation Processes

In this section we again discuss regression analysis of multivariate panel count data, but assume that the underlying recurrent event processes of interest and observation processes may be related as in Chap. 6. In other words, the problem to be investigated is the same as that considered in the previous section, but one needs to take into account the possible correlation between the

7.4 Joint Regression Analysis with Dependent Observation Processes

processes of interest and the observation processes. As in the previous section, we first describe two marginal models, generalizations of models (6.14) and (6.15), for the process of interest and the observation process, respectively. The estimating equation approach is then again employed for estimation of regression parameters of interest. In addition, as for models (6.14) and (6.15), the assessment of new models is discussed and a residual-based goodness-of-fit test procedure is provided. For illustration, we apply the methodology to the bivariate skin cancer panel count data discussed in Sect. 7.2, followed by some remarks on generalizations of the methodology.

7.4.1 Assumptions and Models

Consider a recurrent event study that involves n independent subjects and in which each subject may experience K different types of recurrent events as in the previous section. Also let $N_{ik}(t)$, $t_{ik,j}$, $\tilde{H}_{ik}(t)$, $H_{ik}(t)$, $\boldsymbol{Z}_i$, C_i and $Y_i(t)$ be defined as in the previous section, $j = 1, \ldots, m_{ik}$, $i = 1, \ldots, n$, $k = 1, \ldots, K$, and suppose that the observed data have the form (7.2) or (7.3). That is, we have only panel count data. Note that here again for the simplicity of presentation, we assume that the follow-up time and the covariates are the same for different types of recurrent event processes.

For regression analysis of the observe data, we follow the same idea used in the previous section to focus on the marginal models on the mean functions of both the recurrent event processes of interest and observation processes. Specifically, for the recurrent event process $N_{ik}(t)$, we assume that there exists a positive latent variable u_{ik} and given covariates $\boldsymbol{Z}_i$ and u_{ik}, the marginal mean function of $N_{ik}(t)$ has the form

$$E\{ N_{ik}(t) | \boldsymbol{Z}_i, u_{ik} \} = \mu_k(t)\, g_k(u_{ik})\, \exp(\boldsymbol{Z}_i^T \boldsymbol{\beta}) , \qquad (7.8)$$

$i = 1, \ldots, n$, $k = , 1, \ldots, K$. In the above, $\mu_k(t)$ is an unknown continuous baseline mean function, $g_k(\cdot)$ a completely unspecified positive function, and $\boldsymbol{\beta}$ a vector of regression parameters. Note that here as with model (7.4) and also for simplicity, the covariate effects are assumed to be identical for different types of recurrent events. The estimation procedure given below can be easily generalized to the situation where the effects may differ for different types of recurrent events.

For the underlying observation process $\tilde{H}_{ik}(t)$, we assume that its marginal mean function satisfies

$$E\{ \tilde{H}_{ik}(t) | \boldsymbol{Z}_i, u_{ik} \} = \tilde{\mu}_k(t)\, u_{ik}\, h_k(\boldsymbol{Z}_i) \qquad (7.9)$$

given $\boldsymbol{Z}_i$ and u_{ik}, $i = 1, \ldots, n$, $k = 1, \ldots, K$. Here $\tilde{\mu}_k(t)$ is a completely unknown continuous baseline mean function and $h_k(\cdot)$ is a completely unspecified positive function. It is worth to note that in the model above, the covariates $\boldsymbol{Z}_i$ are allowed to affect the observation process in an arbitrary and different way for different types of recurrent event processes.

It is easy to see if $K = 1$, model (7.8) reduces to model (6.14) and model (7.9) includes model (6.15) as a special case. In the following, it is assumed that for each k, the u_{ik}'s are independent and identically distributed and given u_{ik}, the two processes $N_{ik}(t)$ and $\tilde{H}_{ik}(t)$ are independent. Also it is assumed that one is mainly interested in estimation of the regression parameter $\boldsymbol{\beta}$.

7.4.2 Inference Procedure

For estimation of $\boldsymbol{\beta}$, we present a generalization of the estimation procedure described in Sect. 6.3.2. For this, by following $\tilde{N}_i(t)$ defined in Sect. 5.4.1 and used in Sect. 6.3.2, define

$$\tilde{N}_{ik}(t) = \int_0^t N_{ik}(s)\, dH_{ik}(s), \ t \geq 0.$$

Then we have

$$E\{\tilde{N}_{ik}(t)|\boldsymbol{Z}_i\} = \exp(\boldsymbol{Z}_i^T\boldsymbol{\beta})\, h_k(\boldsymbol{Z}_i)\, E\{g_k(u_{ik})u_{ik}\} \int_0^t \mu_k(s) P(C_i \geq s)\, d\tilde{\mu}_k(s)$$

and

$$E(m_{ik}|\boldsymbol{Z}_i) = E(u_{ik})\, E\{\tilde{\mu}_k(C_i)\}\, h_k(\boldsymbol{Z}_i).$$

These give

$$E\{\tilde{N}_{ik}(t)|\boldsymbol{Z}_i\} = E(m_{ik}|\boldsymbol{Z}_i) \exp\left(\boldsymbol{Z}_i^T\boldsymbol{\beta}\right) \mathcal{A}_k(t) \qquad (7.10)$$

and

$$E\{\tilde{N}_{ik}(\tau)|\boldsymbol{Z}_i\} = E(m_{ik}|\boldsymbol{Z}_i) \exp\left(\boldsymbol{Z}_i^T\boldsymbol{\beta} + \theta_k\right), \qquad (7.11)$$

where τ denotes the length of the study as before,

$$\mathcal{A}_k(t) = \frac{E\{g_k(u_{ik})u_{ik}\}}{E\{u_{ik}\}\, E\{\tilde{\mu}_k(C_i)\}} \int_0^t \mu_k(s)\, P(C_i \geq s)\, d\tilde{\mu}_k(s)$$

and

$$\theta_k = \log\left[\frac{E\{g_k(u_{ik})\, u_{ik}\}}{E(u_{ik})\, E\{\tilde{\mu}_k(C_i)\}} \int_0^\tau \mu_k(t) P(C_i \geq t)\, d\tilde{\mu}_k(t)\right],$$

an unknown parameter, $k = 1, \ldots, K$.

Now we are ready to present the estimating equation for $\boldsymbol{\beta}$. For this, define $\boldsymbol{\beta}_2 = (\boldsymbol{\beta}^T, \theta_1, \ldots, \theta_K)^T$, $\boldsymbol{e}_k$ to be the K-dimensional vector of zeros except its kth entry equal to one, and $\boldsymbol{Z}_{ik} = (\boldsymbol{Z}_i^T, \boldsymbol{e}_k^T)^T$. Then by following the equation given in (6.17) and based on (7.11), it is natural to consider the estimating equation

7.4 Joint Regression Analysis with Dependent Observation Processes

$$U_{MR}(\boldsymbol{\beta}_2) = \sum_{i=1}^{n} \sum_{k=1}^{K} w_{ik} \, \boldsymbol{Z}_{ik} \left\{ \tilde{N}_{ik}(\tau) - m_{ik} \exp\left(\boldsymbol{Z}_{ik}^T \boldsymbol{\beta}_2\right) \right\} = 0 \quad (7.12)$$

for estimation of $\boldsymbol{\beta}_2$. Here the w_{ik}'s are some weights that could depend on covariates $\boldsymbol{Z}_i$. It is easy to see that for $K = 1$, the estimating function $U_{MR}(\boldsymbol{\beta}_2)$ reduces to $U_R(\boldsymbol{\beta}_1)$ defined in (6.17).

Let $\hat{\boldsymbol{\beta}}_{2MR} = (\hat{\boldsymbol{\beta}}_{MR}^T, \hat{\theta}_1, \ldots, \hat{\theta}_K)^T$ denote the estimator of $\boldsymbol{\beta}_2$ given by the solution to the estimating equation (7.12) and $\boldsymbol{\beta}_{20}$ the true value of $\boldsymbol{\beta}_2$. Zhang et al. (2013b) show that under some regularity conditions, $\hat{\boldsymbol{\beta}}_{2MR}$ is consistent. Furthermore, the distribution of $\sqrt{n}\,(\hat{\boldsymbol{\beta}}_{2MR} - \boldsymbol{\beta}_{20})$ can be asymptotically approximated by the normal distribution with mean zero and the covariance matrix $\hat{\Sigma}_{MR} = A_{MR}^{-1} B_{MR} A_{MR}^{-1}$. Here

$$A_{MR} = \frac{1}{n} \sum_{i=1}^{n} \sum_{k=1}^{K} w_{ik} \, \boldsymbol{Z}_{ik}^T \boldsymbol{Z}_{ik} \, m_{ik} \exp\left(\boldsymbol{Z}_{ik}^T \hat{\boldsymbol{\beta}}_{2MR}\right),$$

and

$$B_{MR} = \frac{1}{n} \sum_{i=1}^{n} \hat{\phi}_i \hat{\phi}_i^T$$

with

$$\hat{\phi}_i = \sum_{k=1}^{K} w_{ik} \, \boldsymbol{Z}_{ik} \left\{ \tilde{N}_{ik}(\tau) - m_{ik} \exp\left(\boldsymbol{Z}_{ik}^T \hat{\boldsymbol{\beta}}_{2MR}\right) \right\}.$$

For the determination of $\hat{\boldsymbol{\beta}}_{2MR}$, in general, some iterative algorithms such as the Newton-Raphson algorithm are needed. On the other hand, for the two-sample situation where $Z_i = 0$ or 1, one can easily derive

$$\hat{\beta}_{MR} = \log \left\{ \frac{\sum_{i=1}^{n} \sum_{k=1}^{K} w_{ik} \, Z_i \, \tilde{N}_{ik}(\tau)}{\sum_{i=1}^{n} \sum_{k=1}^{K} w_{ik} \, I(Z_i = 1) \, m_{ik} \exp(\hat{\theta}_k)} \right\}$$

given the $\hat{\theta}_k$'s.

To finish this subsection, we discuss the generalization of the goodness-of-fit test procedure given in Sect. 6.3.2 to the situation considered here. For this, motivated by the residual process $\hat{R}_i(t)$ defined in Sect. 6.3.2 and the Eq. (7.10), we consider the residual process

$$\hat{R}_{ik}(t) = \tilde{N}_{ik}(t) - m_{ik} \exp\left(\boldsymbol{Z}_i^T \hat{\boldsymbol{\beta}}_{MR}\right) \hat{A}_k(t),$$

$i = 1, \ldots, n$, $k = 1, \ldots, K$, where

$$\hat{A}_k(t) = \left\{ \sum_{i=1}^{n} m_{ik} \exp\left(\boldsymbol{Z}_i^T \hat{\boldsymbol{\beta}}_{MR}\right) \right\}^{-1} \sum_{i=1}^{n} \tilde{N}_{ik}(t).$$

It is easy to see that $\hat{R}_{ik}(t)$ represents the difference between the observed and model-predicted numbers of the kth type recurrent events experienced by subject i up to time t. Hence for testing the goodness-of-fit of models (7.8) and (7.9), it is natural to use the statistic

$$\Phi(t, z) = n^{-1/2} \sum_{i=1}^{n} \sum_{k=1}^{K} I(Z_i \leq z) \hat{R}_{ik}(t),$$

the cumulative sum of $\hat{R}_{ik}(t)$ over the values of the Z_i's. Here as before, $I(Z_i \leq z)$ means that each of the components of Z_i is not larger than the corresponding component of z.

To establish the distribution of $\Phi(t, z)$, define

$$S_{k0}(z) = \frac{1}{n} \sum_{i=1}^{n} m_{ik} \exp\left(Z_i^T \hat{\beta}_{MR}\right),$$

$$S_k(z) = \frac{1}{n} \sum_{i=1}^{n} I(Z_i \leq z) m_{ik} \exp\left(Z_i^T \hat{\beta}_{MR}\right),$$

and

$$B(t, z) = \frac{1}{n} \sum_{i=1}^{n} \sum_{k=1}^{K} \left\{ I(Z_i \leq z) - \frac{S_k(z)}{S_{k0}(z)} \right\} Z_i m_{ik} \exp\left(Z_i^T \hat{\beta}_{MR}\right) \hat{A}_k(t).$$

Then one can approximate the distribution of $\Phi(t, z)$ (Zhang et al., 2013b) by that of the zero-mean Gaussian process

$$\hat{\Phi}(t, z) = \frac{1}{\sqrt{n}} \sum_{i=1}^{n} \sum_{k=1}^{K} \left\{ I(Z_i \leq z) - \frac{S_k(z)}{S_{k0}(z)} \right\} \hat{R}_{ik}(t) G_i$$

$$- \frac{1}{\sqrt{n}} B(t, z)^T \sum_{i=1}^{n} \hat{d}_i G_i.$$

In the above, $\hat{d}_i$ is the vector $A_{MR}^{-1} \hat{\phi}_i$ without the last K entries and $(G_1, \ldots, G_n)$ are a simple random sample from the standard normal distribution independent of the observed data. To test the appropriateness of models (7.8) and (7.9), as discussed in Sect. 6.3.2, a common approach is to use the statistic $\sup_{t, z} |\Phi(t, z)|$. For this, based on the results above, the p-value can be determined by comparing the observed value of $\sup_{t, z} |\Phi(t, z)|$ to a large number of realizations of $\sup_{t, z} |\hat{\Phi}(t, z)|$ given by repeatedly generating $(G_1, \ldots, G_n)$.

7.4.3 Analysis of Skin Cancer Chemoprevention Trial

To illustrate the inference procedure described above, we consider the bivariate panel count data arising from the skin cancer chemoprevention trial again. As discussed in Sects. 1.2.4 and 7.2.2, the trial consists of 290 patients who had been suffering two types of skin cancers, basal cell carcinoma and squamous cell carcinoma. There are two treatments involved, placebo and DFMO, and one main objective is to evaluate the effectiveness of the DFMO treatment in reducing the occurrence rates of the two types of skin cancers. In addition, there exist three baseline covariates and they are gender, age at the diagnosis and the number of prior skin cancers of the patients.

Before the analysis, as discussed in Sect. 7.3.3, it is worth to first investigate the correlation between the occurrence processes of skin cancers and the observation process. For this, Fig. 7.4 presents the separate empirical correlation curves for the two types of skin cancers, the pointwise sample correlations between the cumulative numbers of the occurrences of new skin cancers and the total numbers of observations at each observation time. Note that here for the times at which the exact cumulative number is not observed from a patient still under the follow-up, the nearest cumulative number before is used as an approximation. It indicates that the two processes seem to be positively correlated and also the correlations seem to be different for the two types of skin cancers.

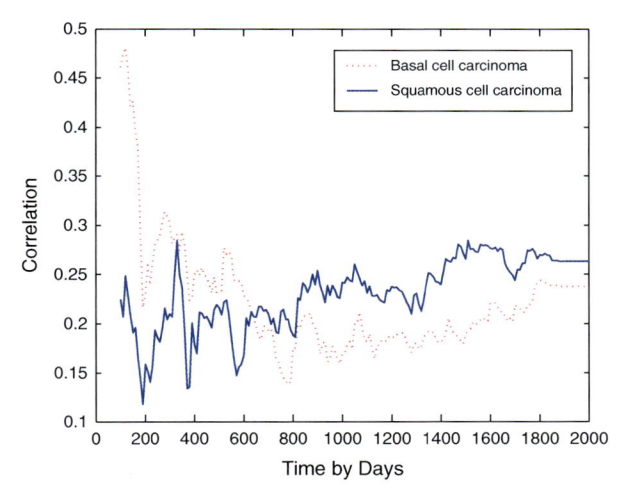

Fig. 7.4. Estimated pointwise correlations between the cancer occurrence process and the observation process for two types of skin cancers

For the analysis, define $N_{i1}(t)$ and $N_{i2}(t)$ to be the underlying counting processes controlling the occurrences of basal cell carcinoma and squamous cell carcinoma from patient i, respectively, $i = 1, \ldots, 290$. Note that for the data considered here, we have $H_{i1}(t) = H_{i2}(t)$. That is, the observation processes are the same for the two types of recurrent events. Also for patient i, define $Z_{i1} = 1$ if the patient was in the DFMO group and 0 otherwise, Z_{i2} and Z_{i3} to be the number of prior skin cancers and the age of the patient, and $Z_{i4} = 1$ if the patient is male and 0 otherwise. The results given by the inference procedure described above are presented in Table 7.2, including the estimated covariate effects as well as the estimated standard errors (SE) and 95% confidence intervals (CI) of the point estimators. They suggest that the DFMO treatment did not seem to have any significant effect on reducing the occurrence rate of the two skin cancers. Also the occurrence rate did not seem to be significantly related to the age and gender of the patient. But the occurrence rate seems to be positively related to the number of the prior skin cancers. Note that the nonparametric test given in Sect. 7.2 suggests that the DFMO treatment may have some mild effect. However, unlike here, the test in Sect. 7.2 assumes that the occurrence process of skin cancers and the observation process are independent.

For comparison, we also apply the estimation procedure discussed in Sect. 7.3 to the data considered here and the obtained results are included in Table 7.2 too. Here it is assumed that $g_N(x) = g_H(x) = x$. It is interesting to see that the analysis gives similar conclusions except that it would indicate that the occurrence rates of skin cancers were significantly different between the male and female patients. In other words, one could get misleading results if ignoring the correlation between the underlying recurrent event processes and the observation process. Finally we apply the goodness-of-fit test procedure described above to the data and obtain the p-value of 0.508 based on 1,000 realizations of $\sup_{t,z} |\hat{\Phi}(t,z)|$. This indicates that models (7.8) and (7.9) seem to be appropriate for the skin cancer data discussed here.

Table 7.2. Estimated covariate effects for the skin cancer chemoprevention trial

Method	$\hat{\beta}_1$ (SE($\hat{\beta}_1$)) 95% CI for β_1	$\hat{\beta}_2$ (SE($\hat{\beta}_2$)) 95% CI for β_2	$\hat{\beta}_3$ (SE($\hat{\beta}_3$)) 95% CI for β_3	$\hat{\beta}_4$ (SE($\hat{\beta}_4$)) 95% CI for β_4
$\hat{\boldsymbol{\beta}}_{MR}$	−0.2253 (0.1831) (−0.5842, 0.1336)	0.0784 (0.0090) (0.0608, 0.0960)	0.0016 (0.0087) (−0.0155, 0.0187)	0.2534 (0.1942) (−0.1272, 0.6340)
$\hat{\boldsymbol{\beta}}_{MI}$	−0.0239 (0.1809) (−0.3785, 0.3307)	0.1440 (0.0212) (0.1024, 0.1856)	−0.0116 (0.0084) (−0.0281, 0.0049)	0.3807 (0.1778) (0.0322, 0.7292)

7.4.4 Discussion

As mentioned above, the methodology discussed in this section can be seen as a generalization of that given in Sect. 6.3. A main advantage of them is the flexibility of the assumed models and in consequence, the resulting estimators of regression parameters are robust. Of course, the efficiency could be an issue and needs to be investigated. Also as discussed before, the illustration above again shows that in the presence of the correlation between the recurrent event process and the observation process, the use of the methods that ignore the correlation could yield misleading or wrong conclusions.

It is straightforward to generalize the inference procedure described above to the general situation where the effects of covariates may be different on different types of recurrent events. In this case, model (7.8) becomes

$$E\{N_{ik}(t)|\mathbf{Z}_i, u_{ik}\} = \mu_k(t) g_k(u_{ik}) \exp\left(\mathbf{Z}_i^T \boldsymbol{\beta}_k\right)$$

or

$$E\{N_{ik}(t)|\mathbf{Z}_{ik}, u_{ik}\} = \mu_k(t) g_k(u_{ik}) \exp\left(\mathbf{Z}_{ik}^T \boldsymbol{\beta}_k\right)$$

with $\boldsymbol{\beta}_k$ being regression parameters, $k = 1, \ldots, K$. Note that the latter case means that covariates also differ for different types of recurrent events. Also for the latter case, as discussed in Sect. 7.3.4, the model above can be equivalently rewritten as

$$E\{N_{ik}(t)|\mathbf{Z}_{ik}^*, u_{ik}\} = \mu_k(t) g_k(u_{ik}) \exp\left(\mathbf{Z}_{ik}^{*T} \boldsymbol{\beta}^*\right).$$

In the above, $\mathbf{Z}_{ik}^*$ and $\boldsymbol{\beta}^*$ are some new and larger vectors of covariates and regression parameters redefined from the original covariates and regression parameters. For the situation, model (7.9) stays the same with $\mathbf{Z}_i$ replaced by $\mathbf{Z}_{ik}$ or $\mathbf{Z}_{ik}^*$.

Another situation that is more general than that discussed above and may occur in practice is that covariates may be time-dependent or their effects are time-dependent. Of course, both can happen at the same time. In this case, model (7.8) should have the form

$$E\{N_{ik}(t)|\mathbf{Z}_i(t), u_{ik}\} = \mu_k(t) g_k(u_{ik}) \exp\left\{\mathbf{Z}_i^T(t) \boldsymbol{\beta}\right\}$$

or

$$E\{N_{ik}(t)|\mathbf{Z}_i(t), u_{ik}\} = \mu_k(t) g_k(u_{ik}) \exp\left\{\mathbf{Z}_i^T(t) \boldsymbol{\beta}(t)\right\}.$$

It is not hard to see that the estimation procedure given above cannot be applied to this latter situation and some new procedures are needed although may not be easy. It is obvious that this is especially the case when covariate effects are time-dependent. More comments on this are given in Sect. 8.6.

7.5 Conditional Regression Analysis with Dependent Observation Processes

For regression analysis of panel count data with dependent observation processes, as discussed before, sometimes one may prefer a conditional analysis rather than a joint analysis. For this, in this section, we generalize the conditional approach discussed in Sect. 6.4 to multivariate panel count data. In particular, instead of models (7.8) and (7.9), we present a class of conditional mean models for the underlying recurrent event processes of interest. The new models are generalizations of the semiparametric transformation model defined in (6.18). With respect to the observation process, the proportional rate model (5.16) is employed as before. For estimation of regression parameters, we follow the idea used in the previous section and present some estimating equations. To give a comparison, the bivariate skin cancer data are used again to illustrate the methodology. It is followed by some remarks on the relationship between the approach discussed here and ones given before as well as on some possible generalizations.

7.5.1 Assumptions and Models

As mentioned above, this section considers exactly the same problem as in the previous section, but from a different point of view. For this, let $N_{ik}(t)$, $t_{ik,j}$, $\tilde{H}_{ik}(t)$, $H_{ik}(t)$, $Z_i(t)$, C_i and $Y_i(t)$ be defined as in the previous section, $j = 1, \ldots, m_{ik}$, $i = 1, \ldots, n$, $k = 1, \ldots, K$, and suppose that one observes the panel count data given in (7.2) or (7.3). Note that here we allow the covariate $Z_i(t)$ to be time-dependent, but still assume that they and the follow-up time C_i are the same for different types of recurrent event processes for the simplicity of presentation.

To describe the conditional regression model for $N_{ik}(t)$, define $\mathcal{F}_{ikt} = \{\tilde{H}_{ik}(s), 0 \leq s < t\}$, the history or filtration of the observation process on subject i and type k recurrent events up to time $t-$, $i = 1, \ldots, n$. In the following, we assume that given $Z_i(t)$ and $\mathcal{F}_{ikt}$, the conditional mean function of $N_{ik}(t)$ has the form

$$E\{N_{ik}(t)|\, Z_i(t), \mathcal{F}_{ikt}\} = g\left\{\mu_{0k}(t)\,\exp\{\boldsymbol{\beta}^T Z_i(t) + \boldsymbol{\alpha}^T Q(\mathcal{F}_{ikt})\}\right\}. \quad (7.13)$$

Here as in model (6.18), g is a known twice continuously differentiable and strictly increasing function, $\mu_{0k}(t)$ denotes an unspecified smooth function of t, $\boldsymbol{\beta}$ and $\boldsymbol{\alpha}$ are vectors of unknown regression parameters, and $\boldsymbol{Q}$ is a vector of known functions of $\mathcal{F}_{ikt}$. It is easy to see that model (7.13) reduces to model (6.18) if $K = 1$ and means that the observation process $H_{ik}(t)$ may be informative or contain relevant information about $N_{ik}(t)$ through the parameter $\boldsymbol{\alpha}$.

7.5 Conditional Regression Analysis with Dependent Observation Processes

The comments given in Sect. 6.4 on the function vector $\boldsymbol{Q}$ apply here. In particular, one simple choice is to let $\boldsymbol{Q}(\mathcal{F}_{ikt}) = \tilde{H}_{ik}(t-)$, meaning that $N_{ik}(t)$ may depend on the total number of the observations before time t on the kth type recurrent event. This could be the case in a medical study in which a patient may pay more visits to their doctors because they feel worse than usual. As discussed before, in addition to the effects on $N_{ik}(t)$, covariates may have effects on the observation process too. For this, following the idea used in Sects. 5.5 and 6.4, we suppose that $\tilde{H}_{ik}(t)$ is a non-homogeneous Poisson process satisfying the proportional rate model

$$E\{d\tilde{H}_{ik}(t) \mid \boldsymbol{Z}_i(t)\} = \exp\{\boldsymbol{\gamma}^T \boldsymbol{Z}_i(t)\} \, d\tilde{\mu}_{0k}(t), \tag{7.14}$$

$i = 1, \ldots, n$, $k = 1, \ldots, K$. In the above, as before, $\boldsymbol{\gamma}$ denotes a vector of unknown regression parameters and $\tilde{\mu}_{0k}(t)$ is an arbitrary, unknown nondecreasing function. In the following, it is assumed that the main goal is to make inference about $\boldsymbol{\beta}$ and $\boldsymbol{\alpha}$.

7.5.2 Estimation Procedure

Now we describe the estimating equations for estimation of $\boldsymbol{\beta}$ and $\boldsymbol{\alpha}$ along with other unknowns. For this, define $\boldsymbol{Z}_{ik}(t) = (\boldsymbol{Z}_i^T(t), \boldsymbol{Q}^T(\mathcal{F}_{ikt}))^T$ and $\boldsymbol{\theta} = (\boldsymbol{\beta}^T, \boldsymbol{\alpha}^T)^T$. Also define

$$M_{ik}(t; \boldsymbol{\theta}, \boldsymbol{\gamma}) = \int_0^t Y_i(s) N_{ik}(s) \, d\tilde{H}_{ik}(s) - \int_0^t Y_i(s) g\left\{\mu_{0k}(s) \exp\{\boldsymbol{\theta}^T \boldsymbol{Z}_{ik}(s)\}\right\} \\ \times \exp\{\boldsymbol{\gamma}^T \boldsymbol{Z}_i(s)\} \, d\tilde{\mu}_{0k}(s),$$

$i = 1, \ldots, n$, $k = 1, \ldots, K$. It is easy to show that under models (7.13) and (7.14), $M_{ik}(t; \boldsymbol{\theta}, \boldsymbol{\gamma})$ is a zero-mean stochastic process for all $1 \leq i \leq n$ and $1 \leq k \leq K$. Thus it is natural to employ the estimating equation

$$\sum_{i=1}^n d\, M_{ik}(t; \boldsymbol{\theta}, \boldsymbol{\gamma}) = \sum_{i=1}^n \left[Y_i(t) \, N_{ik}(t) \, d\tilde{H}_{ik}(t) \right. \\ \left. - Y_i(t) \, g\left\{\mu_{0k}(t) \exp\{\boldsymbol{\theta}^T \boldsymbol{Z}_{ik}(t)\}\right\} \exp\{\boldsymbol{\gamma}^T \boldsymbol{Z}_i(t)\} \, d\tilde{\mu}_{0k}(t) \right] = 0, \tag{7.15}$$

$0 \leq t \leq \tau$, for estimation of $\mu_{0k}(t)$ and the estimating equation

$$U_{MT}(\boldsymbol{\theta}, \boldsymbol{\gamma}) = \sum_{i=1}^n \sum_{k=1}^K \int_0^\tau W(t) \, \boldsymbol{Z}_{ik}(t) \left[Y_i(t) \, N_{ik}(t) \, d\tilde{H}_{ik}(t) \right. \\ \left. - Y_i(t) \, g\left\{\mu_{0k}(t) \exp\{\boldsymbol{\theta}^T \boldsymbol{Z}_{ik}(t)\}\right\} \exp\{\boldsymbol{\gamma}^T \boldsymbol{Z}_i(t)\} \, d\tilde{\mu}_{0k}(t) \right] = 0 \tag{7.16}$$

for estimation of $\boldsymbol{\theta}$ given $\boldsymbol{\gamma}$ and $\tilde{\mu}_{0k}(t)$. In the above, as before, τ denotes the study length and $W(t)$ is a possibly data-dependent weight function.

It is easy to see that the stochastic process $M_{ik}(t;\boldsymbol{\theta},\boldsymbol{\gamma})$ reduces to $M_i^*(\boldsymbol{\theta},\boldsymbol{\gamma})$ defined in (6.19) if $K = 1$, and the estimating function $U_{MT}(\boldsymbol{\theta},\boldsymbol{\gamma})$ is generalizations of the estimating functions $U_T(\boldsymbol{\beta},\boldsymbol{\gamma})$ given in (5.19) and $U_T^*(\boldsymbol{\theta},\boldsymbol{\gamma})$ used in Sect. 6.4.2. To use the estimating equations (7.15) and (7.16), it is apparent that one needs to estimate $\boldsymbol{\gamma}$ and $\tilde{\mu}_{0k}(t)$ first. For this, motivated by the estimating equation (5.20) and the estimator defined in (5.21), it is natural to estimate $\boldsymbol{\gamma}$ based on the estimating equation

$$\sum_{i=1}^{n} \sum_{k=1}^{K} \int_0^\tau Y_i(t) \left\{ \boldsymbol{Z}_i(t) - \frac{S_1(t;\boldsymbol{\gamma})}{S_0(t;\boldsymbol{\gamma})} \right\} d\tilde{H}_{ik}(t) = 0, \qquad (7.17)$$

and $\tilde{\mu}_{0k}(t)$ by

$$\hat{\tilde{\mu}}_{0k}(t;\boldsymbol{\gamma}) = \sum_{i=1}^{n} \int_0^t \frac{Y_i(s)\, d\tilde{H}_{ik}(s)}{n\, S_0(s;\boldsymbol{\gamma})} \qquad (7.18)$$

for given $\boldsymbol{\gamma}$. In the above,

$$S_j(t;\boldsymbol{\gamma}) = \frac{1}{n} \sum_{i=1}^{n} Y_i(t)\, \boldsymbol{Z}_i(t)^j \, \exp\{\boldsymbol{\gamma}^T \boldsymbol{Z}_i(t)\},$$

$j = 0, 1$. Let $\hat{\boldsymbol{\gamma}}_{MT}$ denote the estimator of $\boldsymbol{\gamma}$ given by the solution to (7.17), and $\hat{\mu}_{0k}(t)$ and $\hat{\boldsymbol{\theta}}_{MT} = (\hat{\boldsymbol{\beta}}_{MT}^T, \hat{\boldsymbol{\alpha}}_{MT}^T)^T$ the estimators of $\mu_{0k}(t)$ and $\boldsymbol{\theta}$ given by the solutions to (7.15) and (7.16) with replacing $\boldsymbol{\gamma}$ and $\tilde{\mu}_{0k}(t)$ by $\hat{\boldsymbol{\gamma}}_{MT}$ and $\hat{\tilde{\mu}}_{0k}(t;\hat{\boldsymbol{\gamma}}_{MT})$, respectively. Also let $\boldsymbol{\theta}_0 = (\boldsymbol{\beta}_0^T, \boldsymbol{\alpha}_0^T)^T$ and $\boldsymbol{\gamma}_0$ denote the true values of $\boldsymbol{\theta}$ and $\boldsymbol{\gamma}$. Li et al. (2011) show that asymptotically $\hat{\mu}_{0k}(t)$ and $\hat{\boldsymbol{\theta}}_{MT}$ always exist and are unique and consistent. To give the asymptotic distribution of $\hat{\boldsymbol{\theta}}_{MT}$, define

$$\hat{M}_{ik}(t) = \int_0^t Y_i(s) N_{ik}(s) dH_{ik}(s) - \int_0^t Y_i(s) g\left\{ \hat{\mu}_{0k}(s) \exp\{\hat{\boldsymbol{\theta}}_{MT}^T \boldsymbol{Z}_{ik}(s)\} \right\}$$
$$\times \exp\left\{ \hat{\boldsymbol{\gamma}}_{MT}^T \boldsymbol{Z}_i(s) \right\} d\hat{\tilde{\mu}}_{0k}(t;\hat{\boldsymbol{\gamma}}_{MT}),$$

$$\hat{M}_{ik}^*(t) = \int_0^t Y_i(s) dH_{ik}(s) - \int_0^t Y_i(s) \exp\left\{ \hat{\boldsymbol{\gamma}}_{MT}^T \boldsymbol{Z}_i(s) \right\} d\hat{\tilde{\mu}}_{0k}(s;\hat{\boldsymbol{\gamma}}_{MT}),$$

$$\hat{E}_k(t) = \frac{\sum_{i=1}^n Y_i(t)\, \boldsymbol{Z}_{ik}(t)\, \dot{g}\{\hat{\mu}_{0k}(t)\, e^{\hat{\boldsymbol{\theta}}_{MT}^T \boldsymbol{Z}_{ik}(t)}\}\, e^{\hat{\boldsymbol{\theta}}_{MT}^T \boldsymbol{Z}_{ik}(t) + \hat{\boldsymbol{\gamma}}_{MT}^T \boldsymbol{Z}_i(t)}}{\sum_{i=1}^n Y_i(t)\, \dot{g}\{\hat{\mu}_{0k}(t)\, e^{\hat{\boldsymbol{\theta}}_{MT}^T \boldsymbol{Z}_{ik}(t)}\}\, e^{\hat{\boldsymbol{\theta}}_{MT}^T \boldsymbol{Z}_{ik}(t) + \hat{\boldsymbol{\gamma}}_{MT}^T \boldsymbol{Z}_i(t)}},$$

7.5 Conditional Regression Analysis with Dependent Observation Processes

$$\hat{R}_k(t) = \frac{1}{n} \sum_{i=1}^{n} Y_i(t) \left\{ \boldsymbol{Z}_{ik}(t) - \hat{E}_k(t) \right\} \dot{g} \left\{ \hat{\mu}_{0k}(t) \exp\{\hat{\boldsymbol{\theta}}_{MT}^T \boldsymbol{Z}_{ik}(t)\} \right\}$$
$$\times \exp\left\{ \hat{\boldsymbol{\gamma}}_{MT}^T \boldsymbol{Z}_i(t) \right\},$$

$$\hat{D} = \frac{1}{n} \sum_{i=1}^{n} \sum_{k=1}^{K} \int_{0}^{\tau} Y_i(t) \left\{ \boldsymbol{Z}_i(t) - \frac{S_1(t; \hat{\boldsymbol{\gamma}}_{MT})}{S_0(t; \hat{\boldsymbol{\gamma}}_{MT})} \right\}^{\otimes 2} dH_{ik}(t),$$

and

$$\hat{P} = \frac{1}{n} \sum_{i=1}^{n} \sum_{k=1}^{K} \int_{0}^{\tau} W(t) Y_i(t) \dot{g}\left\{ \hat{\mu}_{0k}(t) \exp\{\hat{\boldsymbol{\theta}}_{MT}^T \boldsymbol{Z}_{ik}(t)\} \right\} \exp\left\{ \hat{\boldsymbol{\gamma}}_{MT}^T \boldsymbol{Z}_i(t) \right\}$$
$$\times \left\{ \boldsymbol{Z}_{ik}(t) - \hat{E}_k(t) \right\} \left\{ \boldsymbol{Z}_i(t) - \frac{S_1(t; \hat{\boldsymbol{\gamma}}_{MT})}{S_0(t; \hat{\boldsymbol{\gamma}}_{MT})} \right\}^T d\hat{\mu}_{0k}(t; \hat{\boldsymbol{\gamma}}_{MT}).$$

In the above $\dot{g}(t) = dg(t)/dt$ and $v^{\otimes 2} = vv^T$ for a vector v. Li et al. (2011) prove that one can asymptotically approximate the distribution of $n^{1/2}(\hat{\boldsymbol{\theta}}_{MT} - \boldsymbol{\theta}_0)$ by the multivariate normal distribution with mean zero and the covariance matrix $\hat{\Sigma}_{MT} = A_{MT}^{-1} B_{MT} A_{MT}^{-1}$. Here

$$A_{MT} = \frac{1}{n} \sum_{i=1}^{n} \sum_{k=1}^{K} \int_{0}^{\tau} W(t) Y_i(t) \dot{g}\left\{ \hat{\mu}_{0k}(t) \exp\{\hat{\boldsymbol{\theta}}_{MT}^T \boldsymbol{Z}_{ik}(t)\} \right\}$$
$$\times \left\{ \boldsymbol{Z}_{ik}(t) - \hat{E}_k(t) \right\}^{\otimes 2} \exp\left\{ \hat{\boldsymbol{\theta}}_{MT}^T \boldsymbol{Z}_{ik}(t) + \hat{\boldsymbol{\gamma}}_{MT}^T \boldsymbol{Z}_i(t) \right\} \hat{\mu}_{0k}(t) d\hat{\mu}_{0k}(t; \hat{\boldsymbol{\gamma}}_{MT})$$

and

$$B_{MT} = \frac{1}{n} \sum_{i=1}^{n} \left[\sum_{k=1}^{K} \int_{0}^{\tau} W(t) \left\{ \boldsymbol{Z}_{ik}(t) - \hat{E}_k(t) \right\} d\hat{M}_{ik}(t) - \sum_{k=1}^{K} \int_{0}^{\tau} \frac{W(t)\hat{R}_k(t)}{S_0(t; \hat{\boldsymbol{\gamma}}_{MT})} \right.$$
$$\left. \times d\hat{M}_{ik}^*(t) - \hat{P}\hat{D}^{-1} \sum_{k=1}^{K} \int_{0}^{\tau} \left\{ \boldsymbol{Z}_i(t) - \frac{S_1(t; \hat{\boldsymbol{\gamma}}_{MT})}{S_0(t; \hat{\boldsymbol{\gamma}}_{MT})} \right\} d\hat{M}_{ik}^*(t) \right]^{\otimes 2}.$$

7.5.3 Determination of Estimators

For the determination of $\hat{\mu}_{0k}(t)$, $\hat{\boldsymbol{\theta}}_{MT}$ and $\hat{\boldsymbol{\gamma}}_{MT}$ or solving the Eqs. (7.15)–(7.17), note that (7.17) involves $\boldsymbol{\gamma}$ only. Thus it is natural to determine $\hat{\boldsymbol{\gamma}}_{MT}$ first, which is also relatively easy as it is based on recurrent event data (Cook and Lawless, 2007). To simplify the Eqs. (7.15) and (7.16), let $s_1 < s_2 < \ldots < s_J$ denote the distinct ordered time points of all observation times $\{t_{ik,l}; l = 1, \ldots, m_{ik}, i = 1, \ldots, n, k = 1, \ldots, K\}$. Then they can be rewritten as

$$\sum_{i=1}^{n} \sum_{l=1}^{m_{ik}} N_{ik}(t_{ik,l}) \, I(t_{ik,l} = s_j) - \sum_{i=1}^{n} Y_i(s_j)$$
$$\times g\left\{\mu_{0k}(s_j) \exp\{\boldsymbol{\beta}^T \boldsymbol{Z}_i(s_j) + \boldsymbol{\alpha}^T \boldsymbol{Q}(\mathcal{F}_{iks_j})\}\right\} \exp\{\boldsymbol{\gamma}^T \boldsymbol{Z}_i(s_j)\} \, d\tilde{\mu}_{0k}(s_j) = 0, \tag{7.19}$$

$j = 1, \ldots, J$, and

$$\sum_{i=1}^{n} \sum_{k=1}^{K} \sum_{j=1}^{m_{ik}} W(t_{ik,j}) \, \boldsymbol{Z}_{ik}(t_{ik,j}) \, N_{ik}(t_{ik,j}) - \sum_{i=1}^{n} \sum_{k=1}^{K} \sum_{j=1}^{J} Y_i(s_j) \, W(s_j) \, \boldsymbol{Z}_{ik}(s_j)$$
$$\times g\left\{\mu_{0k}(s_j) \exp\{\boldsymbol{\beta}^T \boldsymbol{Z}_i(s_j) + \boldsymbol{\alpha}^T \boldsymbol{Q}(\mathcal{F}_{iks_j})\}\right\} \exp\{\boldsymbol{\gamma}^T \boldsymbol{Z}_i(s_j)\} \, d\tilde{\mu}_{0k}(s_j) = 0, \tag{7.20}$$

respectively.

For a set of given data, it is apparent that after obtaining $\hat{\boldsymbol{\gamma}}_{MT}$, one should solve the Eq. (7.19) first to determine $\hat{\mu}_{0k}(t; \boldsymbol{\theta}, \hat{\boldsymbol{\gamma}}_{MT})$ for fixed $\boldsymbol{\theta}$ and by letting $\boldsymbol{\gamma} = \hat{\boldsymbol{\gamma}}_{MT}$. Then $\hat{\boldsymbol{\theta}}_{MT}$ can be determined by solving (7.20) with substituting $\mu_{0k}(t) = \hat{\mu}_{0k}(t; \boldsymbol{\theta}, \hat{\boldsymbol{\gamma}}_{MT})$ and $\boldsymbol{\gamma} = \hat{\boldsymbol{\gamma}}_{MT}$. In general, the closed forms for $\hat{\mu}_{0k}(t; \boldsymbol{\theta}, \hat{\boldsymbol{\gamma}}_{MT})$ and $\hat{\boldsymbol{\theta}}_{MT}$ do not exist and one needs to employ some iterative algorithms. On the other hand, there do exist some situations where their determination is not difficult.

One such situation is when $g(t) = t^\eta$, where η is a positive constant. In this case, the Eqs. (7.15) and (7.16) can be rewritten as

$$g\{\hat{\mu}_{0k}(t; \boldsymbol{\theta}, \boldsymbol{\gamma})\} = \frac{\sum_{i=1}^{n} Y_i(t) \, N_{ik}(t) \, dH_{ik}(t)}{\sum_{i=1}^{n} Y_i(t) \, g\{\exp(\boldsymbol{\theta}^T \boldsymbol{Z}_{ik}(t))\} \, \exp(\boldsymbol{\gamma}^T \boldsymbol{Z}_i(t))} \frac{1}{d\tilde{\mu}_{0k}(t)}$$

and

$$\sum_{i=1}^{n} \sum_{k=1}^{K} \int_0^\tau W(t) \, Y_i(t) \, \{\boldsymbol{Z}_{ik}(t) - \bar{\boldsymbol{Z}}_k(t; \boldsymbol{\theta}, \boldsymbol{\gamma})\} \, N_{ik}(t) \, dH_{ik}(t) = 0,$$

respectively, where

$$\bar{\boldsymbol{Z}}_k(t; \boldsymbol{\theta}, \boldsymbol{\gamma}) = \frac{\sum_{i=1}^{n} Y_i(t) \, \boldsymbol{Z}_{ik}(t) \, g\{\exp(\boldsymbol{\theta}^T \boldsymbol{Z}_{ik}(t))\} \, \exp(\boldsymbol{\gamma}^T \boldsymbol{Z}_i(t))}{\sum_{i=1}^{n} Y_i(t) \, g\{\exp(\boldsymbol{\theta}^T \boldsymbol{Z}_{ik}(t))\} \, \exp(\boldsymbol{\gamma}^T \boldsymbol{Z}_i(t))}.$$

Another situation where the Eqs. (7.15) and (7.16) can be easily solved is when $g(t) = \log(t)$. In this case, we have

$$g\{\hat{\mu}_{0k}(t; \boldsymbol{\theta}, \boldsymbol{\gamma})\} = \frac{\sum_{i=1}^{n} Y_i(t) \, N_{ik}(t) \, dH_{ik}(t)}{\sum_{i=1}^{n} Y_i(t) \, \exp(\boldsymbol{\gamma}^T \boldsymbol{Z}_i(t))} \frac{1}{d\tilde{\mu}_{0k}(t)}$$
$$- \frac{\sum_{i=1}^{n} Y_i(t) \, g\{\exp(\boldsymbol{\theta}^T \boldsymbol{Z}_{ik}(t))\} \, \exp(\boldsymbol{\gamma}^T \boldsymbol{Z}_i(t))}{\sum_{i=1}^{n} Y_i(t) \, \exp(\boldsymbol{\gamma}^T \boldsymbol{Z}_i(t))}$$

7.5 Conditional Regression Analysis with Dependent Observation Processes   183

from the Eq. (7.15). The estimating function $U_{MT}(\boldsymbol{\theta}, \boldsymbol{\gamma})$ becomes

$$U_{MT}(\boldsymbol{\theta}, \boldsymbol{\gamma}) = \sum_{i=1}^{n} \sum_{k=1}^{K} \int_{0}^{\tau} W(t) Y_i(t) \left\{ \boldsymbol{Z}_{ik}(t) - \bar{\boldsymbol{Z}}_k(t; \boldsymbol{\gamma}) \right\} \left[N_{ik}(t) \, dH_{ik}(t) \right.$$
$$\left. - \boldsymbol{\theta}^T \boldsymbol{Z}_{ik}(t) \exp \left\{ \boldsymbol{\gamma}^T \boldsymbol{Z}_i(t) \right\} d\tilde{\mu}_{0k}(t) \right],$$

where

$$\bar{\boldsymbol{Z}}_k(t; \boldsymbol{\gamma}) = \frac{\sum_{i=1}^{n} Y_i(t) \boldsymbol{Z}_{ik}(t) \exp\{\boldsymbol{\gamma}^T \boldsymbol{Z}_i(t)\}}{\sum_{i=1}^{n} Y_i(t) \exp\{\boldsymbol{\gamma}^T \boldsymbol{Z}_i(t)\}}.$$

It follows that

$$\hat{\boldsymbol{\theta}}_{MT} = \left\{ \sum_{i=1}^{n} \sum_{k=1}^{K} \int_{0}^{\tau} W(t) Y_i(t) \left\{ \boldsymbol{Z}_{ik}(t) - \bar{\boldsymbol{Z}}_k(t; \boldsymbol{\gamma}) \right\} \boldsymbol{Z}_{ik}^T(t) \exp \left\{ \boldsymbol{\gamma}^T \boldsymbol{Z}_i(t) \right\} \right.$$
$$\left. \times d\tilde{\mu}_{0k}(t) \right\}^{-1} \sum_{i=1}^{n} \sum_{k=1}^{K} \int_{0}^{\tau} W(t) Y_i(t) \left\{ \boldsymbol{Z}_{ik}(t) - \bar{\boldsymbol{Z}}_k(t; \boldsymbol{\gamma}) \right\} N_{ik}(t) dH_{ik}(t).$$

with replacing $\boldsymbol{\gamma}$ and $\tilde{\mu}_{0k}(t)$ by $\hat{\boldsymbol{\gamma}}_{MT}$ and $\hat{\tilde{\mu}}_{0k}(t; \hat{\boldsymbol{\gamma}}_{MT})$, respectively.

7.5.4 Reanalysis of Skin Cancer Chemoprevention Trial

For illustration and comparison, we now reanalyze the bivariate panel count data on the occurrence rates of two types of non-melanoma skin cancers discussed in Sect. 7.4.3. As described before, for each of 290 patients, the observed data include a sequence of observation or clinic visit times and the numbers of occurrences of basal cell carcinoma and squamous cell carcinoma between the observation times. There is also information on four baseline covariates, treatment indicator (placebo or DFMO), patient's gender and age at the diagnosis, and the number of prior skin cancers from the first diagnosis to randomization. In addition, among the 290 patients, the number of observations ranges from 1 to 17. With respect to the occurrences of new skin cancers, the number of basal cell carcinoma ranges from 0 to 16, while the number of squamous cell carcinoma ranges from 0 to 23. As discussed in Sect. 7.4.3, the occurrence processes between the two types of skin cancers seem to be correlated.

To apply the conditional regression tool given above, let $N_{i1}(t)$ and $N_{i2}(t)$ as well as $H_{i1}(t)$ and $H_{i2}(t)$ be defined as in Sect. 7.4.3. Note that the two observation processes $H_{i1}(t)$ and $H_{i2}(t)$ are the same for the data. With respect to the covariates, also let $\boldsymbol{Z}_i = (Z_{i1}, Z_{i2}, Z_{i3}, Z_{i4})^T$ be defined as in Sect. 7.4.3. To apply the methodology, we need to choose the link functions g and Q. For this, following the discussion in Sects. 6.4.3 and 6.5.3, we consider three choices for g, $g(t) = t$, $g(t) = t^2$ and $g(t) = \log(t)$, and two choices for

Table 7.3. Estimated regression parameters with $Q(\mathcal{F}_{it}) = \tilde{H}_i(t-)$

Function $g(t)$	$\hat{\beta}_{MT,1}$ SE($\hat{\beta}_{MT,1}$) CI($\hat{\beta}_{MT,1}$)	$\hat{\beta}_{MT,2}$ SE($\hat{\beta}_{MT,2}$) CI($\hat{\beta}_{MT,2}$)	$\hat{\beta}_{MT,3}$ SE($\hat{\beta}_{MT,3}$) CI($\hat{\beta}_{MT,3}$)	$\hat{\beta}_{MT,4}$ SE($\hat{\beta}_{MT,4}$) CI($\hat{\beta}_{MT,4}$)	$\hat{\alpha}_{MT}$ SE($\hat{\alpha}_{MT}$) CI($\hat{\alpha}_{MT}$)
$g(t) = t$	−0.2629 0.1849 (−0.63,0.10)	0.0697 0.0080 (0.05,0.09)	−0.0016 0.0085 (−0.02,0.02)	0.2419 0.1896 (−0.13,0.61)	0.1657 0.0469 (0.07,0.26)
$g(t) = t^2$	−0.1314 0.0924 (−0.31, 0.05)	0.0348 0.0040 (0.03,0.04)	−0.0008 0.0043 (−0.01,0.01)	0.1210 0.0948 (−0.06, 0.31)	0.0828 0.0234 (0.04,0.13)
$g(t) = \log(t)$	−0.1107 0.1111 (−0.33,0.11)	0.0981 0.0223 (0.05,0.14)	−0.0035 0.0047 (−0.01,0.01)	0.1478 0.1106 (−0.07,0.36)	0.1718 0.0736 (0.03,0.32)

Table 7.4. Estimated regression parameters with $Q(\mathcal{F}_{it}) = \tilde{H}_i(t-) - \tilde{H}_i(t-100)$

Function $g(t)$	$\hat{\beta}_{MT,1}$ SE($\hat{\beta}_{MT,1}$) CI($\hat{\beta}_{MT,1}$)	$\hat{\beta}_{MT,2}$ SE($\hat{\beta}_{MT,2}$) CI($\hat{\beta}_{MT,2}$)	$\hat{\beta}_{MT,3}$ SE($\hat{\beta}_{MT,3}$) CI($\hat{\beta}_{MT,3}$)	$\hat{\beta}_{MT,4}$ SE($\hat{\beta}_{MT,4}$) CI($\hat{\beta}_{MT,4}$)	$\hat{\alpha}_{MT}$ SE($\hat{\alpha}_{MT}$) CI($\hat{\alpha}_{MT}$)
$g(t) = t$	−0.3863 0.2116 (−0.80,0.03)	0.0774 0.0095 (0.06,0.10)	0.0044 0.0094 (−0.02,0.02)	0.2050 0.2060 (−0.20,0.61)	−0.7768 0.2744 (−1.31,−0.24)
$g(t) = t^2$	−0.1932 0.1058 (−0.40,0.01)	0.0387 0.0048 (0.03,0.05)	0.0022 0.0047 (−0.01,0.01)	0.1025 0.1030 (−0.10,0.30)	−0.3884 0.1372 (−0.66,−0.12)
$g(t) = \log(t)$	−0.1418 0.1146 (−0.37,0.08)	0.1060 0.0247 (0.06,0.15)	−0.0008 0.0048 (−0.01,0.01)	0.1149 0.1108 (−0.10,0.33)	−0.4621 0.0983 (−0.65,−0.27)

Q, $Q(\mathcal{F}_{ikt}) = H_{ik}(t-)$ and $Q(\mathcal{F}_{ikt}) = H_{ik}(t-) - H_{ik}(t-100)$. The former Q assumes that the occurrence rate of skin cancers may depend on the total number of patient's visits. On the other hand, the latter Q supposes that the occurrence rate may depend only on the number of patient's visits during the 100-day period before.

Tables 7.3 and 7.4 present the estimated effects of the covariates given by the estimation procedure with $W(t) = 1$ described above. One is for the case with $Q(\mathcal{F}_{ikt}) = H_{ik}(t-)$ and the other corresponds to $Q(\mathcal{F}_{ikt}) = H_{ik}(t-) - H_{ik}(t-100)$. They include the estimated parameters $\hat{\boldsymbol{\beta}}_{MT}$ and $\hat{\boldsymbol{\alpha}}_{MT}$, their estimated standard errors (SE), and the estimated 95% confidence intervals (CI). One can see from the two tables that the analyses essentially give the same conclusions as those obtained in Sect. 7.4.3 based on the joint analysis procedure. More specifically, all results indicate that the DFMO treatment did not seem to have a significant effect on the occurrence rates of the two types of skin cancers. Also the occurrence rate did not seem to be significantly related to either the age or gender of the patient. But it seems that the number of prior skin cancers can be used as a predictor for

7.5 Conditional Regression Analysis with Dependent Observation Processes

the occurrence rate. It is worth noting that the results are consistent with respect to the choices of both g and $\boldsymbol{Q}(\mathcal{F}_{ikt})$.

With respect to the correlation between the recurrent event process of interest and the observation process, it is interesting to see from Tables 7.3 and 7.4 that both analyses suggest that they are indeed correlated. In other words, the patient's visit process does seem to contain some relevant information about the occurrence process of the skin cancer, but the correlation may depend on the time or follow-up period. More specifically, the analyses indicate that a higher number of the observations or clinical visits in total could mean a higher occurrence rate of the skin cancer. On the other hand, a higher number of the observations or clinical visits over a short period before a particular time point could mean a lower occurrence rate. One possible explanation is that within a short period, the higher number of the visits may leave no time for the occurrence of new skin cancers.

7.5.5 Discussion

From the point of the relationship between the underlying recurrent event processes of interest and observation processes, the approach discussed in this section is a conditional procedure. In contrast, the approach described in the previous section is a joint procedure. On the other hand, from the modeling point of view, both methods are marginal approaches as the method presented in Sect. 7.2. This is because they all are based on the models on the mean functions of the event processes of interest. From the relationship point of view, an alternative to models (7.13) and (7.14) is to model the marginal mean or rate function of the event process of interest and the conditional mean or rate function of the observation process given the event process. One may prefer this alternative if the observation process is the main target. This can be the case if the observation and event processes are, for example, a hospitalization process of the patients with certain disease and some marker process related to the disease.

As discussed before, a major advantage of marginal approaches is that they leave the correlation between different types of recurrent event processes arbitrary. This method is usually preferred if the main goal of a study is on estimation of covariate effects. An alternative is to directly model the correlation structure or make specific assumptions on the underlying event processes like the Poisson process assumption. It is obvious that the alternative would be appealing if the correlation is of main interest or the efficiency is a major concern. In this case, of course, the model verification could be much more difficult than that for the marginal approach discussed above among other aspects.

Also as mentioned above, the conditional procedure discussed above is a generalization of the method described in Sect. 6.4. In particular, model (7.13) is a generalization of model (6.18). Actually, one could also generalize model (6.18) to

$$E\{N_{ik}(t)|\,Z_i(t),\mathcal{F}_{ikt}\} = g_k\left\{\mu_{0k}(t)\,\exp\{\boldsymbol{\beta}^T\boldsymbol{Z}_i(t)+\boldsymbol{\alpha}^T\boldsymbol{Q}_k(\mathcal{F}_{ikt})\}\right\}$$

by allowing both link functions g_k and $\boldsymbol{Q}_k$ to depend on the type of recurrent events. In this situation, it is straightforward to develop an estimation procedure similar to that given above. Of course, sometimes one may also want to generalize model (7.13) or the model above to allow covariate effects being time-dependent or different for different types of recurrent events as discussed in Sect. 7.4.4.

There exist other generalizations that one may be of interest or are useful sometimes. For example, in the discussion above, it has been assumed that the observation process $\tilde{H}_{ik}(t)$ is a non-homogeneous Poisson process. It is clear that this may not be true in practice as discussed before and in this case, one needs some other estimation procedures rather than the one discussed above. Another direction for more research is to develop some procedures or generalize the procedures described in Sects. 5.5.4 and 6.4.2 to perform the goodness-of-fit test on model (7.13). Note that although the analysis results in Sect. 7.5.4 are consistent with respect to different g, this may not be the case in general. In order to make the approach less sensitive against the selection of g, one could allow g to belong to some class of functions characterized by, say, some link parameters. Some estimation procedures are then needed for both regression parameters and the link parameters.

7.6 Bibliography, Discussion, and Remarks

As mentioned before, the literature on statistical analysis of multivariate panel count data is relatively thin. One relatively earlier reference on this is given by Chen et al. (2005), followed by He et al. (2008). Both investigated regression analysis of multivariate panel count data for the case with independent observation processes. The differences between the two include that the former is a parametric procedure in nature and the latter is a semiparametric one. Li et al. (2011) and Zhang et al. (2013b) also studied the regression analysis problem, but their approaches allow the dependence between the recurrent event processes of interest and the observation processes. In addition, Lee (2008) considered the same situation as the one discussed in Chen et al. (2005) and He et al. (2008) and gave some simple parametric methods. Zhao et al. (2013c) proposed a class of nonparametric test procedures for the two-sample comparison based on multivariate panel count data.

For regression analysis of multivariate panel count data, the focus in this chapter has been on marginal modeling-based or estimating equation-based approaches. As remarked before, an alternative to these approaches is likelihood-based methods such as those discussed in Sect. 5.2. A key issue for

7.6 Bibliography, Discussion, and Remarks

the latter, which does not exist for univariate panel count data, is to specify or model the correlation structure between different types of recurrent event processes, which may not be easy. For this, of course, a natural way is to employ some frailty or latent variables as in Sect. 6.3. Such approaches have been commonly used for regression analysis of recurrent event data or longitudinal data with informative follow-ups (Huang and Wang, 2004; Jin et al., 2006; Liu et al., 2008; Tsiatis and Davidian, 2004; Ye et al., 2007) . On the other hand, the resulting methods would usually be complicated in both computation and the derivation of theoretical properties. The assessment of the assumed correlation structure would be hard too.

For the analysis of multivariate panel count data, one could ask many questions that have been asked and investigated for the analysis of univariate panel count data but have not been touched for the multivariate case. One such question is regression analysis of multivariate panel count data in the presence of dependent follow-up process or terminal events. As discussed in Sect. 6.5, this can often happen in the studies yielding panel count data, and one common example of such terminal events is the death caused by something related to the recurrent event of interest. To be more specific, consider the set-up discussed in Sect. 7.5 but with a dependent terminal event. Let D_i and $\mathcal{Z}_i(t)$ be defined as in Sect. 6.5, denoting the time to the terminal event and the history of the covariate process, respectively, $i = 1, \ldots, n$. Also let $N^*_{dik}(t)$ be defined as $N^*_{di}(t)$ in Sect. 6.5 but for type k recurrent events considered here, $k = 1, \ldots, K$. Then for regression analysis, following model (6.20), one could consider the following conditional mean model

$$E\{ N^*_{dik}(t) \mid \mathcal{Z}_i(t), \mathcal{F}_{ikt}, D_i \geq t \} = \mu_{0k}(t) + \boldsymbol{\beta}^T \boldsymbol{Z}_i(t) + \boldsymbol{\alpha}^T \boldsymbol{Q}(\mathcal{F}_{ikt})$$

or

$$E\{ N^*_{dik}(t) \mid \mathcal{Z}_i(t), \mathcal{F}_{ikt}, D_i \geq t \} = g\left\{ \mu_{0k}(t) \exp\{\boldsymbol{\beta}^T \boldsymbol{Z}_i(t) + \boldsymbol{\alpha}^T \boldsymbol{Q}(\mathcal{F}_{ikt})\} \right\}$$

for the terminal event-adjusted recurrent event process $N^*_{dik}(t)$. Corresponding to the model above, one may want to impose some models similar to models (6.21) and (6.22) on the observation process and the terminal event too, respectively. Actually Zhao et al. (2013b) recently investigated this problem under model (6.21) and developed an estimating equation procedure for estimation of regression parameters. In their method, they assumed that observation processes are non-homogeneous Poisson processes and follow the proportional rate model (6.21). Furthermore, the D's were assumed to follow the proportional hazards model (6.22) as in Sect. 6.5.

8
Other Topics

8.1 Introduction

In addition to what discussed in the previous chapters, there exist some other issues or topics about the analysis of panel count data that have been investigated in the literature or could occur in practice. In conducting regression analysis, for example, one can always ask which or if all covariate variables are important or significant enough to be included in the final model for the response variable of interest. That is, one faces a variable selection problem. For the problem, two situations usually occur. One is that the number of covariate variables is fixed and smaller than the sample size as in usual linear or nonlinear regression analysis (Johnson and Wichern, 2002). The other is that the number of covariate or predictor variables is much larger than the sample size and could be over several thousands or hundred thousands. The latter has become a huge and important topic in statistical genetic analysis as well as some other related areas (Beebe et al., 1998; Lee, 2004).

In this chapter, we discuss several topics that have not been touched in the previous chapters, including variable selection, the analysis of mixed recurrent event and panel count data, and the analysis of panel count data arising from multi-state models. In addition, some discussions are also given on Bayesian approaches for the analysis of panel count data and the analysis of panel count data arising from mixture models or with measurement errors. First in Sect. 8.2 we consider the variable selection problem mentioned above with the focus on the first situation mentioned above. It is assumed that the goal is to choose relevant and important covariates or risk factors among the observed ones in terms of their effects on the underlying event history or recurrent event process of interest. More specifically, we confine the discussion to the multivariate panel count data generated from models (7.4) and (7.5). A general variable selection procedure is introduced that is developed based on the estimating equation theory and the idea behind the penalized likelihood approach. It selects variables and estimates regression coefficients simultaneously, and the resulting estimators of regression parameters have the so-called oracle properties.

As discussed above, the literature on event history studies of recurrent events or recurrent event studies mainly focuses on two types of data, recurrent event data and panel count data. In practice, however, a third type of data can occur that involve both recurrent event data and panel count data. That is, we have mixed recurrent event and panel count data (Zhu et al., 2013). This happens if study subjects are observed continuously over some time periods but only at discrete time points over other time periods. In other words, we have complete information about the occurrences of the event of interest over some time periods but only incomplete information about the occurrences over other time periods. In Sect. 8.3, we discuss some issues related to the analysis of such mixed recurrent event and panel count data. A procedure for regression analysis of the data is described. Also one set of such data, arising from a Childhood Cancer Survivor Study, is discussed and analyzed.

So far the focus has been on the panel count data concerning the occurrence patterns or rates of certain recurrent events of interest or the recurrent event processes that control the occurrences of the recurrent events. In practice, a different type of panel count data may occur that concern how long study subjects stay in certain states and how often they move from one state to another state. An example of the states could be different stages of a disease. Here by panel count data, as above, we mean that the observations on study subjects occur only at discrete time points. Such data are also often referred to as panel count data from multi-state models (Bartholomew, 1983; Kalbfleisch and Lawless, 1985; Singer and Spilerman, 1976a,b; Wasserman, 1980). In Sect. 8.4, we discuss some inference procedures for the analysis of such panel count data from continuous-time finite state Markov models.

Section 8.5 briefly considers three other topics related to the analysis of panel count data that have not been touched in the previous chapters. They are Bayesian approaches for the analysis of panel count data, the analysis of panel count data with measurement errors, and the analysis of panel count data arising from mixture models. Here by measurement errors, we mean that the covariates or risk factors of interest cannot be measured or observed exactly, while the mixture model means that the underlying recurrent event process of interest is a mixed point process. Finally, Sect. 8.6 concludes this chapter and the book with some comments and discussions on the issues related to the analysis of panel count data that are beyond this book. In addition, some discussions on a few directions for future research are also provided.

8.2 Variable Selection with Panel Count Data

Variable selection is an important topic in all regression analyses and many procedures have been developed for it such as the commonly used stepwise and subset selection procedures. Other commonly used general procedures

8.2 Variable Selection with Panel Count Data

include AIC (Akaike, 1973), Mallow's C_p (Mallows, 1973) and BIC (Schwartz, 1978). Among those developed more recently, a general type of procedures is the penalized procedure that adds a penalty function to an objective function such as a likelihood function (Fan and Li, 2001, 2004; Tibshirani, 1996, 1997). The advantages of penalized procedures over traditional procedures include easy implementation, stability and flexibility in controlling the structure of resulting models (Breiman, 1996; Fan and Peng, 2004). In this section, we discuss such a procedure for the variable selection when one faces multivariate panel count data. To begin with, we first describe some commonly used penalty functions after introducing some notation and assumptions. A penalized estimating function is then derived for both estimation of regression parameters and variable selection together. In addition, the properties of the resulting estimators and their determination are discussed. Finally the methodology is illustrated by using the skin cancer data discussed in Chap. 8, which is followed by some general discussion.

8.2.1 Assumptions and Penalty Functions

Consider an event history study that involves n independent subjects and in which each subject may experience K different types of recurrent events as in Sect. 7.3. Also let the $N_{ik}(t)$, $t_{ik,j}$, $\tilde{H}_{ik}(t)$, $H_{ik}(t)$, $\boldsymbol{Z}_i$, C_i and $Y_i(t)$ be defined as in Sect. 7.3, $j = 1, \ldots, m_{ik}$, $i = 1, \ldots, n$, $k = 1, \ldots, K$, and suppose that one only observes multivariate panel count data given in (7.2) or (7.3). Furthermore, assume that the effects of covariates on the recurrent event process of interest $N_{ik}(t)$ and the observation process $\tilde{H}_{ik}(t)$ can be described by models (7.4) and (7.5), respectively. In the following, we use p to denote the dimension of $\boldsymbol{Z}_i$ and assume that p is fixed. Some comments on this are given below. Also we use $\Omega = \{\, j; \beta_j \neq 0 \,\}$ to denote the true model or the set of indices of the regression parameters that are not zero, and let $s = |\Omega|$, the size of the true model.

To select significant covariate variables or determine Ω, as mentioned above, a general type of procedures is the penalized approach that adds a penalty function to an existing objective function. For this, many penalty functions have been proposed in the literature (Fan and Lv, 2010). Among them, an early one is given by Tibshirani (1996) as $p_\lambda(|\theta|) = \lambda|\theta|$, which leads to the well-known least absolute shrinkage and selection operator (LASSO) approach. Here λ is a tuning parameter and θ denotes the regression parameter of interest. Following Tibshirani (1996), Zou (2006) suggests to use a more general penalty function given by $p_\lambda(|\theta|) = \lambda \omega |\theta|$ (ALASSO), where ω is a data-dependent weight. Also following Tibshirani (1996), Fan and Li (2001) give the so-called SCAD penalty function defined as

$$\dot{p}_\lambda(|\theta|) = \lambda \operatorname{sgn}(\theta) \left\{ I(|\theta| \leq \lambda) + \frac{\max(a\lambda - |\theta|, 0)}{(a-1)\lambda} I(|\theta| > \lambda) \right\}$$

for $\theta \neq 0$. In the above, it is assumed that $p_\lambda(0) = 0$, $a > 2$ is a tuning parameter as λ, and $\dot{p}_\lambda(\cdot)$ denotes the first derivative of $p_\lambda(\cdot)$. More recently, Zhang (2010) gives another penalty function, which he refers to as the minimax concave penalty (MC+) and has the form

$$p_{\lambda,\delta}(|\theta|) = \lambda \left\{ |\theta| - \frac{|\theta|^2}{2\delta\lambda} \right\} I(0 \leq |\theta| < \delta\lambda) + \frac{\lambda^2 \delta}{2} I(|\theta| \geq \delta\lambda).$$

Here the parameter $\delta > 0$ is used to control the concavity of the function.

In addition to these described above, one could also employ the so-called seamless-L_0 (SELO) penalty function defined as

$$p_{\lambda_1,\lambda_2}(|\theta|) = \frac{\lambda_1}{\log(2)} \log\left(\frac{|\theta|}{|\theta| + \lambda_2} + 1 \right). \tag{8.1}$$

In the above, $\lambda_1 > 0$ and $\lambda_2 > 0$ are tuning parameters as before with $p_{\lambda_1,\lambda_2}(\theta) \approx \lambda_1 I_{\{\theta \neq 0\}}$ for small λ_2. The function above is proposed by Dicker et al. (2012) in the context of fitting the linear model $\boldsymbol{Y} = \boldsymbol{Z\theta} + \epsilon$. Here, $\boldsymbol{Y}$ is a vector of the observed values of the response variable, $\boldsymbol{Z}$ a design matrix, $\boldsymbol{\theta} = (\theta_1, \ldots, \theta_d)^T$ a vector of unknown parameters, and ϵ a vector of measurement errors with mean zero. For estimation of $\boldsymbol{\theta}$, they suggest to minimize the penalized function

$$\frac{1}{2n} \|\boldsymbol{Y} - \boldsymbol{Z\theta}\|^2 + \sum_{j=1}^{d} p_{\lambda_1,\lambda_2}(|\theta_j|).$$

Furthermore they argue that the SELO penalty function usually gives a stable and computationally feasible penalized procedure. Also they show through numerical studies that it can outperform the procedures based on other penalty functions by various metrics.

It is worth to point out that all penalty functions discussed above as well as the resulting penalized procedures are for general regression, which is quite different from the problem discussed here. In the next subsection, we introduce a general penalized procedure for multivariate panel count data with the focus on the use of the SELO penalty function. However, the approach is applicable or still valid if any other penalty function is used as shown in Sect. 8.2.3 below.

8.2.2 Variable Section Procedure

To derive an estimation and variable selection procedure using the penalized approach, first we need to have an objective function. For this, let $\bar{N}_{ik}$ be defined as in Sect. 7.3.2. Then motivated by the estimating function $U_{MI}(\boldsymbol{\beta}, \boldsymbol{\gamma})$ given in (7.6), it is natural to consider

8.2 Variable Selection with Panel Count Data

$$l(\boldsymbol{\beta}, \boldsymbol{\gamma}) = -\sum_{k=1}^{K}\sum_{i=1}^{n} \boldsymbol{Z}_i \, \bar{N}_{ik} \left\{ g_H(\boldsymbol{Z}_i^T \boldsymbol{\gamma}) \right\}^{-1} \int \left\{ g_N(\boldsymbol{Z}_i^T \boldsymbol{\beta}) \right\}^{-1} d\boldsymbol{\beta}$$

as the objective function. It thus follows that for estimation of $\boldsymbol{\beta}$, we can minimize the penalized function

$$l_p(\boldsymbol{\beta}, \boldsymbol{\gamma}; \lambda_1, \lambda_2) = l(\boldsymbol{\beta}, \boldsymbol{\gamma}) + n \sum_{j=1}^{p} p_{\lambda_1, \lambda_2}(|\beta_j|) \tag{8.2}$$

based on the SELO penalty function given in (8.1). It is easy to see that the derivative of $l(\boldsymbol{\beta}, \boldsymbol{\gamma})$ with respect to $\boldsymbol{\beta}$ gives $-\sqrt{n}\, U_{MI}(\boldsymbol{\beta}, \boldsymbol{\gamma})$. Furthermore, the procedure described above with letting the penalty being zero would yield the same estimator as that defined in Sect. 7.3.2.

For the implementation of the estimation procedure above, of course, we need to estimate $\boldsymbol{\gamma}$ as well as λ_1 and λ_2. For $\boldsymbol{\gamma}$, it is apparent that we can employ the approach discussed in Sect. 7.3.2 and the estimation of λ_1 and λ_2 is discussed below. Let $\hat{\boldsymbol{\gamma}}_M$ denote the estimator of $\boldsymbol{\gamma}$ defined in Sect. 7.3.2. Then it is natural to define the penalized estimator of $\boldsymbol{\beta}$ as

$$\hat{\boldsymbol{\beta}}_v = \arg\min_{\boldsymbol{\beta}} l_p(\boldsymbol{\beta}, \hat{\boldsymbol{\gamma}}_M; \lambda_1, \lambda_2). \tag{8.3}$$

Let $\boldsymbol{\beta}_0$ denote the true value of $\boldsymbol{\beta}$ and suppose that it can be written as $\boldsymbol{\beta}_0 = (\beta_{01}, \ldots, \beta_{0p})^T = (\boldsymbol{\beta}_{01}^T, \boldsymbol{\beta}_{02}^T)^T$, where $\boldsymbol{\beta}_{01}$ and $\boldsymbol{\beta}_{02}$ denote the nonzero and zero components of $\boldsymbol{\beta}_0$, respectively. Also suppose that we can write $\hat{\boldsymbol{\beta}}_v = (\hat{\beta}_{v1}, \ldots, \hat{\beta}_{vp})^T = (\hat{\boldsymbol{\beta}}_{v1}^T, \hat{\boldsymbol{\beta}}_{v2}^T)^T$, the same as $\boldsymbol{\beta}_0$. Let s denote the dimension of $\boldsymbol{\beta}_{01}$ and $\hat{\boldsymbol{\beta}}_{v1}$, and assume that the tuning parameters λ_1 and λ_2 are chosen such that $\lambda_1 = O(n^\rho)$ and $\lambda_2 = O(n^{-\rho - 1/2})$ with $-1/2 < \rho < 0$. Then under some regularity conditions, Zhang et al. (2013a) show that $\hat{\boldsymbol{\beta}}_v$ exists, it is $\sqrt{n}$-consistent and $Pr\{\hat{\boldsymbol{\beta}}_{v2} = 0\} \to 1$ as $n \to \infty$. Note that this latter fact is often referred to as the sparsity property in the variable selection literature.

In addition, Zhang et al. (2013a) show that under the same conditions above, the distribution of $\hat{\boldsymbol{\beta}}_{v1}$ can be asymptotically approximated by the multivariate normal distribution with mean $\boldsymbol{\beta}_{01}$ and the covariance matrix

$$\hat{\Sigma}_{v1}(\lambda_1, \lambda_2) = \frac{1}{n} \left\{ \hat{A}_{v1} + \hat{B}_{v1}(\lambda_1, \lambda_2) \right\}^{-1} \hat{\Gamma}_{v1} \left\{ \hat{A}_{v1} + \hat{B}_{v1}(\lambda_1, \lambda_2) \right\}^{-1}$$

with replacing λ_1 and λ_2 by their estimators given below. In the above, $\hat{A}_{v1}$, $\hat{B}_{v1}(\lambda, \tau)$ and $\hat{\Gamma}_{v1}$ are the upper-left $s \times s$ submatrices of

$$\hat{A}_v = \frac{1}{n}\sum_{i=1}^{n}\sum_{k=1}^{K} \bar{N}_{ik} \boldsymbol{Z}_i \boldsymbol{Z}_i^T \, \dot{g}_N(\boldsymbol{Z}_i^T \hat{\boldsymbol{\beta}}_v) \left\{ g_N(\boldsymbol{Z}_i^T \hat{\boldsymbol{\beta}}_v) \right\}^{-2} \left\{ g_H(\boldsymbol{Z}_i^T \hat{\boldsymbol{\gamma}}_M) \right\}^{-1}, \tag{8.4}$$

$$\hat{B}_v(\lambda_1, \lambda_2) = \text{diag}\left\{\dot{p}_{\lambda_1,\lambda_2}(|\hat{\beta}_{v1}|)/|\hat{\beta}_{v1}|, \ldots, \dot{p}_{\lambda_1,\lambda_2}(|\hat{\beta}_{vd}|)/|\hat{\beta}_{vd}|\right\}, \quad (8.5)$$

and

$$\hat{\Gamma}_v = (I_d, -\hat{C}_v \hat{D}_v^{-1})\hat{\Phi}(I_d, -\hat{C}_v \hat{D}_v^{-1})^T,$$

respectively. Here

$$\hat{C}_v = \frac{1}{n}\sum_{i=1}^{n}\sum_{k=1}^{K} \bar{N}_{ik} \boldsymbol{Z}_i \boldsymbol{Z}_i^T \left\{g_N(\boldsymbol{Z}_i^T \hat{\boldsymbol{\beta}}_v)\right\}^{-1} \dot{g}_H(\boldsymbol{Z}_i^T \hat{\boldsymbol{\gamma}}_M) \left\{g_H(\boldsymbol{Z}_i^T \hat{\boldsymbol{\gamma}}_M)\right\}^{-2},$$

$$\hat{D}_v = \frac{1}{n}\sum_{i=1}^{n}\sum_{k=1}^{K} \int_0^\tau V_k(t; \hat{\boldsymbol{\gamma}}_M)\, dH_{ik}(t),$$

and

$$\hat{\boldsymbol{\Phi}} = \begin{pmatrix} \hat{\boldsymbol{\Phi}}_U & \hat{\boldsymbol{\Phi}}_{UH} \\ \hat{\boldsymbol{\Phi}}_{UH}^T & \hat{\boldsymbol{\Phi}}_H \end{pmatrix},$$

where

$$\hat{\boldsymbol{\Phi}}_U = \frac{1}{n}\sum_{i=1}^{n}\left[\sum_{k=1}^{K} \bar{N}_{ik} \boldsymbol{Z}_i \left\{g_N(\boldsymbol{Z}_i^T \hat{\boldsymbol{\beta}}_v)\right\}^{-1}\left\{g_H(\boldsymbol{Z}_i^T \hat{\boldsymbol{\gamma}}_M)\right\}^{-1}\right]^{\otimes 2},$$

$$\hat{\boldsymbol{\Phi}}_H = \frac{1}{n}\sum_{i=1}^{n}\left[\sum_{k=1}^{K}\int_0^\tau \left\{\boldsymbol{Z}_i \frac{\dot{g}_H(\boldsymbol{Z}_i^T \hat{\boldsymbol{\gamma}}_M)}{g_H(\boldsymbol{Z}_i^T \hat{\boldsymbol{\gamma}}_M)} - E_k(t; \hat{\boldsymbol{\gamma}}_M)\right\} dM_{ik}(t; \hat{\boldsymbol{\gamma}}_M)\right]^{\otimes 2},$$

$$\hat{\boldsymbol{\Phi}}_{UH} = \frac{1}{n}\sum_{i=1}^{n}\left[\sum_{k=1}^{K} \bar{N}_{ik} \boldsymbol{Z}_i \left\{g_N(\boldsymbol{Z}_i^T \hat{\boldsymbol{\beta}}_v)\right\}^{-1}\left\{g_H(\boldsymbol{Z}_i^T \hat{\boldsymbol{\gamma}}_M)\right\}^{-1}\right]$$
$$\times \left[\sum_{k=1}^{K}\int_0^\tau \left\{\boldsymbol{Z}_i \frac{\dot{g}_H(\boldsymbol{Z}_i^T \hat{\boldsymbol{\gamma}}_M)}{g_H(\boldsymbol{Z}_i^T \hat{\boldsymbol{\gamma}}_M)} - E_k(t; \hat{\boldsymbol{\gamma}}_M)\right\} dM_{ik}(t; \hat{\boldsymbol{\gamma}}_M)\right]',$$

and $V_k(t; \boldsymbol{\gamma})$, $E_k(t; \boldsymbol{\gamma})$ and $dM_{ik}(t; \boldsymbol{\gamma})$ are defined as in Sect. 7.3.2.

For the determination of $\hat{\boldsymbol{\beta}}_v$ for given λ_1 and λ_2, by following Fan and Li (2001), Zhang et al. (2013a) suggest to use the following Newton-Raphson algorithm. Let $\boldsymbol{\beta}^{(0)} = (\beta_1^{(0)}, \ldots, \beta_p^{(0)})^T$ denote an initial estimator of $\boldsymbol{\beta}$ that is assumed to be close to the true value $\boldsymbol{\beta}_0$. The algorithm is based on the following two facts. One is that in solving the estimating equation

$$U_v(\boldsymbol{\beta}) = \frac{\partial l_p(\boldsymbol{\beta}, \hat{\boldsymbol{\gamma}}_M; \lambda_1, \lambda_2)}{\partial \boldsymbol{\beta}} = 0,$$

the penalty function $p_{\lambda_1,\lambda_2}(|\beta_j|)$ can be irregular at the origin and thus may not have a second derivative at the origin. To address this, one way is to use

8.2 Variable Selection with Panel Count Data

the linear function approximation. Specifically, for each j, if $\beta_j^{(0)}$ is not close to zero, we can use

$$\dot{p}_{\lambda_1,\lambda_2}(|\beta_j|)\,\text{sgn}(\beta_j) \approx \frac{\dot{p}_{\lambda_1,\lambda_2}(|\beta_j^{(0)}|)}{|\beta_j^{(0)}|}\beta_j$$

and otherwise, set the updated estimator $\beta_j^{(1)} = 0$. The other fact is that when $\boldsymbol{\beta}$ is close to $\boldsymbol{\beta}^{(0)}$, we have

$$U_v(\boldsymbol{\beta}) \approx U_v(\boldsymbol{\beta}^{(0)}) + \dot{U}_v(\boldsymbol{\beta}^{(0)})(\boldsymbol{\beta} - \boldsymbol{\beta}^{(0)})$$
$$\approx U_v(\boldsymbol{\beta}^{(0)}) + n\,\hat{A}_v(\boldsymbol{\beta}^{(0)})\,(\boldsymbol{\beta} - \boldsymbol{\beta}^{(0)}) + n\,\hat{B}_v(\boldsymbol{\beta}^{(0)};\lambda_1,\lambda_2)\,(\boldsymbol{\beta} - \boldsymbol{\beta}^{(0)}).$$

In the above, $\hat{A}_v(\boldsymbol{\beta}^{(0)})$ and $\hat{B}_v(\boldsymbol{\beta}^{(0)};\lambda_1,\lambda_2)$ are the matrices $\hat{A}_v$ and $\hat{B}_v$ defined in (8.4) and (8.5), respectively, with replacing $\hat{\boldsymbol{\beta}}_v$ by $\boldsymbol{\beta}^{(0)}$. It thus follows from these two facts that for given λ_1 and λ_2 and the estimator $\boldsymbol{\beta}^{(k)}$ at the kth step, one can define the updated estimator as

$$\boldsymbol{\beta}^{(k+1)} = \boldsymbol{\beta}^{(k)} - \left\{n\,\hat{A}_v(\boldsymbol{\beta}^{(k)}) + n\,\hat{B}_v(\boldsymbol{\beta}^{(k)};\lambda_1,\lambda_2)\right\}^{-1} U_v(\boldsymbol{\beta}^{(k)}),$$

and continue this process until convergence.

Now we discuss the determination of the tuning parameters λ_1 and λ_2. For this, a few general procedures are available. Among them, one, by following Dicker et al. (2012), is to minimize the BIC statistic

$$\text{BIC}(\lambda_1,\lambda_2) = \log\left(\frac{-\sum_{i=1}^n \sum_{k=1}^K \bar{N}_{ik} \mathbf{Z}_i \int \left\{g_N(\mathbf{Z}_i^T \hat{\boldsymbol{\beta}}_v(\lambda_1,\lambda_2))\right\}^{-1} d\hat{\boldsymbol{\beta}}_v(\lambda_1,\lambda_2)}{n - \hat{s}(\lambda_1,\lambda_2)}\right)$$
$$+ \frac{\log(n)}{n}\,\hat{s}(\lambda_1,\lambda_2).$$

In the above, $\hat{\boldsymbol{\beta}}_v(\lambda_1,\lambda_2)$ denotes the estimator defined in (8.3) for given λ_1 and λ_2, and $\hat{s}(\lambda_1,\lambda_2)$ the number of the non-zero components of $\hat{\boldsymbol{\beta}}_v(\lambda_1,\lambda_2)$.

8.2.3 An Illustration

To illustrate the variable selection procedure described above, we apply it to the bivariate panel count data on the occurrence rates of two types of non-melanoma skin cancers analyzed in Sects. 7.2.2, 7.4.3 and 7.5.4. As described before, the data are from a double-blinded and placebo-controlled randomized Phase III clinical trial on the patients with a history of non-melanoma skin cancers. The primary objective of the trial is to evaluate the effectiveness of DFMO in reducing the recurrence rates of two types of skin cancers, basal cell carcinoma and squamous cell carcinoma. In addition to the treatment indicator, for each patient, there exist three baseline covariates, gender, age at

Table 8.1. Analysis results of the skin cancer chemoprevention trial

Link function	Method	β_{01} (SE)	β_{02} (SE)	β_{03} (SE)	β_{04} (SE)
	LASSO	0	0.13758	−0.01030	0
		(−)	(0.01871)	(0.00837)	(−)
	ALASSO	0	0.12719	0	0
		(−)	(0.01673)	(−)	(−)
	SCAD	0	0.13758	−0.01030	0
		(−)	(0.01844)	(0.00837)	(−)
$\exp(t)$	MC+	0	0.13816	−0.01036	0
		(−)	(0.01871)	(0.00837)	(−)
	SELO	0	0.14411	0	0
		(−)	(0.01789)	(−)	(−)
	Best subset	0	0.14397	0	0.38246
		(−)	(0.02226)	(−)	(0.18900)
	$\hat{\beta}_{MI}$	−0.02391	0.14395	−0.01158	0.38068
		(0.18086)	(0.02121)	(0.00836)	(0.17779)
	LASSO	0	0.20668	0	0
		(−)	(0.04572)	(−)	(−)
	ALASSO	0	0.24682	0	0
		(−)	(0.04909)	(−)	(−)
	SCAD	0	0.20676	0	0
		(−)	(0.04572)	(−)	(−)
$\log\{1+\exp(t)\}$	MC+	0	0.20739	0	0
		(−)	(0.04571)	(−)	(−)
	SELO	0	0.25009	0	0
		(−)	(0.04939)	(−)	(−)
	Best subset	0	0.26888	0	0.57559
		(−)	(0.05129)	(−)	(0.31230)
	$\hat{\beta}_{MI}$	−0.04181	0.26718	−0.01692	0.56942
		(0.30139)	(0.04929)	(0.01378)	(0.29818)

the diagnosis, and the number of prior skin cancers. The main goal here is to determine which of these covariates have significant effects on the recurrence rate.

For the analysis, as in Sect. 7.4.3, for patient i, let $N_{i1}(t)$ and $N_{i2}(t)$ denote the total numbers of the occurrences of basal cell carcinoma and squamous cell carcinoma, respectively, up to time t, $i = 1, \ldots, 290$. Also as in Sect. 7.4.3, for patient i, define $Z_{i1} = 1$ if the patient is in the DFMO group and 0 otherwise, Z_{i2} and Z_{i3} to represent the number of prior skin cancers and the age of the patient, and $Z_{i4} = 1$ if the patient is male and 0 otherwise. With respect to the penalty function, in addition to the penalty function SELO, a few other penalty functions are also employed for comparison, including the LASSO, ALASSO, SCAD and MC+. Also for comparison, the best subset selection procedure and the estimation procedure given in Sect. 7.3, which does not employ any penalty function, are considered.

8.2 Variable Selection with Panel Count Data

Table 8.1 gives the estimated covariate effects obtained by all procedures discussed above along with their estimated standard errors (SE). The top half of the table is for the case with the use of the link functions $g_N(t) = g_H(t) = \exp(t)$, while the bottom half for the situation with the use of the link functions $g_N(t) = g_H(t) = \log\{1 + \exp(t)\}$. It is easy to see that all penalized procedures essentially give similar results and suggest that the DFMO treatment seems to have no significant effect on reducing the recurrence rates of both types of skin cancers. Also the recurrence rates did not seem to be significantly related to the age and gender of the patient. On the other hand, the recurrence process of the skin cancers seems to be positively related to the number of prior skin cancers. Note that these conclusions are similar to those given by Tables 7.2–7.4. In contrast, the best subset procedure and the procedure in Sect. 7.3 indicate that the gender may have some effects on the recurrence rate of the skin cancers. Note that the results given by the procedure in Sect. 7.3 are similar to those given in Table 7.2 based on the same approach with different link functions.

8.2.4 Discussion

As mentioned above, variable selection based on panel count data is a relatively new topic and there exists only limited literature on it. In addition to Zhang et al. (2013a), the only other existing reference on it is given by Tong et al. (2009) on the univariate panel count data arising from the proportional mean model (1.4). Actually the procedure described above can be seen as a generalization of that proposed in Tong et al. (2009), which has the same structure as $l_p(\boldsymbol{\beta}, \boldsymbol{\gamma}, \lambda_1, \lambda_2)$ defined in (8.2). Note that the development of the penalized function $l_p(\boldsymbol{\beta}, \boldsymbol{\gamma}, \lambda_1, \lambda_2)$ is based on the estimating function $U_{MI}(\boldsymbol{\beta}, \boldsymbol{\gamma})$ given in Sect. 7.3. Alternatively one can develop similar penalized functions and variable selection procedure by using other estimating functions.

It is easy to see that one advantage of the statistical procedure given above is that it selects variables and estimates covariate effects simultaneously. In particular, the approach has the oracle property in that it yields estimators as if the correct submodel was known. Another advantage of the proposed method is that it leaves the correlation among different types of recurrent events arbitrary. On the other hand, it is apparent that the method may not be efficient if some knowledge about the correlation is known. This is similar to the situation that one faces with respect to the generalized estimating equation. If some structure of the correlation can be reasonably assumed, one may want to incorporate or make use of it to construct more efficient estimating equations. Of course, in general, the correlation structure may be unknown.

Penalized estimation procedures are usually employed for the situations where there exists a large number of covariates or regression coefficients. It is well-known that one main reason for this is to address the collinearity that commonly exists in these cases. At the same time, it is apparent that the collinearity can exist too with the small number of covariates, which is one of the motivations for the development of the penalized procedure given above. It is worth noting that although the dimension p of covariates is assumed to be fixed in the approach above, it can be any number smaller than n.

To apply the variable selection procedure given above, one needs to choose a penalty function. Although the different penalty functions considered in Sect. 8.2.3 give similar results, this may not be true in general. Actually Zhang et al. (2013a) give some simulation results for comparing the performance of the procedures based on these penalty functions plus the best subset procedure. They suggest that although all procedures tend to overestimate the true model in terms of the model size, the SELO-based procedure seems to have the highest percentage to select the correct model. On the other hand, with respect to the false positive and negative rates, the SELO-based procedure tends to be conservative and always to choose smaller models than the others. Furthermore, in terms of the bias and efficiency of the estimated covariate effects, the SELO-based procedure also tends to outperform the others although no procedure is uniformly better than the others.

More research is needed for the topic discussed in this section. One direction for future research is to generalize the variable selection procedure discussed above to the case where there exist some type-specific covariates. That is, covariate effects on different types of recurrent events are different. For this, the discussion and generalized models given in Sect. 7.3.4 apply here. A similar situation is that unlike in models (7.4) and (7.5), covariates may be time-dependent or their effects are time-varying, and for this, it is apparent that one also needs new variable selection procedures. In the procedure given above, it has been assumed that the censoring or follow-up time C_i is independent of covariates. As discussed before, this may not be true in practice, and it would be useful to generalize the procedure to the situation where C_i may depend on covariates. Note that for this, a common approach is to specify a regression model such as the proportional hazards model (5.5) for the dependence. Another assumption used above is the independence between the underlying event history process of interest and the observation process. As discussed in Chap. 6, this can be questionable in practice and one may want to generalize the procedure above to this situation too.

8.3 Analysis of Mixed Recurrent Event and Panel Count Data

8.3.1 Introduction

As described above, in addition to recurrent event data and panel count data, sometimes event history studies concerning some recurrent events may yield a third type of data, mixed recurrent event and panel count data (Zhu et al., 2013). Such data occur when study subjects are observed continuously over some observation periods, but only at discrete time points over other observation periods. That is, we have recurrent event data over some observation periods, but panel count data over other observation periods. One situation that yields such data is the long-term follow-up study on, for example, health conditions, in which some patients are always observed continuously, while others are only monitored or observed periodically. Another example of mixed data is given by the chronic disease study on, for example, medication adherence, in which the adherence is observed daily (continuously) when the patients are in the hospital, but may be observed only monthly (discretely) otherwise. Note that in the first example, we have relatively a simple situation and the study subjects can be classified into two groups, these giving recurrent event data and these giving only panel count data. Sometimes we refer such data as to type I mixed data and otherwise, the data such as these in the second example are referred to as type II mixed data (Zhu et al., 2013).

A third, more specific example of mixed data is given by a Childhood Cancer Survivor Study (CCSS), a multi-center longitudinal cohort study (Robison et al., 2002). Starting in 1996, the study distributed a baseline summary questionnaire to more than 13,000 childhood cancer survivors who were diagnosed between 1970 and 1986 and had survived more than 5 years since diagnosis. The questionnaire was also sent to a random sample of the siblings of the survivors, who served as a control group. The follow-up summary questionnaires were sent periodically thereafter. The information asked in these questionnaires includes reports of all pregnancies, the age range at the beginning of each pregnancy and the outcome. If a pregnancy was reported in any summary questionnaire, a detailed pregnancy questionnaires would be sent to the person to ask for the precise age at pregnancy and other information. Among others, one objective of the study is to determine the long-term effects, if any, of childhood cancer and cancer treatments on the subsequent reproductive function. With respect to the pregnancy, some patients answered the detailed pregnancy questionnaire and thus provided complete recurrent event data for the pregnancy process, while some others only returned the summary questionnaire and gave incomplete panel count data for the process. Also there are some patients who provided detailed pregnancy and thus the recurrent event data during some periods, but only panel count data during some other periods. Note that these periods differ from subject to subject.

In other words, we only have mixed recurrent event and panel count data on the pregnancy process, both types I and II mixed data.

For the analysis of type I mixed recurrent event and panel count data, it is apparent that a simple and naive approach would be to base the analysis on the subjects giving recurrent event data or panel count data only. Another naive approach would be to treat the observed data as panel count data or to generate recurrent event data by using, for example, some imputation procedures. It is easy to see that both methods could either give biased results or be less efficient. In the following, we discuss an estimating equation approach for regression analysis of mixed data that makes use of all available information but does not rely on the imputation. The approach is illustrated by the mixed CCSS data discussed above, followed by some discussions.

8.3.2 Regression Analysis of Mixed Data

As before, consider an event history study that concerns some recurrent events and involves n independent subjects. Also as before, let $N_i(t)$ denote the total number of the recurrent events that subject i has experienced up to time t, and $\boldsymbol{Z}_i$ and C_i the vector of covariates and the follow-up time associated with subject i, respectively, $i = 1, \ldots, n$. Suppose that for each subject, there exists a sequence of intervals $\{(t_{i,j-1}, t_{i,j}]; j = 1, \ldots, m_i\}$ with $t_{i,0} = 0 < t_{i,1} < \cdots < t_{i,m_i}$ during which the subject is observed either continuously or only at discrete times over each interval. Also suppose that the main goal is to estimate covariate effects on the $N_i(t)$'s.

For subject i, define $r_i(t) = 1$ for $t \in (t_{i,j-1}, t_{i,j}]$ if the subject is observed continuously over $(t_{i,j-1}, t_{i,j}]$ and 0 otherwise. Also define $\tilde{H}_i(t) = \sum_{j=1}^{m_i} I(t \geq t_{i,j})$, $H_i(t) = \tilde{H}_i(t \wedge C_i)$ and $Y_i(t) = I(t \leq C_i)$, $i = 1, \ldots, n$. That is, $r_i(t)$ is the data type indicator function. It is easy to see that for type I mixed data, we have that either $r_i(t) = 0$ or 1 for all t. Furthermore, one has recurrent event data if $r_i(t) = 1$ for all t and i and panel count data if $r_i(t) = 0$ for all t and i. Note that the time points $t_{i,j}$'s and the process $\tilde{H}_i(t)$ defined here have different meanings compared to those defined in the previous chapters. They become the same if mixed data reduce to panel count data. In the following, we assume that the mean function of $N_i(t)$ satisfies the proportional mean model (1.4), and both the observation process $\tilde{H}_i(t)$ and the data type indicator function $r_i(t)$ are independent of $N_i(t)$ and C_i given $\boldsymbol{Z}_i$.

For estimation of regression parameter $\boldsymbol{\beta}$ in model (1.4), define $Y_i^*(t) = I(t \leq t_{i,m_i})$, $\tilde{N}_i(t) = \int_0^t Y_i^*(s) N_i(s) dH_i(s)$, $\Gamma_0(t) = \int_0^t \mu_0(s) dE\{H_i(s)\}$, and

$$M_i(t; \boldsymbol{\beta}, \mu_0, \Gamma_0) = r_i(t) M_{ir}(t; \boldsymbol{\beta}, \mu_0) + \{1 - r_i(t)\} M_{ip}(t; \boldsymbol{\beta}, \Gamma_0).$$

8.3 Analysis of Mixed Recurrent Event and Panel Count Data

In the above,

$$M_{ir}(t;\boldsymbol{\beta},\mu_0) = Y_i(t)\,N_i(t) - \int_0^t Y_i(s)\exp\left(\boldsymbol{\beta}^T \boldsymbol{Z}_i\right) d\mu_0(s)$$

and

$$M_{ip}(t;\boldsymbol{\beta},\Gamma_0) = \tilde{N}_i(t) - \int_0^t Y_i^*(s)\exp\left(\boldsymbol{\beta}^T \boldsymbol{Z}_i\right) d\Gamma_0(s).$$

One can easily show that $E\{M_i(t;\boldsymbol{\beta},\mu_0,\Gamma_0)\}=0$. That is, the $M_i(t;\boldsymbol{\beta},\mu_0,\Gamma_0)$'s are zero-mean processes. Thus for estimation of $\boldsymbol{\beta}$ as well as $\mu_0(t)$ and $\Gamma_0(t)$, it is natural to consider the following estimating equations

$$\sum_{i=1}^n r_i(t)\,dM_i(t;\boldsymbol{\beta},\mu_0,\Gamma_0) = 0, \tag{8.6}$$

$$\sum_{i=1}^n \{1 - r_i(t)\}\,dM_i(t;\boldsymbol{\beta},\mu_0,\Gamma_0) = 0, \tag{8.7}$$

and

$$\sum_{i=1}^n \int_0^\tau \boldsymbol{Z}_i\,dM_i(t;\boldsymbol{\beta},\mu_0,\Gamma_0) = 0, \tag{8.8}$$

where τ denotes the longest follow-up time as before.

For given $\boldsymbol{\beta}$, the solving of Eqs. (8.6) and (8.7) gives

$$\hat{\mu}_0(t;\boldsymbol{\beta}) = \int_0^t \frac{\sum_{i=1}^n r_i(s)\,Y_i(s)\,dN_i(s)}{S_r^{(0)}(s;\boldsymbol{\beta})} \tag{8.9}$$

and

$$\hat{\Gamma}_0(t;\boldsymbol{\beta}) = \int_0^t \frac{\sum_{i=1}^n \{1 - r_i(s)\}\,d\tilde{N}_i(s)}{S_p^{(0)}(s;\boldsymbol{\beta})}, \tag{8.10}$$

where

$$S_r^{(j)}(t;\boldsymbol{\beta}) = \sum_{i=1}^n r_i(t)\,Y_i(t)\exp\left(\boldsymbol{\beta}^T \boldsymbol{Z}_i\right)\boldsymbol{Z}_i^{\otimes j}$$

and

$$S_p^{(j)}(t;\boldsymbol{\beta}) = \sum_{i=1}^n \{1 - r_i(t)\}\,Y_i^*(t)\exp\left(\boldsymbol{\beta}^T \boldsymbol{Z}_i\right)\boldsymbol{Z}_i^{\otimes j}$$

for $j = 0, 1, 2$. By plugging the estimators given in (8.9) and (8.10) into the Eq. (8.8), we obtain

$$U_{\text{mix}}(\boldsymbol{\beta}) = \sum_{i=1}^n \int_0^\tau r_i(t)\,\{\boldsymbol{Z}_i - \bar{\boldsymbol{Z}}_r(t;\boldsymbol{\beta})\}\,Y_i(t)\,dN_i(t)$$

$$+ \int_0^\tau \{1 - r_i(t)\}\,\{\boldsymbol{Z}_i - \bar{\boldsymbol{Z}}_p(t;\boldsymbol{\beta})\}\,d\tilde{N}_i(t) = 0, \tag{8.11}$$

where

$$\bar{Z}_r(t;\boldsymbol{\beta}) = \frac{S_r^{(1)}(t;\boldsymbol{\beta})}{S_r^{(0)}(t;\boldsymbol{\beta})}, \quad \bar{Z}_p(t;\boldsymbol{\beta}) = \frac{S_p^{(1)}(t;\boldsymbol{\beta})}{S_p^{(0)}(t;\boldsymbol{\beta})}.$$

Note that it is easy to see that if one observes recurrent event data, the estimating function $U_{\mathrm{mix}}(\boldsymbol{\beta})$ and the estimator given in (8.9) reduce to the estimating function $U(\tau;\boldsymbol{\beta})$ and the estimator given in (1.9) and (1.10), respectively. In the case of panel count data, $U_{\mathrm{mix}}(\boldsymbol{\beta})$ reduces to the estimating function used in Cheng and Wei (2000), similar to that given in (5.11).

Let $\hat{\boldsymbol{\beta}}_{\mathrm{mix}}$ denote the estimator of $\boldsymbol{\beta}$ given by the solution to the Eq. (8.11). Zhu et al. (2013) show that under some regularity conditions, $\hat{\boldsymbol{\beta}}_{\mathrm{mix}}$ is consistent and one can approximate the distribution of $\sqrt{n}\,(\hat{\boldsymbol{\beta}}_{\mathrm{mix}} - \boldsymbol{\beta}_0)$ by the multivariate normal distribution with mean zero and the covariance matrix $\hat{\Sigma}_{\mathrm{mix}}^{-1}(\hat{\boldsymbol{\beta}}_{\mathrm{mix}})\,\hat{\Gamma}_{\mathrm{mix}}(\hat{\boldsymbol{\beta}}_{\mathrm{mix}})\,\hat{\Sigma}_{\mathrm{mix}}^{-1}(\hat{\boldsymbol{\beta}}_{\mathrm{mix}})$. Here $\boldsymbol{\beta}_0$ denotes the true value of $\boldsymbol{\beta}$ as before,

$$\hat{\Sigma}_{\mathrm{mix}}(\boldsymbol{\beta}) = \frac{1}{n}\sum_{i=1}^{n}\left[\int_0^{\tau} r_i(t)\left\{\mathbf{Z}_i - \bar{Z}_r(t;\boldsymbol{\beta})\right\}^{\otimes 2} Y_i(t)dN_i(t) \right. $$
$$\left. + \int_0^{\tau} \{1 - r_i(t)\}\left\{\mathbf{Z}_i - \bar{Z}_p(t;\boldsymbol{\beta})\right\}^{\otimes 2} d\tilde{N}_i(t)\right],$$

and

$$\hat{\Gamma}_{\mathrm{mix}}(\boldsymbol{\beta}) = \frac{1}{n}\sum_{i=1}^{n}\left[\int_0^{\tau} r_i(t)\left\{\mathbf{Z}_i - \bar{Z}_r(t;\boldsymbol{\beta})\right\} d\hat{M}_{ir}(t) \right. $$
$$\left. + \int_0^{\tau} \{1 - r_i(t)\}\left\{\mathbf{Z}_i - \bar{Z}_p(t;\boldsymbol{\beta})\right\} d\hat{M}_{ip}(t)\right]^{\otimes 2},$$

where

$$\hat{M}_{ir}(t) = M_{ir}(t;\hat{\boldsymbol{\beta}}_{\mathrm{mix}}, \hat{\mu}_0(t;\hat{\boldsymbol{\beta}}_{\mathrm{mix}})), \quad \hat{M}_{ip}(t) = M_{ip}(t;\hat{\boldsymbol{\beta}}_{\mathrm{mix}}, \hat{\Gamma}_0(t;\hat{\boldsymbol{\beta}}_{\mathrm{mix}})).$$

8.3.3 Analysis of the Childhood Cancer Survivor Study

Now we apply the estimation procedure discussed in the previous subsection to the mixed data arising from the CCSS described above. For the analysis, we confine ourselves to a subgroup of the female participants who were at least 25 years old in 1996. It includes 3,966 participants in total, with 2,765 being childhood cancer survivors and the others being their siblings. For the pregnancy process, there exist some subjects who provided only one type data, either recurrent event data or panel count data. Also there exist some subjects who provided recurrent event data over some periods but panel count data over other periods. That is, we have type II mixed data. However, for the data collected before 2001, all participant provided only one type of

8.3 Analysis of Mixed Recurrent Event and Panel Count Data

Table 8.2. Frequencies of the pregnancy counts of the participants in the CCSS

# of pregnancy	0 (%)	1 (%)	2 (%)	≥ 3 (%)
	All observed data			
Survivors ($n = 2{,}765$)	1,057 (38.23)	389 (14.07)	501 (18.12)	818 (29.58)
Siblings ($n = 1{,}201$)	216 (17.99)	151 (12.57)	319 (26.56)	515 (42.88)
All subjects ($n = 3{,}966$)	1,273 (32.10)	540 (13.62)	820 (20.68)	1,333 (33.61)
	The observed data before 2011			
Survivors ($n = 2{,}765$)	1,146 (41.45)	406 (14.68)	530 (19.17)	683 (24.70)
Siblings ($n = 1{,}201$)	275 (22.90)	181 (15.07)	338 (28.14)	407 (33.89)
All subjects ($n = 3{,}966$)	1,421 (35.83)	587 (14.80)	868 (21.89)	1,090 (27.48)

data, either recurrent event data or panel count data. That is, we have type I mixed data before 2001. In the following, we consider both parts of the data for comparison. Also it is assumed that one is interested in comparing the pregnancy processes between the cancer survivors and the siblings.

To give an idea about the observed data and the difference between the two groups, Table 8.2 presents the frequencies of the pregnancy counts among the survivors and the siblings. The top part of the table is for the whole data and the bottom part is for the data before 2001. For the whole data, the average numbers of the pregnancy per subject are 1.684 and 2.403 for the cancer survivors and the siblings, respectively. The corresponding numbers for the data before 2001 are 1.498 and 2.049, respectively. These suggest that the siblings seem to have a higher pregnancy rate than the survivors.

For the comparison of the pregnancy rates between the cancer survivors and the siblings, define $Z_i = 1$ if the ith subject is a survivor and 0 otherwise. The application of the estimation procedure discussed above to the whole data yields $\hat{\beta}_{\text{mix}} = -0.247$ with the estimated standard error being 0.032. This gives a p-value close to zero for testing no difference between the two groups. If we only consider the data before 2001, the estimated difference and the associated standard error are $\hat{\beta}_{\text{mix}} = -0.128$ and 0.034, respectively, yielding a p-value of 0.0002 for testing the no difference. Both analyses indicate that as discussed above, the cancer survivors seem to have a significantly lower pregnancy rate than their siblings. In other words, the childhood cancer and its treatments indeed seem to have some significantly negative effect on the subsequent reproductive function.

To give a graphical presentation about the difference between the pregnancy rates, we display in Fig. 8.1 the separate estimated cumulative average numbers of the pregnancy for the two groups given by (8.9) with setting $\beta = 0$. Again it suggests that the siblings had much higher pregnancy rate than the cancer survivors. On the other hand, one may want to be careful to interpret these results due to several factors. One is the significantly different numbers of the subjects in the two groups. Another factor is that the estimation procedure assumes that all participants or subjects are independent. But it is apparent that the survivors and their siblings could be related although the correlation may not be strong.

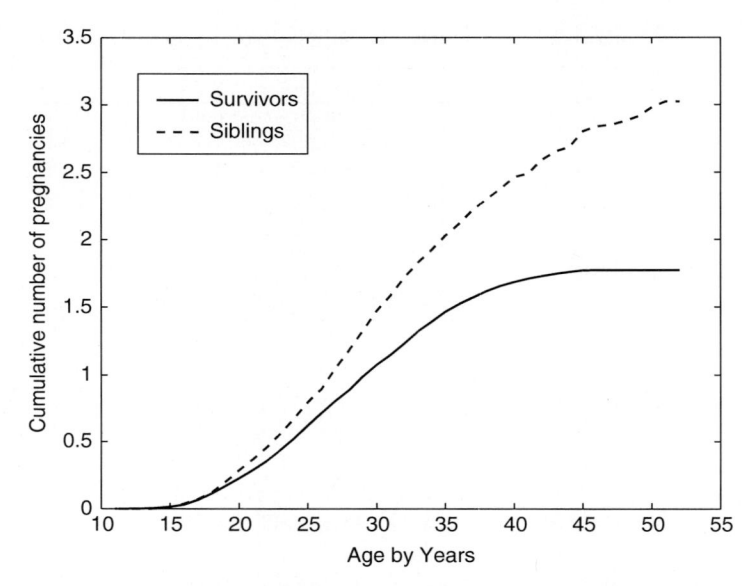

Fig. 8.1. Estimators of the cumulative average numbers of pregnancies

8.3.4 Discussion

As remarked above, the literature on mixed recurrent event and panel count data is quite limited compared to that for either recurrent event data or panel count data. In other words, more research remains to be done. One direction for future research is the development of more efficient estimation procedures than that discussed above. To see that, note that the estimating function $U_{\mathrm{mix}}(\boldsymbol{\beta})$ given in (8.11) is essentially a simple combination of the estimating functions used for recurrent event data and panel count data, respectively. It is possible to derive some other more efficient estimating functions and thus the more efficient estimators of regression parameters. The same is actually true for nonparametric estimation of the mean function of the underlying recurrent event process of interest too. For this, as pointed out in Sect. 8.3.3, one could employ the estimator given in (8.9) with setting $\boldsymbol{\beta} = 0$. However, it is easy to see that this estimator only makes use of the observed information over the continuously observed periods. One can expect to obtain more efficient estimators if all observed information can be used.

In the estimation procedure described above, it is assumed that the mean function of the underlying event process satisfies the proportional mean model (1.4). As discussed in Chaps. 5 and 6, the model can be generalized in different ways. One is to consider the semiparametric transformation model defined in (5.15) assuming that covariates are time-dependent. Furthermore, one could also consider the model

$$E\{\,N_i(t)|\mathbf{Z}_i\,\} \;=\; g\left\{\,\mu_0(t)\,\exp\{\boldsymbol{\beta}^T(t)\,\mathbf{Z}_i(t)\}\,\right\}$$

to allow time-varying covariate effects. Under the model above, it is easy to see that the development of estimation procedures may not be straightforward.

Another assumption used in the estimation procedure above is that the underlying recurrent event process $N_i(t)$ of interest and the observation process $\tilde{H}_i(t)$ are independent given covariates. As discussed in Chap. 6, this may not be true in reality. Also the process $N_i(t)$ could be related to the follow-up time C_i and/or there exists a dependent terminal event such as death. It is clear that one needs to develop new and different inference procedures for these situations as well as for the analysis of multivariate mixed recurrent event and panel count data.

8.4 Analysis of Panel Count Data from Multi-state Models

8.4.1 Introduction

So far up to this section, the focus has been on panel count data on counting processes or the recurrent event processes of interest with incomplete or interval-censored observations. In this section, we discuss another type of panel count data that concern transitions among possible finite states with the focus on continuous-time finite state Markov models. In other words, we consider the analysis of the finite state Markov models with incomplete or interval-censored observations (Chen et al., 2010; Joly et al., 2009; Kalbfleisch and Lawless, 1985; Titman, 2011).

Multi-state models or Markov models are commonly used in many fields including engineering, medical research and social sciences (Andersen and Klein, 2004). In these situations, a main objective is usually to make inference about the transition probabilities or intensities. In other words, we are interested in how long a study subject stays or occupies a state among finite possible states and how often the study subject moves or transfers from one to another state. Among the commonly used multi-state models, the survival model can perhaps be seen as the simplest one with two states, a transient state *alive* and an absorbing state *death*. Another simple multi-state model that has been intensively used and investigated is the three-state or illness-death model that consists of three states, heath, illness and death. In this case, one can only transit from health state to illness or death state, or from illness state to death state (Hsieh et al., 2002; Joly and Commenges, 1999; Joly et al., 2002). Among others, the illness-death model is commonly used in tumorigenicity experiments, and in this case, the three states correspond to tumor-free, tumor-onset and death (French and Ibrahim, 2002; Lagakos and Louis, 1988; Lindsey and Ryan, 1993).

A more complicated and specific multi-state model is shown in Fig. 8.2, reproduced from Andersen and Klein (2007). The model was designed to describe the recovery process of the patients given a haematopoietic stem cell transplant or bone marrow transplant (BMT) for leukaemia. Here it is supposed that an infusion of donor cells or the Donor Leuco-cyte infusion (DLI) is given to the patients who relapse to use the graft versus tumor effect of BMT to induce a second remission. The model has six states in total and three transient states, alive in the first post-BMT remission, alive in the first relapse and alive in the second remission following DLI. For such studies, one of the variables of interest is the current leukaemia-free survival function, the probability that a patient stays in state 0 or 4.

A well-known example of panel count data from a multi-state model is given in Kalbfleisch and Lawless (1985), arising from a survey study of public school students on their smoking behavior. In the study, the students starting their sixth grade in two Ontario counties (Canada) were surveyed four times during about a 2-year period. At each time point, the smoking status of each student was asked or recorded, which is that the child has never smoked, is currently a smoker or has smoked but has now quit. That is, we have a three-state model like the illness-death model mentioned above. There are two groups, control group and treatment group consisting of the students who received educational material on smoking during the first 2 months of the study. One of the objectives is to compare the two groups to assess the effect of the training on smoking. One can find another example of panel count data from the multi-state model in Chen et al. (2010) and Gladman et al. (1995). They analyzed the panel count data on psoriatic arthritis discussed in Sect. 7.3.3 by using a four-state Markov model. The states were defined based on the number of damaged joints determined by the clinical assessment, corresponding to no damage, mild, moderate and severe damage, respectively.

For the analysis of panel count data from multi-state models, a common and general procedure is to apply the maximum likelihood approach. In the following, we first consider the situation where the data arise from continuous-time, homogeneous finite state Markov models and present the maximum likelihood procedure. Other situations including non-homogeneous finite state

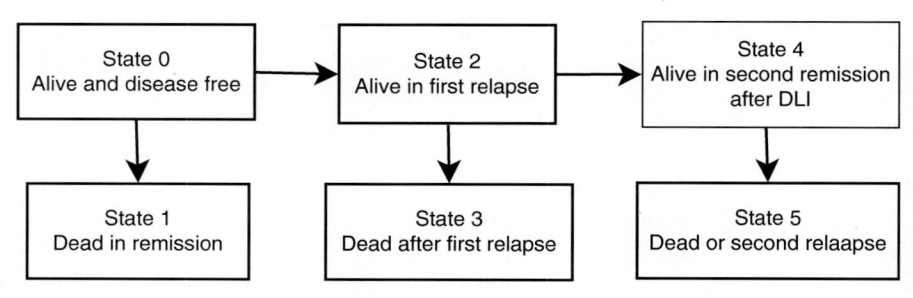

Fig. 8.2. A multi-state model for the recovery process of the patients given BMT

8.4 Analysis of Panel Count Data from Multi-state Models

Markov models and regression analysis are then briefly discussed. In this section, we assume that the observation process is independent and some comments on informative observation processes are provided at the end of the section.

8.4.2 Maximum Likelihood Estimation with Homogeneous Finite State Markov Models

Consider a follow-up study involving n independent subjects and in which each subject can stay at one of or move among m possible states denoted by $1, \ldots, m$. For subject i, let $X_i(t)$ denote the state where the subject occupies at time t and suppose that $\{X_i(t) : t \geq 0\}$ is a continuous-time Markov Chain as defined in Sect. 1.3.2, $i = 1, \ldots, n$. Also for $0 \leq s \leq t$, let $P(s,t) = \{p_{jl}(s,t)\}$ denote the $m \times m$ transition probability matrix with

$$p_{jl}(s,t) = P\{X_i(t) = l | X_i(s) = j\},$$

and $Q(t) = \{q_{jl}(t)\}$ the $m \times m$ transition intensity matrix, respectively, $j, l = 1, \ldots, m$. Then we have

$$q_{jl}(t) = \lim_{\Delta t \to 0} \frac{p_{jl}(t, t + \Delta t)}{\Delta t}, \; j \neq l.$$

In the following, we assume that the processes $X_i(t)$'s are time-homogeneous. That is, $Q(t) = Q = (q_{jl})$ is independent of t and $X_i(t)$ is stationary. Then we have

$$P(t) = P(s, s+t) = P(0,t)$$

and

$$P(t) = \exp(Qt) = \sum_{u=0}^{\infty} \frac{Q^u t^l}{u!}$$

(Cox and Miller, 1965).

For the estimation of the transition intensity matrix Q, suppose that the transition intensity $q_{jl} = q_{jl}(\boldsymbol{\theta})$ is known up to p functionally independent parameters $\theta_1, \ldots, \theta_p$, where $\boldsymbol{\theta} = (\theta_1, \ldots, \theta_p)^T$. Also suppose that each study subject is observed only at $k+1$ distinct time points $t_0 < t_1 < \cdots < t_k$. That is, we only know the states where each subject occupies at these time points but do not know when the transitions happen. Usually we set $t_0 = 0$. Define n_{jlu} to be the number of subjects in state j at time t_{u-1} and state l at time t_u, $u = 1, \ldots, k$. Then it is easy to show that conditional on the distribution of the state at time t_0, the log likelihood function of $\boldsymbol{\theta}$ has the form

$$\log L(\boldsymbol{\theta}) = \sum_{u=1}^{k} \sum_{j,l=1}^{m} n_{jlu} \log\{p_{jl}(w_u; \boldsymbol{\theta})\}, \tag{8.12}$$

where $w_u = t_u - t_{u-1}$. Thus it is natural to estimate $\boldsymbol{\theta}$ by maximizing the log likelihood function given above.

Let $\hat{\boldsymbol{\theta}}$ denote the maximum likelihood estimator of $\boldsymbol{\theta}$ defined above. It is easy to see that the determination of $\hat{\boldsymbol{\theta}}$ is not straightforward in general due to the complicated relationship between the $p_{jl}(w_u; \boldsymbol{\theta})$ and $q_{jl}(\boldsymbol{\theta})$'s. For this, several algorithms have been developed and in the following, we describe the quasi-Newton procedure originally given in Kalbfleisch and Lawless (1985).

To obtain $\hat{\boldsymbol{\theta}}$, first we need

$$S_v(\boldsymbol{\theta}) = \frac{\partial \log L(\boldsymbol{\theta})}{\partial \theta_v} = \sum_{u=1}^{k} \sum_{j,l=1}^{m} n_{jlu} \frac{\partial p_{jl}(w_u; \boldsymbol{\theta})/\partial \theta_v}{p_{jl}(w_u; \boldsymbol{\theta})},$$

$v = 1, \ldots, p$, and

$$\frac{\partial^2 \log L(\boldsymbol{\theta})}{\partial \theta_{v_1} \partial \theta_{v_2}} = \sum_{u=1}^{k} \sum_{j,l=1}^{m} n_{jlu}$$

$$\times \left\{ \frac{\partial^2 p_{jl}(w_u; \boldsymbol{\theta})/\partial \theta_{v_1} \partial \theta_{v_2}}{p_{jl}(w_u; \boldsymbol{\theta})} - \frac{\partial p_{jl}(w_u; \boldsymbol{\theta})/partial \theta_{v_1} \partial p_{jl}(w_u; \boldsymbol{\theta})/\partial \theta_{v_2}}{p_{jl}^2(w_u; \boldsymbol{\theta})} \right\}.$$

To finish the calculation above, suppose that for a given $\boldsymbol{\theta}$, the transition intensity matrix $Q(\boldsymbol{\theta})$ has m distinct eigenvalues $d_1(\boldsymbol{\theta}), \ldots, d_m(\boldsymbol{\theta})$. Then we have the canonical decomposition $Q(\boldsymbol{\theta}) = A(\boldsymbol{\theta}) D^{-1}(\boldsymbol{\theta}) A^{-1}(\boldsymbol{\theta})$, where $D(\boldsymbol{\theta}) = \text{diag}\{d_1(\boldsymbol{\theta}), \ldots, d_m(\boldsymbol{\theta})\}$ and $A(\boldsymbol{\theta})$ is the $m \times m$ matrix whose jth column is a right eigenvector of $Q(\boldsymbol{\theta})$ corresponding to $d_j(\boldsymbol{\theta})$. This along with the fact that $P(t; \boldsymbol{\theta}) = \exp\{Q(\boldsymbol{\theta}) t\}$ gives

$$P(t; \boldsymbol{\theta}) = A(\boldsymbol{\theta}) \, \text{diag} \left\{ \exp(d_1(\boldsymbol{\theta})t), \ldots, \exp(d_m(\boldsymbol{\theta})t) \right\} A^{-1}(\boldsymbol{\theta}). \tag{8.13}$$

It follows that

$$\frac{\partial P(t; \boldsymbol{\theta})}{\partial \theta_v} = A(\boldsymbol{\theta}) \, V_v \, A^{-1}(\boldsymbol{\theta}),$$

$v = 1, \ldots, p$, where V_v is the $m \times m$ matrix with the (j, l) element given by

$$\frac{g_{jl}^{(v)} \{\exp(d_j(\boldsymbol{\theta})t) - \exp(d_l(\boldsymbol{\theta})t)\}}{d_j(\boldsymbol{\theta}) - d_l(\boldsymbol{\theta})}, \quad j \neq l,$$

$$g_{jj}^{(v)} \, t \exp(d_j(\boldsymbol{\theta})t), \quad j = l.$$

In the above, $g_{jl}^{(v)}$ is the (j, l) element in

$$G^{(v)} = A^{-1}(\boldsymbol{\theta}) \frac{\partial Q(\boldsymbol{\theta})}{\partial \theta_v} A(\boldsymbol{\theta}).$$

8.4 Analysis of Panel Count Data from Multi-state Models

Note that given $S_v(\boldsymbol{\theta})$ and $\partial^2 \log L(\boldsymbol{\theta})/\partial \theta_{v_1} \partial \theta_{v_2}$, one could employ the Newton-Raphson algorithm for the determination of $\hat{\boldsymbol{\theta}}$. It is apparent, however, that this would not be easy as it involves the computations of the second derivatives. To avoid this, define $n_{j.u} = \sum_{l=1}^{k} n_{jlu}$, the number of the subjects in state j at time t_{u-1}. By using the fact that

$$\frac{\partial^2 p_{jl}(w_u; \boldsymbol{\theta})}{\partial \theta_{v_1} \partial \theta_{v_2}} = 0,$$

we have

$$E\left\{-\frac{\partial^2 \log L(\boldsymbol{\theta})}{\partial \theta_{v_1} \partial \theta_{v_2}}\right\} = \sum_{u=1}^{k} \sum_{j,l=1}^{m} \frac{E\{n_{j.u}\}}{p_{jl}(w_u; \boldsymbol{\theta})} \frac{\partial p_{jl}(w_u; \boldsymbol{\theta})}{\partial \theta_{v_1}} \frac{\partial p_{jl}(w_u; \boldsymbol{\theta})}{\partial \theta_{v_2}}.$$

It is obvious that the expectation above can be estimated by

$$\sigma_{v_1 v_2}(\boldsymbol{\theta}) = \sum_{u=1}^{k} \sum_{j,l=1}^{m} \frac{n_{j.u}}{p_{jl}(w_u; \boldsymbol{\theta})} \frac{\partial p_{jl}(w_u; \boldsymbol{\theta})}{\partial \theta_{v_1}} \frac{\partial p_{jl}(w_u; j.u)}{\partial \theta_{v_2}}.$$

This suggests the following iterative estimation procedure.

Let $\boldsymbol{\theta}^{(b-1)}$ denote the estimator of $\boldsymbol{\theta}$ obtained at the $(b-1)$ iteration, and define $S(\boldsymbol{\theta}) = (S_1(\boldsymbol{\theta}), \ldots, S_p(\boldsymbol{\theta}))^T$ and $\Sigma(\boldsymbol{\theta}) = (\sigma_{v_1 v_2})$, a $p \times p$ matrix. Then one can obtain the updated estimator of $\boldsymbol{\theta}$ by

$$\boldsymbol{\theta}^{(b)} = \boldsymbol{\theta}^{(b-1)} + \Sigma^{-1}(\boldsymbol{\theta}^{(b-1)}) S(\boldsymbol{\theta}^{(b-1)}) \tag{8.14}$$

and continue the process above until the convergence. Suppose that the true value, denoted by $\boldsymbol{\theta}_0$, of $\boldsymbol{\theta}$ is an interior point of the parameter space. Then it can be shown that $\sqrt{n}\,(\hat{\boldsymbol{\theta}} - \boldsymbol{\theta}_0)$ asymptotically follows the multivariate normal distribution with mean zero and the covariance matrix that can be consistently estimated by $\Sigma^{-1}(\hat{\boldsymbol{\theta}})/n$.

Note that in the discussion above, for simplicity, it has been assumed that the observation times for all subjects are the same. The approach described actually applies to the general situation where the observation times differ from subject to subject. More specifically, let $t_{i,0} < t_{i,1} < \cdots < t_{i,k_i}$ denote the observation times on the process $X_i(t)$. In this case, the log likelihood function of $\boldsymbol{\theta}$ has the form

$$\log L^*(\boldsymbol{\theta}) = \sum_{i=1}^{n} \sum_{u=1}^{k_i} \sum_{r,s=1}^{m} I\{X_i(t_{i,u-1}) = r, X_i(t_{i,u}) = s\}\, p_{rs}(w_{i,u}; \boldsymbol{\theta}),$$

where $w_{i,u} = t_{i,u} - t_{i,u-1}$. Furthermore, we have

$$E\left\{-\frac{\partial^2 \log L^*(\boldsymbol{\theta})}{\partial \theta_{v_1} \partial \theta_{v_2}}\right\} = \sum_{i=1}^{n} \sum_{u=1}^{k_i} \sum_{r,s=1}^{m} \frac{E\{\delta_{iur}\}}{p_{rs}(w_{i,u}; \boldsymbol{\theta})} \frac{\partial p_{rs}(w_{i,u}; \boldsymbol{\theta})}{\partial \theta_{v_1}} \frac{\partial p_{rs}(w_{i,u}; \boldsymbol{\theta})}{\partial \theta_{v_2}},$$

which can be estimated by

$$\sigma^*_{v_1 v_2}(\boldsymbol{\theta}) = \sum_{i=1}^{n} \sum_{u=1}^{k_i} \sum_{r,s=1}^{m} \frac{\delta_{iur}}{p_{rs}(w_{i,u};\boldsymbol{\theta})} \frac{\partial p_{rs}(w_{i,u};\boldsymbol{\theta})}{\partial \theta_{v_1}} \frac{\partial p_{rs}(w_{i,u};\boldsymbol{\theta})}{\partial \theta_{v_2}},$$

where $\delta_{ijr} = I(X_i(t_{i,j-1}) = r)$. It follows that one can obtain the maximum likelihood estimator of $\boldsymbol{\theta}$ based on $L^*(\boldsymbol{\theta})$ by using the iterative algorithm similar to that given in (8.14) (Gentlemen et al., 1994). Note that one advantage of the algorithms discussed above is that they only involve the first derivatives of the log likelihood function.

8.4.3 Discussion

In the previous subsection, it has been assumed that the $X_i(t)$'s are homogeneous Markov processes and it is apparent that this may not be true in practice. In other words, the transition intensity matrix $Q(t)$ may depend on time t and the $X_i(t)$'s are non-homogeneous. Assume that the $X_i(t)$'s are continuous-time non-homogeneous Markov processes and $Q(t) = Q(t;\boldsymbol{\theta})$ is known up to the vector of unknown parameters $\boldsymbol{\theta}$. Let $t_{i,0} < t_{i,1} < \cdots < t_{i,k_i}$ denote the observation times on subject i, $i = 1, \ldots, n$. Then the likelihood function of $\boldsymbol{\theta}$ has the form

$$\prod_{i=1}^{n} \prod_{u=1}^{k_i} P\left\{ X_i(t_{i,u}) = x_{i,u} | X_i(t_{i,u-1}) = x_{i,u-1} \right\},$$

where $x_{i,0}, x_{i,1}, \ldots, x_{i,k_i}$ denote the states that subject i occupies at times $t_{i,0} < t_{i,1} < \cdots < t_{i,k_i}$, respectively. Thus it is natural to estimate $\boldsymbol{\theta}$ by maximizing the likelihood function above.

On the other hand, the maximization above is usually quite difficult due to the relationship between the transition probability matrix $P(s,t)$ and the transition intensity matrix $Q(t)$. More specifically, for the situation, we need to solve the following Kolmogorov Forward Equations (KFE)

$$\frac{dP(t_0,t)}{dt} = P(t_0,t)\,Q(t)$$

subject to the initial condition $P(t_0,t_0) = I$ (Cox and Miller, 1965). The general solution to the KFE above is given by

$$P(t_0,t) = \sum_{k=0}^{\infty} \int_{t_1-t_0}^{t} \int_{t_2-t_1}^{t} \cdots \int_{t_l-t_{l-1}}^{t} Q(t_1)\,Q(t_2) \cdots Q(t_l)\,dt_1 dt_2 \cdots dt_l,$$

8.4 Analysis of Panel Count Data from Multi-state Models

where l represents the number of jumps made by the Markov chain between t_0 and t, and $t_1, \ldots, t_l$ denote the times of these jumps.

It is easy to see that unlike (8.13) for the homogeneous Markov process, the relationship above is very difficult or intractable in general. There exist two exceptions to this. One is that the transition intensities can be assumed to be piecewise constant functions (Kay, 1986; Titman, 2011). As commented before, the use of the piecewise constant function allows considerable flexibility in the form of the time dependence. On the other hand, this implies deterministic discontinuities in the hazard functions, which may not be viewed as biologically plausible. The other situation where the KFE have an analytic solution is that the transition intensity matrix has the form

$$Q(t) = Q_0 \, g(t; \lambda).$$

Here Q_0 is a time-independent and unknown intensity matrix and $g(t; \lambda)$ is a known, nonnegative function with the parameter λ. For given λ, define $s = \int_0^t g(u; \lambda) \, du$ and the stochastic process $Y(s) = X(t)$. Then one can show that the process $\{Y(s) : s \geq 0\}$ is a homogeneous Markov process with intensity matrix Q_0. It follows that if λ is known and Q_0 is known up to a vector of unknown parameters, one can estimate Q_0 by using the maximum likelihood procedure described in the previous subsection. If λ is unknown, one may apply the profile likelihood approach to estimate it.

For estimation of non-homogeneous Markov processes in general, one approach is to employ the discrete-time approximation (Aalen, 1975; Bacchetti et al., 2010). However, it may not be practical in some situations since it assumes that there exists only a single possible jump within a time period. Titman (2011) gives another approach developed based on numerical solutions to differential equations and the use of B-splines to approximate the transition intensities. It is more flexible than the time transformation method mentioned above. Also it is biologically more plausible than the piecewise constant intensity method commented before. Although the approach makes use of only the first derivatives as that described in the previous subsection, it is still computationally intensive in nature.

As discussed in the previous sections, in many situations, there may exist some covariates, and one may be interested in estimating or making inference about the relationship between these covariates and the transition intensities $q_{jl}(t)$'s. In this case, as the proportional hazards model in failure time data analysis or the proportional rate model (1.3), a commonly used model is given by

$$q_{jl}(t; \boldsymbol{Z}) = \exp\left(\boldsymbol{\beta}_{jl}^T \boldsymbol{Z}\right)$$

for a homogeneous Markov process (Kalbfleisch and Lawless, 1985; Tuma and Robins, 1980). In the above, $\boldsymbol{\beta}_{jl}$ is a vector of unknown regression parameters and $\boldsymbol{Z}$ denotes the vector of covariates as before but with the first component being equal to one. One advantage of the model above is its analytical

convenience. On the other hand, for a particular application, a different model such as
$$q_{jl}(t; \boldsymbol{Z}) = q_{jl} + \boldsymbol{\beta}_{jl}^T \boldsymbol{Z}$$
may be more appropriate.

Throughout this section, it has been assumed that the observation process or the process generating the observation times $t_{i,u}$'s is noninformative or independent of the Markov process of interest. As discussed in Chap. 6, this may not be true sometimes. An example of panel count data with informative observation processes is discussed in Chen et al. (2010) with the data arising from a progressive multi-state model. By the progressive multi-state model, also sometimes referred to as the irreversible multi-state model, we mean that study subjects can transfer from one to another state in one direction only (Hsieh et al., 2002; Joly and Commenges, 1999; Joly et al., 2002). An example of such models is the illness-death model discussed above. In the case of informative observation processes, one complicated factor is that one cannot simply construct the likelihood function conditional on the observation times as above.

8.5 Bayesian Analysis and Analysis of Nonstandard Panel Count Data

In this section, we briefly discuss three topics related to panel count data that have not been touched previously. First we consider the Bayesian analysis of panel count data with the focus on nonparametric estimation. Regression analysis of panel count data is then investigated when parts of the covariates of interest are measured or observed with some errors. That is, we do not know the exact values of some covariates. In this case, it is apparent that the use of the regression procedures described before may yield biased results or conclusions, and thus new regression procedures are needed (Carroll et al., 1995; Kim, 2007; Lin et al., 1993; Prentice, 1982; Zhou and Pepe, 1995). Finally, we discuss the situation in which instead of only one underlying recurrent event process, the observed panel count data may arise from one of several possible underlying recurrent event processes. That is, one faces mixture models (Mclachlan and Peel, 2000; Nielsen and Dean, 2008; Rosen et al., 2000; Wang et al., 1996).

8.5.1 Bayesian Analysis of Panel Count Data

Bayesian approach is commonly used in many fields including failure time data analysis (Gómez et al., 2004; Ibrahim et al., 2001). However, only limited literature exists on the use of Bayesian approach for the analysis of panel count data. In the case of parametric analysis, it is apparent that the

8.5 Bayesian Analysis and Analysis of Nonstandard Panel Count Data

application of Bayesian approaches is straightforward at least in theory. In the following, we confine the discussion to nonparametric estimation of panel count data.

Consider a recurrent event study that yields panel count data given in (3.1), and suppose that one is mainly interested in the nonparametric estimation problem considered in Sect. 3.2. In the following, we use the same notation as those used in Sect. 3.2. To apply the Bayesian approach, one needs to specify a prior distribution or process. For the current situation, a natural way is clearly to directly impose a prior process such as Dirichlet or gamma process on the intensity or cumulative intensity process of the recurrent event processes $N_i(t)$'s. Another approach, briefly discussed below and given by Ishwaran and James (2004), is to assume that the mean function $\mu(t)$ has the form

$$\mu(t|P) = \int_{\mathcal{S}} \int_0^t K(s,v)\, ds\, P(dv)$$

and impose a prior process on P. In the above, $K(s,v)$ denotes a prespecified kernel function and P is a finite measure over a measurable space $(\mathcal{S}, \mathcal{A})$. To describe the approach, for each i, define $A_{i,j} = (t_{i,j-1}, t_{i,j}]$ and $A_i = (0, t_{i,m_i}]$, $j = 1, \ldots, m_i$, $i = 1, \ldots, n$. Motivated by the likelihood function given in (3.3), Ishwaran and James (2004) suggest to consider the likelihood function

$$L(P) = \exp\left\{-\sum_{i=1}^n \int_{\mathcal{S}} \int_0^\infty Y_i(t)\, F(dt|v)\, P(dv)\right\}$$

$$\times \prod_{i=1}^n \prod_{j=1}^{m_i} \prod_{l=1}^{\Delta n_{i,j}} \int_{\mathcal{S}} F(A_{i,j}|v_{i,j,l})\, P(dv_{i,j,l}).$$

In the above, $F(A|v) = \int_A K(s,v)\, ds$ for each Borel-measurable set A, $Y_i(t) = I(t \in A_i)$, $\Delta n_{i,j} = n_{i,j} - n_{i,j-1}$, and the $v_{i,j,l}$'s can be viewed as missing observations.

For the specification of a prior process on P and the determination of the resulting posterior process, define $\mathbf{v} = (v_{i,j,l}\ l = 1, \ldots, \Delta n_{i,j}, j = 1, \ldots, m_i, i = 1, \ldots, n)$ and

$$\pi(d\mathbf{v}|P) = \prod_{i=1}^n \prod_{j=1}^{m_i} \prod_{l=1}^{\Delta n_{i,j}} P(dv_{i,j,l}),$$

a conditional measure of $\mathbf{v}$ given P. Assume that P has a weighted gamma prior process denoted by $\mathcal{G}(\cdot|\alpha, \beta)$. More specifically, for each Borel-measurable set $A \in \mathcal{A}$, a measure P in $\mathcal{G}(\cdot|\alpha, \beta)$ has the form

$$P(A) = \int_A \beta(s)\, \gamma_\alpha(ds),$$

where $\beta(s)$ is a positive integrable function over $\mathcal{S}$ and γ_α is a gamma process over $\mathcal{S}$ with shape measure α. That is, for a Borel-measurable set $A \in \mathcal{A}$, $\gamma_\alpha(A)$ is a gamma random variable with mean $\alpha(A)$ and variance $\alpha(A)$. Then it follows from Theorem 3 of James (2003) that for any integrable function $g(\mathbf{v}, P)$, the resulting posterior is given by

$$\int g(\mathbf{v}, P)\, \pi(d\mathbf{v}, dP|\mathbf{D})$$

$$\int \int g(\mathbf{v}, P)\, \mathcal{G}\left(dP\Big|\alpha + \sum_{i=1}^n \sum_{j=1}^{m_i} \sum_{l=1}^{\Delta n_{i,j}} \delta_{v_{i,j,l}}, \beta^*\right) \pi(d\mathbf{v}|\mathbf{D}).$$

In the above, $\mathbf{D}$ represents the observed data, δ_v denotes a discrete measure concentrated at v,

$$\pi(d\mathbf{v}|\mathbf{D}) \propto m_0(d\mathbf{v}) \prod_{i=1}^n \prod_{j=1}^{m_i} \prod_{l=1}^{\Delta n_{i,j}} \beta^*(v_{i,j,l})\, F(A_{i,j}|v_{i,j,l}),$$

where

$$\beta^*(v) = \frac{\beta(v)}{1 + \beta(v) \sum_{i=1}^n F(A_i|v)},$$

and

$$m_0(d\mathbf{v}) = \int \prod_{i=1}^n \prod_{j=1}^{m_i} \prod_{l=1}^{\Delta n_{i,j}} M(v_{i,j,l})\, \mathcal{P}(dM|\alpha),$$

the Pólya urn density for a Dirichlet process $\mathcal{P}(\cdot|\alpha)$ (Ferguson, 1973, 1974).

It is apparent that there is no close form for the posterior given above for the function $g(\mathbf{v}, P)$ and some approximation has to be used. One approach is to apply the Blocked Gibbs sampling and one can find the details on this in Ishwaran and James (2004).

8.5.2 Analysis of Panel Count Data with Measurement Errors

This subsection discusses regression analysis of panel count data as in Chap. 5. However, we assume that some components of the covariates of interest cannot be measured or observed exactly. That is, there exist measurement errors on covariates. The problems related to measurement errors occur and have been discussed in many fields including failure time data analysis (Lin et al., 1993; Prentice, 1982; Zhou and Pepe, 1995), longitudinal data analysis (Tsiatis et al., 1995; Wulfsohn and Tsiatis, 1997), and recurrent event data analysis (Yi and Lawless, 2012). In the following, we use the same notation as those defined in Sect. 5.2 and discuss the generalization of the estimation procedure given there to the situation with measurement errors.

Consider a recurrent event study with n independent subjects as in Sect. 5.2. Also let the $N_i(t)$'s, $\mathbf{Z}_i$'s, $t_{i,j}$'s, $n_{i,j}$'s, and m_i's be defined as

8.5 Bayesian Analysis and Analysis of Nonstandard Panel Count Data

there, and suppose that one only observes the data given in (5.1). In the following, we assume that the covariate $\mathbf{Z}_i$ can be written in two parts as $\mathbf{Z}_i = (\mathbf{Z}_{i1}^T, \mathbf{Z}_{i2}^T)^T$. Here $\mathbf{Z}_{i1}$ denotes the components that can be observed exactly and $\mathbf{Z}_{i2}$ the components that may be measured or observed with errors. Also we assume that for $\mathbf{Z}_{i2}$, there exists an auxiliary variable W_i and the recurrent event processes $N_i(t)$'s follow the proportional mean model (1.4). Then we have

$$E\{N_i(t)|\mathbf{Z}_i\} = \mu_0(t) \exp\left(\boldsymbol{\beta}_1^T \mathbf{Z}_{i1} + \boldsymbol{\beta}_2^T \mathbf{Z}_{i2}\right),$$

where $\mu_0(t)$ and $\boldsymbol{\beta} = (\boldsymbol{\beta}_1^T, \boldsymbol{\beta}_2^T)^T$ are defined as before. Here it is supposed that $\boldsymbol{\beta}$ is partitioned in the same way as $\mathbf{Z}_i$. Define

$$V = \{i : \mathbf{Z}_{i2} \text{ is observed without errors}\},$$

which is usually referred to as the validation set, and let $\bar{V}$ denotes the complement of V. Also in the following, it is assumed that the observation process is independent and given $\mathbf{Z}_{i2}$, W_i is independent of both the recurrent event process N_i and the observation process.

For estimation of $\boldsymbol{\beta}$, we assume that the $N_i(t)$'s are non-homogeneous Poisson processes as in Sect. 5.2. Then the log pseudo-likelihood function $l_p(\mu_0, \boldsymbol{\beta})$ given in (5.2) has the form

$$l_p(\mu_0, \boldsymbol{\beta}) = \sum_{i=1}^{n} \sum_{j=1}^{m_i} \left\{ n_{i,j} \log \mu_0(t_{i,j}) + n_{i,j} (\boldsymbol{\beta}_1^T \mathbf{Z}_{i1} + \boldsymbol{\beta}_2^T \mathbf{Z}_{i2}) \right.$$
$$\left. - \mu_0(t_{i,j}) \exp(\boldsymbol{\beta}^T \mathbf{Z}_{i1} + \boldsymbol{\beta}_2^T \mathbf{Z}_{i2}) \right\}$$
$$= \sum_{l=1}^{m} w_l \left\{ \bar{n}_l \log \mu_0(s_l) - \bar{a}_l(\boldsymbol{\beta}) \mu_0(s_l) + \bar{b}_l(\boldsymbol{\beta}) \right\}.$$

In the above, the s_l's, w_l's, $\bar{n}_l$'s, $\bar{a}_l(\boldsymbol{\beta})$'s and $\bar{b}_l(\boldsymbol{\beta})$'s are defined as in Sect. 5.2 with the latter two terms having the forms

$$\bar{a}_l(\boldsymbol{\beta}) = \frac{1}{w_l} \sum_{i=1}^{n} \sum_{j=1}^{m_i} \exp(\boldsymbol{\beta}_1^T \mathbf{Z}_{i1} + \boldsymbol{\beta}_2^T \mathbf{Z}_{i2}) I(t_{i,j} = s_l),$$

and

$$\bar{b}_l(\boldsymbol{\beta}) = \frac{1}{w_l} \sum_{i=1}^{n} \sum_{j=1}^{m_i} n_{i,j} (\boldsymbol{\beta}_1^T \mathbf{Z}_{i1} + \boldsymbol{\beta}_2^T \mathbf{Z}_{i2}) I(t_{i,j} = s_l),$$

respectively, $l = 1, \ldots, m$.

It is obvious that for the current situation, the log pseudo-likelihood function $l_p(\mu_0, \boldsymbol{\beta})$ is not available due to the measurement errors. To see this more closely, note that we can rewrite $\bar{a}_l(\boldsymbol{\beta})$ and $\bar{b}_l(\boldsymbol{\beta})$ as

$$\bar{a}_l(\boldsymbol{\beta}) = \frac{1}{w_l} \sum_{i \in V} \sum_{j=1}^{m_i} \exp(\boldsymbol{\beta}_1^T \mathbf{Z}_{i1} + \boldsymbol{\beta}_2^T \mathbf{Z}_{i2}) I(t_{i,j} = s_l)$$

$$+ \frac{1}{w_l} \sum_{i \in \bar{V}} \sum_{j=1}^{m_i} \exp(\boldsymbol{\beta}_1^T \boldsymbol{Z}_{i1} + \boldsymbol{\beta}_2^T \boldsymbol{Z}_{i2}) I(t_{i,j} = s_l),$$

and

$$\bar{b}_l(\boldsymbol{\beta}) = \frac{1}{w_l} \sum_{i \in V} \sum_{j=1}^{m_i} n_{i,j} (\boldsymbol{\beta}_1^T \boldsymbol{Z}_{i1} + \boldsymbol{\beta}_2^T \boldsymbol{Z}_{i2}) I(t_{i,j} = s_l)$$

$$+ \frac{1}{w_l} \sum_{i \in \bar{V}} \sum_{j=1}^{m_i} n_{i,j} (\boldsymbol{\beta}_1^T \boldsymbol{Z}_{i1} + \boldsymbol{\beta}_2^T \boldsymbol{Z}_{i2}) I(t_{i,j} = s_l),$$

respectively. That is, for $i \in \bar{V}$, we have an unobserved quantity $h(\boldsymbol{\beta}_2^T \boldsymbol{Z}_{i2})$ which needs to be estimated in order to use $l_p(\mu_0, \boldsymbol{\beta})$, where $h(x) = x$ or $\exp(x)$. If the auxiliary covariates W_i's are categorical variables, at $t_{i,j} = s_l$, Kim (2007) suggests to estimate $h(\boldsymbol{\beta}_2^T \boldsymbol{Z}_{i2})$ by

$$\hat{h}(\boldsymbol{\beta}_2^T \boldsymbol{Z}_{i2}) = \frac{\sum_{k \in V} I(t_{k,m_k} \geq s_l) I(W_k = W_i) h(\boldsymbol{\beta}_2^T \boldsymbol{Z}_{k2})}{\sum_{k \in V} I(t_{k,m_k} \geq s_l) I(W_k = W_i)}.$$

For the continuous W_i's, she gives the following kernel estimator

$$\hat{h}(\boldsymbol{\beta}_2^T \boldsymbol{Z}_{i2}) = \frac{\sum_{k \in V} I(t_{k,m_k} \geq s_l) K_h(W_k = W_i) h(\boldsymbol{\beta}_2^T \boldsymbol{Z}_{k2})}{\sum_{k \in V} I(t_{k,m_k} \geq s_l) I(W_k = W_i)}$$

for $h(\boldsymbol{\beta}_2^T \boldsymbol{Z}_{i2})$, where $K_h(t) = K(t/h)$ with $K(t)$ being some kernel function satisfying $\int K(t) dt = 1$ and $\int t K(t) dt = 0$, and $h > 0$ is a bandwidth, some positive constant. Similar estimators can be found in other fields such as failure time data analysis.

Define $\hat{a}_l(\boldsymbol{\beta})$ and $\hat{b}_l(\boldsymbol{\beta})$ to be $\bar{a}_l(\boldsymbol{\beta})$ and $\bar{b}_l(\boldsymbol{\beta})$ defined above with $h(\boldsymbol{\beta}_2^T \boldsymbol{Z}_{i2})$ replaced by $\hat{h}(\boldsymbol{\beta}_2^T \boldsymbol{Z}_{i2})$. Also define

$$\hat{l}_p(\mu_0, \boldsymbol{\beta}) = \sum_{l=1}^{m} w_l \left\{ \bar{n}_l \log \mu_0(s_l) - \hat{a}_l(\boldsymbol{\beta}) \mu_0(s_l) + \hat{b}_l(\boldsymbol{\beta}) \right\}.$$

Then it is natural to estimate $\mu_0(t)$ and $\boldsymbol{\beta}$ by maximizing the estimated log pseudo-likelihood function $\hat{l}_p(\mu_0, \boldsymbol{\beta})$ with the use of the two-step algorithm described in Sect. 5.2. As in Sect. 5.2, one can estimate the values of $\mu_0(t)$ only at the s_l's and the resulting estimator of $\mu_0(t)$ is a non-decreasing step function with possible jumps only at the s_l's.

Note that in the discussion above, for the simplicity, it has been assumed that the $N_i(t)$'s are non-homogeneous Poisson processes. As commented before, this assumption may not hold in practice. On the other hand, it is not difficult to see that it is straightforward to apply the idea discussed here to other regression procedures described in Chap. 5. Also note that in the above, no relationship between $\boldsymbol{Z}_{i2}$'s and W_i's has been assumed. In practice,

8.5 Bayesian Analysis and Analysis of Nonstandard Panel Count Data 217

sometimes it may be reasonable to impose some relationship between $\boldsymbol{Z}_{i2}$'s and W_i's (Carroll et al., 1995).

A situation that is closely related to the situation discussed above is that no auxiliary variable exists. In other words, we have no information about the $\boldsymbol{Z}_{i2}$'s for $i \in \bar{V}$ or the $\boldsymbol{Z}_{i2}$'s are completely missing for some subjects. It does not seem that there exists any established method for the analysis of such panel count data.

8.5.3 Analysis of Panel Count Data from Mixture Models

Mixture models are often used in many fields to describe heterogeneity (Chen and Li, 2009; Chen and Tan, 2009; Rosen et al., 2000; Susko et al., 1998). A common way to formulate the mixture model problem is to assume that the population density function has the form

$$f(\boldsymbol{x}; H) = \int f(\boldsymbol{x}; \boldsymbol{\theta}) \, d\, H(\boldsymbol{\theta}) \,.$$

In the above, $f(\boldsymbol{x}; \boldsymbol{\theta})$ denotes a density function for given $\boldsymbol{\theta}$ and $H(\boldsymbol{\theta})$ is a mixing cumulative distribution function, which can be discrete or continuous. A simple example of mixture models is that H is discrete and $f(\boldsymbol{x}; \boldsymbol{\theta})$ is a normal density function (Chen and Li, 2009). That is, the overall population is the mixture of several normal subpopulations. In this subsection, we briefly discuss the use of the mixture models for the analysis of panel count data.

Consider a recurrent event study that consists of n independent subjects and let $N_i(t)$ be defined as before, the recurrent event process given by subject i, $i = 1, \ldots, n$. In the following, we assume that there exist G subprocesses or clusters denoted by $\mathcal{G}_1, \ldots, \mathcal{G}_G$, and $N_i(t)$ can be written as

$$N_i(t) = \sum_{g=1}^{G} \delta_{gi} \, C_{gi}(t) \,. \tag{8.15}$$

In the above, $\delta_{gi} = I(i \in \mathcal{G}_g)$, the indicator function assumed to be unobservable, and $C_{gi}(t)$ denotes the subprocess corresponding to $\mathcal{G}_g$, $g = 1, \ldots, G$. Furthermore, we assume that there exist independent latent variables $\{V_{gi}\}$ and given V_{gi} and the vector of covariates $\boldsymbol{Z}_i = (Z_{i1}, \ldots, Z_{ip})^T$, $C_{gi}(t)$ is a non-homogeneous Poisson process with the rate function $V_{gi} \lambda_{gi}(t|\boldsymbol{Z}_i)$. Here $\lambda_{gi}(t|\boldsymbol{Z}_i)$ is supposed to have the form

$$\lambda_{gi}(t|\boldsymbol{Z}_i) = \exp\left\{ \phi_{g0}(t) + \sum_{k=1}^{p} \phi_{gk}(t) \, Z_{ik} \right\}$$

with $\phi_{gk}(t) = \boldsymbol{\alpha}_{gk}^T \boldsymbol{B}(t)$, $k = 0, 1, \ldots, p$. In the above, $\boldsymbol{B}(t)$ is the vector of cubic B-spline basis functions, and $\boldsymbol{\alpha}_{gk}$ is a vector of group-specific, unknown coefficients.

Suppose that one only observes panel count data, and let the $t_{i,0} = 0 < t_{i,1} < \cdots < t_{i,m_i}$ denote the observation times on subject i and the $n_{i,j}$'s be defined as before, $i = 1, \ldots, n$. Also suppose that the V_{gi}'s have the density function $h_g(\nu)$ with mean 1 and unknown variance σ_g^2, $g = 1, \ldots, G$. Then under the assumptions above, the vector $\mathbf{N}_i = (n_{i,1}, n_{i,2} - n_{i,3}, \ldots, n_{i,m_i-1} - n_{i,m_i})^T$ has the marginal distribution

$$P(\mathbf{N}_i) = \sum_{g=1}^{G} p_g \, P_g(\mathbf{N}_i).$$

In the above, $p_g = P(i \in G_g)$ and

$$P_g(\mathbf{N}_i) = \int \prod_{j=1}^{m_i} P_g(N_{i,j}|V_{gi} = v_{gi}) \, h_g(v_{gi}) \, dv_{gi}$$

with $P_g(N_{ij}|V_{gi} = v_{gi})$ denoting the Poisson distribution with the mean $v_{gi}\,\mu_{gij}$, where

$$\mu_{gij} = \Lambda_{gi}(t_{i,j}) - \Lambda_{gi}(t_{i,j-1}) = \int_{t_{i,j-1}}^{t_{i,j}} \lambda_{gi}(t|\mathbf{Z}_i) \, dt.$$

Let $\boldsymbol{\theta} = (\boldsymbol{\psi}^T, \mathbf{p}^T)^T$, denoting all unknown parameters, where $\boldsymbol{\psi} = (\boldsymbol{\psi}_1^T, \ldots, \boldsymbol{\psi}_G^T)^T$ with $\boldsymbol{\psi}_g = (\boldsymbol{\alpha}_g^T, \sigma_g^2)^T$ and $\boldsymbol{\alpha}_g = (\boldsymbol{\alpha}_{g0}^T, \ldots, \boldsymbol{\alpha}_{Gp}^T)^T$, and $\mathbf{p} = (p_1, \ldots, p_G)^T$. For estimation of $\boldsymbol{\theta}$, it is apparent that a natural approach would be to maximize the likelihood function $\prod_{i=1}^{n} P(\mathbf{N}_i)$. On the other hand, it is easy to see that this is not straightforward. In the following, we describe the estimating equation procedure given by Nielsen and Dean (2008) assuming that G, the number of hidden subprocesses or clusters, is known.

For each $i = 1, \ldots, n$ and $g = 1, \ldots, G$, define

$$\boldsymbol{\mu}_{gi} = (\mu_{gi1}, \ldots, \mu_{gim_i})^T, \quad D_{gi} = \frac{\partial \boldsymbol{\mu}_{gi}}{\partial \boldsymbol{\alpha}_g^T},$$

$$\Gamma_{gi}^{-1} = \text{diag}\left(\frac{1}{\mu_{gij}}\right)_{m_i \times m_i} - \frac{\sigma_g^2}{1 + \sigma_g^2 \mu_{gi+}} J_{m_i},$$

and $r_{gi} = \text{tr}(\delta_{gi} R_g)$. In the above, J_{m_i} denotes the $m_i \times m_i$ matrix with all elements equal to 1, $\mu_{gi+} = \sum_{j=1}^{m_i} \mu_{gij}$,

$$R_g = \left(\sum_{i=1}^{n} \delta_{gi} D_{gi}^T \Gamma_{gi}^{-1} D_{gi} + \text{diag}\{\xi_g\} \otimes A \right)^{-1} \left(\sum_{i=1}^{n} \delta_{gi} D_{gi}^T \Gamma_{gi}^{-1} D_{gi} \right),$$

$$A = \int_0^{\max\{t_{i,m_i}\}} \mathbf{b}(t) \, \mathbf{b}^T(t) \, dt$$

8.5 Bayesian Analysis and Analysis of Nonstandard Panel Count Data

with $\mathbf{b}(t) = \partial \mathbf{B}(t)/\partial t$, and $\boldsymbol{\xi}_g = (\xi_{g0}, \xi_{g1}, \ldots, \xi_{gp})^T$ are some unknown parameters satisfying

$$\xi_{gl} = \frac{\text{tr}(R_g)}{\boldsymbol{\alpha}_{gk}^T A \boldsymbol{\alpha}_{gk}}.$$

To estimate $\boldsymbol{\theta}$, assuming that $h_g(\nu)$ is the gamma density function, Nielsen and Dean (2008) give the following estimating equations:

$$U_{\boldsymbol{\alpha}_g} = \sum_{i=1}^{n} \delta_{gi} D_{gi}^T \Gamma_{gi}^{-1} (\mathbf{N}_i - \boldsymbol{\mu}_{gi}) - (\text{diag}\{\boldsymbol{\xi}_g\} \otimes A) \boldsymbol{\alpha}_g = 0, \quad (8.16)$$

$$U_{\sigma_g^2} = \sum_{i=1}^{n} \delta_{gi} \frac{(n_{i,j} - \mu_{gi+})^2 - \mu_{gi+}(1 + \sigma_g^2 \mu_{gi+}) + r_{gi}}{(1 + \sigma_g^2 \mu_{gi+})^2} = 0, \quad (8.17)$$

and

$$U_{p_g} = \sum_{i=1}^{n} \left(\frac{\delta_{gi}^*}{p_g} - \frac{\delta_{Gi}^*}{p_G} \right) = 0, \quad (8.18)$$

where

$$\delta_{gi}^* = \frac{p_g P_g(\mathbf{N}_i)}{\sum_{l=1}^{G} p_l P_l(\mathbf{N}_i)}.$$

Note that each of the Eqs. (8.16) and (8.17) involves G independent functions ($g = 1, \ldots, G$), while the Eq. (8.18) involves only $G - 1$ independent functions ($g = 1, \ldots, G-1$). It is easy to see that there are no direct solutions to the equations above and one has to employ some iterative algorithms. Also it is easy to see that the Eq. (8.18) is equivalent to

$$p_g = \frac{1}{n} \sum_{i=1}^{n} \delta_{gi}^*.$$

Let $\hat{\boldsymbol{\theta}}$ denote the estimator of $\boldsymbol{\theta}$ given by the Eqs. (8.16)–(8.18) and $\boldsymbol{\theta}_0$ the true value of $\boldsymbol{\theta}$. Then it follows from the estimating equation theory (Nielsen and Dean, 2008; White, 1982) that $\sqrt{n}(\hat{\boldsymbol{\theta}} - \boldsymbol{\theta}_0)$ asymptotically follows a multivariate normal distribution with mean zero and the covariance matrix that can be estimated by

$$E\left(\frac{\partial U_{\boldsymbol{\theta}}}{\partial \boldsymbol{\theta}^T}\right)^{-1} \left(\sum_{i=1}^{n} U_{i,\boldsymbol{\theta}} U_{i,\boldsymbol{\theta}}^T\right) E\left(\frac{\partial U_{\boldsymbol{\theta}}^T}{\partial \boldsymbol{\theta}}\right)^{-1} \Big|_{\boldsymbol{\theta}=\hat{\boldsymbol{\theta}}}.$$

In the above,

$$U_{\boldsymbol{\theta}} = \left(U_{\boldsymbol{\alpha}_1}^T, U_{\sigma_1^2}, \ldots, U_{\boldsymbol{\alpha}_G}^T, U_{\sigma_G^2}, U_{p_1}, \ldots, U_{p_{G-1}} \right)^T,$$

and $U_{i,\boldsymbol{\theta}}$ denotes $U_{\boldsymbol{\theta}}$ based only on the observed information from subject i, $i = 1,\ldots,n$.

Note that in the estimation procedure above, it has been assumed that G is known and in practice, this may not be true. Some discussion on the case where G is unknown can be found in Nielsen and Dean (2008). Another assumption used above is that the $C_{gi}(t)$'s are non-homogeneous Poisson processes. It is apparent that this may also not be true in practice. That is, the recurrent event process defined in (8.15) does not have to be a mixture of Poisson processes.

8.6 Concluding Remarks

The analysis of panel count data is still a relatively new and growing field and there exist many open problems. Before discussing these open problems or directions for future research, it is worth to emphasize again that most of the approaches described in this book are for panel count data with unbalanced structures. In other words, both observation and follow-up times differ from subject to subject, and they can be regarded as realizations of some underlying observation and follow-up processes, respectively. For the situation where observation times or intervals are the same for all subjects, it is easy to see that the data can be regarded as multivariate data. Hence any method that accommodates multivariate positive integer-valued response variables can be used for the analysis. This holds even though some subjects may miss some intermediate observations and/or drop out of the study early. In this case, the resulting data can be seen as multivariate data with missing values. On the other hand, it is apparent that the procedures discussed above are much more appropriate for the analysis of panel count data than multivariate data analysis procedures in general.

Similar to treating panel count data as multivariate data, one can also regard them as a special case of longitudinal data and apply the methods developed for longitudinal data. However, as mentioned before, these methods may not be able to take into account the special structure of panel count data and thus would be less efficient. In addition, some questions of interest regarding the analysis of panel count data may not appropriately or cannot be answered from the longitudinal data point of view.

Another general point that has been discussed above and is worth to be emphasized again is the use of the mean function of underlying recurrent event processes in modeling and analyzing panel count data. As mentioned before, a key reason for this is the structure of panel count data and the amount of observed information. In addition, the mean function is often also the target of interest similarly as the mean or expectation of a population. Of course, a drawback is that the mean function itself cannot uniquely determine the processes in general. An example of this is the nonparametric comparison

8.6 Concluding Remarks

of recurrent event processes discussed in Chap. 4. Also as commented before, if needed, one could directly model the intensity process or rate function of the recurrent event processes as often done for the analysis of recurrent event data. However, one usually has to make certain assumptions about the shape of the intensity process or rate function such as approximating them by some smooth functions. In addition, inference procedures would be much harder or more complicated (Ishwaran and James, 2004; Lawless and Zhan, 1998; Staniswalls et al., 1997; Sun and Matthews, 1997; Sun and Rai, 2001).

With respect to the directions for future research, it is apparent that in theory, one could ask almost any question imposed on recurrent event data. On the other hand, of course, some of them may not make sense or have no practical meaning. One topic that has been investigated by many authors in the case of recurrent event data is the gap time of the event, the time between successive occurrences of the event (Darlington and Dixon, 2013; Huang and Liu, 2007; Park, 2005; Sun et al., 2006; Wang and Chen, 2000; Zhao and Zhou, 2012; Zhao et al., 2012). In this case, instead of the occurrence rate of recurrent events, the distribution of the gap time is usually the target for inference. However, there seems to exist little research on this in the case of panel count data. Note that in the literature, the term gap time could also mean the time between two successive failure events in multivariate failure time data analysis (Lin and Ying, 2001; Schaubel and Cai, 2004), or the observation gap in recurrent event data analysis (Zhao and Sun, 2006).

For all regression models discussed in this book, a basic assumption is that covariate effects are time-independent. As mentioned before, this may not be true in reality as, for example, the effects of treatments or medicines for a disease may change, or be more or less effective as time changes. The topic of regression analysis with time-varying covariate effects has been considered in many areas. They include longitudinal data analysis (Song and Wang, 2008; Sun et al., 2005; Sun and Wu, 2005), failure time data analysis (Cai and Sun, 2003; Scheike and Martinussen, 2004; Yan and Huang, 2012), and recurrent event data analysis (Sun et al., 2009b; Zhao et al., 2011b). For the case of panel count data, one reference on it is given by Sun et al. (2009a), who generalized the proportional mean model (1.4) to

$$E\{\,N(t)|\boldsymbol{Z}_1(t), \boldsymbol{Z}_2(t)\,\} \;=\; \mu_0(t)\,\exp\left\{\,\boldsymbol{\beta}_1^T(t)\boldsymbol{Z}_1(t) \;+\; \boldsymbol{\beta}_2^T\boldsymbol{Z}_2(t)\,\right\}\;.$$

In the above, $\mu_0(t)$ is defined as in model (1.4), $\boldsymbol{Z}_1(t)$ and $\boldsymbol{Z}_2(t)$ represent the parts of covariates whose effects are time-dependent and time-independent, respectively, and $\boldsymbol{\beta}_1(t)$ and $\boldsymbol{\beta}_2$ denote the corresponding effects. Furthermore, they developed an estimating equation procedure for estimation of $\boldsymbol{\beta}_1(t) = \int_0^t \boldsymbol{\beta}_1(s)\,ds$ and $\boldsymbol{\beta}_2$. It is easy to see that more work needs to be done in this area. For example, as discussed above, the proportional mean model may not fit panel count data well sometimes. Another issue is that Sun et al. (2009a) only considered the situation where the observation process is independent, and again as discussed above, this may not be true in practice.

Again on regression analysis of panel count data, another basic assumption behind all methods discussed in this book is that accurate and complete data on covariates are available. One exception is the procedure described in Sect. 8.5.2, which allows measurement errors on covariates. In reality, sometimes covariates may have missing values (Chen and Little, 1999; Little and Rubin, 1987). Also they could suffer some censoring (Gómez et al., 2003; Langohr et al., 2004). For example, Chen and Cook (2003) considered regression analysis of recurrent event data where the observations on covariates are interval-censored. More specifically, the covariate considered there is actually a marker process and also a recurrent event process. On the other hand, there does not seem to exist an established method for regression analysis of panel count data under these situations.

Software for and the implementation of the existing methods are always an important issue in almost every statistical area. For the analysis of panel count data, unfortunately, there does not seem to exist any specifically developed R or SAS package yet although there exists some effort. For example, two R packages were developed but are not available at the time when the book is written. They are the packages *panel* and *spef*. The former aims to implement the maximum likelihood estimation procedure discussed in Sect. 8.4.2, while the latter aims to implement some regression procedures discussed in Chap. 5. On the other hand, two R functions, *isoreg* and *monoreg*, can be used for the determination of the IRE discussed in Sect. 3.3. The latter belongs to the package *fdrtool*.

9
Some Sets of Data

The following sets of data are used for the examples and discussion at various places of the book.

Data set I, given in Table 9.1, arises from the National Cooperative Gallstone Study. It is a 10-year, multicenter, double-blinded, placebo-controlled clinical trial of the use of the natural bile acid chenodeoxycholic acid (cheno) for the dissolution of cholesterol gallstones. The data are discussed in Sect. 1.2.2 and analyzed in Sects. 3.3–3.5, 4.4 and 5.6. The table includes the successive visit times in study weeks and the associated counts of episodes of nausea for the 113 patients in the high-dose cheno and placebo groups during the first 52 weeks of the study.

Data set II, given in Table 9.2, arises from a bladder cancer study conducted by the Veterans Administration Cooperative Urological Research Group. It is discussed in Sect. 1.2.3 and analyzed in Sects. 2.4, 4.5, and 6.3–6.5. In the table, dot means no visit and the number represents the number of bladder tumors that occurred between the previous and current visits. The second column gives the size of the largest initial tumor, and the number of initial tumors (at month 0) is given in column 3.

Data set III, given in Table 9.3, arises from a skin cancer chemoprevention trial conducted by the University of Wisconsin Comprehensive Cancer Center in Madison, Wisconsin. It is a double-blinded and placebo-controlled randomized phase III clinical trial to evaluate the effectiveness of $0.5\,\text{g/m}^2/\text{day}$ PO difluoromethylornithine in reducing new skin cancers in a population of the patients with a history of non-melanoma skin cancers. The data are discussed in Sect. 1.2.4 and analyzed in Sects. 7.2, 7.4, 7.5, and 8.2. In the table, t denotes the observation time, $N_1(t)$ and $N_2(t)$ represent the numbers of the occurrences of basal cell carcinoma and quamous cell carcinoma, respectively, between the observations. The column Covariates refers to three covariates, the number of prior skin cancers, age and gender.

Table 9.1. Data set I—Visit times in weeks and the observed counts of episodes of nausea for 113 patients with floating gallstones in the National Cooperation Gallstone Study

Patient ID	t_1	N_1	t_2	N_2	t_3	N_3	t_4	N_4	t_5	N_5	t_6	N_6	t_7	N_7	t_8	N_8	t_9	N_9
High-dose cheno group																	
1	4	0	8	0	13	0	26	0	38	0	51	0	.	.	.	.	.	.
2	4	0	9	3	13	0	26	0	39	0	51	0	.	.	.	.	.	.
3	4	0	8	0	12	0	24	0	38	0	51	0	.	.	.	.	.	.
4	4	0	8	0	12	0	26	0	38	0	51	0	.	.	.	.	.	.
5	4	0	8	0	13	0	26	0	38	0	52	0	.	.	.	.	.	.
6	4	0	8	0	12	0	25	0	39	0	51	0	.	.	.	.	.	.
7	4	0	9	0	14	0	26	0	39	0	52	0	.	.	.	.	.	.
8	4	0	9	0	14	0	28	0	39	0	.	.	.	.	.	.	.	.
9	4	0	9	1	14	0	27	1	38	1	.	.	.	.	.	.	.	.
10	4	0	9	0	13	0	17	0	22	0	26	0	38	0	43	0	.	.
11	3	0	8	0	13	0	26	0	40	4	.	.	.	.	.	.	.	.
12	4	0	8	0	13	1	27	0	39	0	52	0	.	.	.	.	.	.
13	4	20	10	2	14	2	17	10	28	0	41	0	.	.	.	.	.	.
14	5	1	9	0	13	0	26	0	38	0	52	0	.	.	.	.	.	.
15	5	0	9	0	15	0	27	0	39	0	51	0	.	.	.	.	.	.
16	4	0	9	0	13	0	26	0	38	0	52	0	.	.	.	.	.	.
17	4	0	8	0	12	0	27	0	39	0	51	0	.	.	.	.	.	.
18	4	0	8	0	12	0	26	0	37	0	48	0	.	.	.	.	.	.
19	4	0	9	0	14	0	28	0	38	0	52	0	.	.	.	.	.	.
20	9	0	22	0	31	0	38	0	.	0	.	.	.	.	.	.	.	.
21	5	0	10	0	13	0	25	0	50	2	.	.	.	.	.	.	.	.
22	4	0	9	0	12	0	25	0	39	0	50	0	.	.	.	.	.	.
23	5	0	8	0	13	0	25	0	40	0	.	.	.	.	.	.	.	.
24	4	0	9	0	13	0	26	0	38	0	51	0	.	.	.	.	.	.
25	4	0	9	0	13	0	26	0	38	0	52	99	.	.	.	.	.	.
26	4	0	9	1	13	0	26	0	39	0	.	.	.	.	.	.	.	.
27	3	0	8	0	13	1	25	0	40	0	51	0	.	.	.	.	.	.
28	4	0	8	0	13	0	24	0	38	0	52	0	.	.	.	.	.	.
29	3	0	9	0	12	5	26	0	38	0	50	0	.	.	.	.	.	.
30	4	0	10	0	15	1	28	0	41	0	.	.	.	.	.	.	.	.
31	3	0	8	0	13	0	26	0	39	0	52	0	.	.	.	.	.	.
32	3	1	9	3	13	0	26	0	38	0	52	0	.	.	.	.	.	.
33	4	0	10	0	16	0	29	0	41	0	.	6	.	.	.	.	.	.
34	3	0	7	0	12	0	25	0	38	0	51	0	.	.	.	.	.	.
35	4	0	9	0	13	0	26	0	39	0	51	0	.	.	.	.	.	.
36	5	0	9	2	13	0	26	0	39	0	51	0	.	.	.	.	.	.
37	6	0	12	6	16	0	28	0	41	0	.	.	.	.	.	.	.	.
38	4	0	9	0	13	0	25	0	38	0	51	0	.	.	.	.	.	.
39	4	0	8	0	12	0	26	0	40	0	.	.	.	.	.	.	.	.
40	4	0	8	0	12	10	26	0	39	0	52	0	.	.	.	.	.	.

9 Some Sets of Data

Data set I (Continued)

Patient ID	t_1	N_1	t_2	N_2	t_3	N_3	t_4	N_4	t_5	N_5	t_6	N_6	t_7	N_7	t_8	N_8	t_9	N_9
41	5	0	9	0	14	0	27	0	39	0	52	0	.	.	.	.	.	.
42	5	0	9	0	13	0	26	0	36	2	38	0	51	0	.	.	.	.
43	4	0	10	0	14	0	26	0	39	0	53	0	.	.	.	.	.	.
44	4	0	9	0	16	2	28	4	39	0	51	0	.	.	.	.	.	.
45	5	0	10	0	15	0	29	0	40	0	55	0	.	.	.	.	.	.
46	4	0	9	0	13	0	26	0	37	0	51	0	.	.	.	.	.	.
47	4	0	8	0	13	0	26	0	38	0	51	0	.	.	.	.	.	.
48	5	0	10	0	13	0	25	0	39	0	.	.	.	.	.	.	.	.
49	3	0	7	0	13	2	25	0	36	5	49	3	.	.	.	.	.	.
50	3	0	8	0	13	0	25	8	37	20	.	.	.	.	.	.	.	.
51	6	0	9	0	13	0	26	0	40	0	51	0	.	.	.	.	.	.
52	5	0	8	0	12	0	25	0	38	0	51	0	.	.	.	.	.	.
53	4	0	8	0	13	0	25	0	41	0	.	.	.	.	.	.	.	.
54	4	0	8	0	15	0	27	0	40	0	51	10	.	.	.	.	.	.
55	4	0	8	1	12	0	27	0	41	0	.	.	.	.	.	.	.	.
56	5	0	12	0	16	0	29	0	41	0	52	0	.	.	.	.	.	.
57	5	0	11	4	16	0	30	5	44	24	51	40	.	.	.	.	.	.
58	3	0	9	0	14	0	26	0	.	.	.	.	.	.	.	.	.	.
59	3	0	.	.	.	.	.	.	.	.	.	.	.	.	.	.	.	.
60	3	0	.	.	.	.	.	.	.	.	.	.	.	.	.	.	.	.
61	4	0	9	0	13	0	25	0	38	0	.	.	.	.	.	.	.	.
62	4	0	8	0	14	0	18	0	20	0	.	.	.	.	.	.	.	.
63	4	0	8	0	13	0	17	0	23	0	27	0	32	0	.	.	.	.
64	3	0	10	0	26	0	.	.	.	.	.	.	.	.	.	.	.	.
65	8	5	19	0	28	0	.	.	.	.	.	.	.	.	.	.	.	.
Placebo group																		
66	4	0	8	0	12	0	25	0	38	0	52	0	.	.	.	.	.	.
67	4	0	8	0	13	0	27	0	40	0	44	0	.	.	.	.	.	.
68	4	0	11	0	14	0	26	0	39	0	52	0	.	.	.	.	.	.
69	4	0	9	0	12	0	25	0	40	0	52	0	.	.	.	.	.	.
70	4	0	8	0	14	0	27	0	40	0	52	0	.	.	.	.	.	.
71	5	1	9	0	13	0	26	1	40	0	.	.	.	.	.	.	.	.
72	4	0	8	0	13	0	24	0	37	0	50	0	.	.	.	.	.	.
73	4	1	9	0	14	4	28	3	41	1	.	.	.	.	.	.	.	.
74	3	0	9	0	13	0	25	0	38	0	50	0	.	.	.	.	.	.
75	5	0	9	0	13	0	27	0	38	0	51	0	.	.	.	.	.	.
76	4	0	8	0	13	0	27	0	38	0	51	0	.	.	.	.	.	.
77	4	3	9	0	14	0	25	0	39	0	51	0	.	.	.	.	.	.
78	3	8	8	0	11	1	17	4	24	0	38	2	42	0	46	0	51	20
79	4	0	9	0	13	0	25	0	39	0	51	0	.	.	.	.	.	.
80	4	0	8	0	13	0	24	0	38	0	51	0	.	.	.	.	.	.
81	4	0	9	0	13	0	26	0	40	0	51	0	.	.	.	.	.	.
82	4	0	9	0	14	0	28	0	40	0	51	0	.	.	.	.	.	.

Data set I (Continued)

Patient ID	t_1	N_1	t_2	N_2	t_3	N_3	t_4	N_4	t_5	N_5	t_6	N_6	t_7	N_7	t_8	N_8	t_9	N_9
							Placebo group											
83	5	0	8	0	16	0	28	0	36	0	.	.	.	.	.	.	.	.
84	5	0	7	0	12	0	25	2	38	0	.	.	.	.	.	.	.	.
85	5	0	10	0	15	0	29	0	41	0	.	.	.	.	.	.	.	.
86	4	0	9	0	13	0	25	0	35	0	.	.	.	.	.	.	.	.
87	4	0	9	0	13	0	28	0	39	0	.	.	.	.	.	.	.	.
88	4	0	9	3	12	0	24	0	37	0	51	0	.	.	.	.	.	.
89	4	0	8	60	13	0	24	0	40	1	.	.	.	.	.	.	.	.
90	3	0	8	1	14	0	26	0	38	0	.	.	.	.	.	.	.	.
91	5	0	9	0	13	0	27	0	40	0	.	.	.	.	.	.	.	.
92	3	0	8	0	11	0	25	0	37	0	51	0	.	.	.	.	.	.
93	3	1	7	4	11	0	24	0	38	0	.	.	.	.	.	.	.	.
94	3	5	8	0	13	0	25	0	38	0	52	0	.	.	.	.	.	.
95	4	0	9	0	13	0	26	3	39	0	52	0	.	.	.	.	.	.
96	4	0	9	0	14	0	26	0	39	0	52	0	.	.	.	.	.	.
97	4	6	9	0	18	1	28	0	39	0	54	0	.	.	.	.	.	.
98	5	0	9	0	15	0	27	0	39	0	.	.	.	.	.	.	.	.
99	4	0	9	0	13	2	25	0	38	0	50	0	.	.	.	.	.	.
100	3	3	7	0	12	0	25	6	38	0	52	0	.	.	.	.	.	.
101	4	0	7	0	12	0	25	0	38	1	.	.	.	.	.	.	.	.
102	4	0	8	0	13	0	26	0	39	0	51	0	.	.	.	.	.	.
103	4	0	8	0	13	0	26	0	40	0	52	0	.	.	.	.	.	.
104	4	3	.	.	.	.	.	.	.	.	.	.	.	.	.	.	.	.
105	4	0	8	2	.	.	.	.	.	.	.	.	.	.	.	.	.	.
106	5	0	9	0	13	0	17	0	21	0	28	1	39	1	.	.	.	.
107	3	0	.	.	.	.	.	.	.	.	.	.	.	.	.	.	.	.
108	6	0	.	.	.	.	.	.	.	.	.	.	.	.	.	.	.	.
109	3	25	8	30	14	20	.	.	.	.	.	.	.	.	.	.	.	.
110	4	0	9	0	13	12	.	.	.	.	.	.	.	.	.	.	.	.
111	4	0	9	0	13	1	.	.	.	.	.	.	.	.	.	.	.	.
112	5	0	9	0	14	0	26	0	.	.	.	.	.	.	.	.	.	.
113	4	0	9	0	14	0	25	0	.	.	.	.	.	.	.	.	.	.

9 Some Sets of Data

Table 9.2. Data set II—Observed numbers of bladder tumors along with the numbers of initial tumors and the size of the largest initial tumor from a bladder cancer study

```
Patient Size                           Months
   ID     0            10              20              30
                         Placebo group
    1     3   1 0 . . . . . . . . . . . . . . . . . . . . . . . . . . . . . .
    2     1   2 0 . . . 0 . . . . . . . . . . . . . . . . . . . . . . . . . .
    3     1   1 . . . . . . . 0 . . . . . . . . . . . . . . . . . . . . . . .
    4     1   5 . . 0 . . . . . 0 0 . . . . . . . . . . . . . . . . . . . . .
    5     1   4 0 . . 0 . 1 0 . . . 0 . . . . . . . . . . . . . . . . . . . .
    6     1   1 . 0 . . . . . . 0 . . . 0 . . . . . . . . . . . . . . . . . .
    7     1   1 . 0 . . . . . . 0 . 2 . . . 3 . 0 . . . . . . . . . . . . . .
    8     1   1 . . 0 . . . . . . . . . . 0 . . . 0 . . . . . . . . . . . . .
    9     3   1 . . . . 2 . . . . 0 . 0 . . . . . 0 . . . . . . . . . . . . .
   10     3   1 . . 0 . . . 0 . . 6 . . . . 3 . . . 0 . . . 0 . . . . . . . .
   11     1   1 0 . 8 . . . . 0 . 0 . . 0 . . 8 . . 0 . . . 8 . . . . . . . .
   12     1   3 . . 1 . . 0 . . 1 0 . . 0 . 0 . 0 . . 0 8 . 0 . . . . . . . .
   13     3   3 . . 0 . . . 0 . . 0 . 0 . . 0 . . . 0 . . . . 0 . . . . . . .
   14     3   2 . . 0 . . . 8 . . 7 . . 0 . 5 . . . . . . . 7 . . . . . .
   15     1   1 . . 1 . . 0 . . 0 . . 0 . . 1 0 . . 0 . 0 . . 3 . . . . .
   16     1   8 8 . . 0 . . . 0 . . . 0 . . 0 . . . 0 . . . . 0 0 . . . .
   17     4   1 . 4 . . . 0 . . . . . . . . . . . . . . . . . . . . 8 . . .
   18     2   1 . . 0 . . 0 . . . . . . . 0 . . 0 . . . . 0 0 . . . 0 . . . .
   19     2   1 . . . . . . 0 . . . . . . . . . . . . . . . . . 3 . . . 0 . .
   20     4   1 . . . . 0 . . 0 . . . . . . . . . 0 . . . . . . . . . . . 0 .
   21     2   1 . . 0 . . 0 . . . . . . . . 0 . . . . . . . . . . . . . . 0 .
   22     1   4 . 0 . . 0 . . 0 . . 0 . . . . . . 0 . . . . 0 . . . . 0 .
   23     5   1 . 4 . . . . . . . 0 . . . . . . 2 . . . 4 0 . . . . . 0 . 0
   24     1   2 . . 1 . . 3 . 3 . . . 3 0 . 0 0 0 0 . . . 0 0 . . 3 . . . 0
   25     6   1 . 0 . . 0 0 . . 0 . . . 0 . . . . . . . . . 0 . . . . . 2 . 1
   26     3   1 0 . 0 0 . 0 . . . 0 . . 2 . . 3 . . 0 . . . . 1 . . . 0 . .
   27     2   1 . . 0 . . 0 . . 0 . . . 0 . 0 . . 0 . . 0 . . . . . 0 . . . .
   28     1   2 . . . 0 . . . 0 . 0 . . . 0 . . . . . . 0 . . . . . . . . 0
   29     1   2 . . 0 . . 0 . . 0 . 0 . . 0 . . 0 . . 0 . . 0 . . . . . . 0
   30     1   3 . . . . . . . . 0 . . . . . . . . 0 . . . . . . . . . 8 .
   31     2   1 0 . . 0 . . . . . 0 . . . . . . 0 . . . . . 0 . . . . . .
   32     1   4 . 0 . . . . . . 8 . . . . 0 . 2 . . . 5 . 1 . . . . 0 . .
   33     1   5 . 0 . 0 0 . . . 0 . . 0 . . . 0 1 . . 8 . . . 1 . . 0 . . 2 .
   34     2   1 . . 0 . . 0 . . 0 . 0 . . 0 . . 0 . . 0 . . 0 . . 0 . . 0 .
   35     1   1 . . 3 . 0 . 0 . . 0 . . . 0 . . . . . 0 . . . . . . 0 . . 0
   36     6   2 . . 0 . . 1 0 0 . . 0 . . 0 . 0 0 . . 0 . . 0 . . . . . . .
   37     1   2 . . 5 . 0 3 . . 4 . . . . 0 . . 0 . . 0 . . 0 . . . 0 . . 0
   38     1   1 . 0 . . . 0 . 1 . 3 . 0 . . . 0 . . 1 . . 0 . . 4 . . . 3
   39     1   1 . . 0 . . 0 . . 0 . 0 . . . 0 . . 1 . . 0 . . 0 . . 0 . .
   40     3   1 . . . . . . 0 . 0 . . . 0 . . . . 0 . . . . . 0 . . . . . 0
   41     1   3 . 0 . . 0 . . . . . 0 . . . . . 0 . . . . . 0 . . . . 0 .
   42     7   1 . . 0 . . . . . . . 0 . . 0 0 . . 1 . . . 0 . . 0 . . 0 . . 0
```

Data set II (Continued)

```
Patient  Size                         Months
ID              0              10              20              30
 43      1   3 . . 7 . . . . . . . 0 . . . 2 . . . . . . . . . . 0 . . . .
 44      1   1 0 . . 0 . . 0 . . 0 . . 0 . . 0 . . 0 . . 0 . . . . . 0 . .
 45      2   3 . 1 . . 0 . 0 . . 0 . . 0 . 3 . . . 0 . . . . 4 . . 0 . . 3
 46      3   1 . 0 . . . 3 . . 0 . . . 0 . . 4 . . . 0 2 0 . . . 0 . . . 5 . 0 .
 47      3   2 . 1 . . 0 . . . 3 . . . 6 2 . . . 2 . . 1 . 0 0 . . 0 . . 0
                                 Thiotepa group
 48      3   1 0 . . . . . . . . . . . . . . . . . . . . . . . . . . . . .
 49      1   1 0 . . . . . . . . . . . . . . . . . . . . . . . . . . . . .
 50      1   8 . . . . 8 . . . . . . . . . . . . . . . . . . . . . . . . .
 51      2   1 0 0 0 0 0 0 0 0 0 . . . . . . . . . . . . . . . . . . . . .
 52      1   1 . . . . . 0 . . . 0 . . . . . . . . . . . . . . . . . . . .
 53      1   1 . . 0 . . . . . . . . . 0 . . . . . . . . . . . . . . . . .
 54      6   2 . . 1 . 0 . . . 0 . 0 . . 0 . . . . . . . . . . . . . . . .
 55      3   5 5 . 2 . 5 . 2 . . 2 . . 0 . . 0 0 . . . . . . . . . . . . .
 56      3   1 . . . . 0 . . . . . 0 . . . . 2 0 . . . . . . . . . . . . .
 57      1   5 . . . . . . . . . . . . . . . . . 0 . . . . . . . . . . . .
 58      1   5 0 2 0 . . . . . . . . . . . . . . . . . 0 . . . . . . . . .
 59      1   1 0 0 0 0 0 0 0 0 0 . . . 0 0 0 0 1 . 1 . 0 . . . . . . . . .
 60      1   1 . 0 . . 0 . . . . 0 . . . . 0 . . 0 . . . 0 . . . . . . . .
 61      3   1 0 0 0 . . . . . 0 . . . 0 . . . . . 0 . . 0 . . . 0 . . . .
 62      5   1 0 . . . . . . . . 0 . 0 . . . . . . . . 0 . . . . . 0 . . .
 63      1   1 0 0 0 0 0 0 0 0 0 . 0 . 0 0 . . 0 0 . . . 0 0 . 0 . . . . .
 64      1   1 0 0 0 0 0 2 . . . 0 0 3 1 . . . . . . . 0 . . 0 . . 0 . . .
 65      1   1 0 . 0 . . 1 . . . 0 . . 0 . . 0 . . . . 0 . . . . . 0 . . .
 66      1   2 . 2 . . . . . . . . . . . . . . . . . . . . . . . . . . 0 .
 67      3   8 . . 0 . . 0 . . 0 . . . . . . . . . . . 0 . 0 0 . . 3 . . 0 .
 68      1   1 0 0 0 0 0 0 0 0 0 0 0 0 0 0 . 0 0 0 0 . 0 0 0 . 0 0 . . . .
 69      1   6 0 0 0 1 . . 0 0 0 0 0 0 0 0 . 3 . 0 0 . 0 0 3 . 0 0 3 . 0 .
 70      1   1 0 0 0 0 0 0 0 0 0 0 0 0 . 0 0 0 . 0 0 0 0 . 2 1 0 0 . 2 0 . .
 71      1   3 . . . . 0 . . . . . . . 0 . . 0 . . . . . . 3 . 2 . . 1 .
 72      2   3 0 0 0 0 0 0 0 0 . 0 0 0 0 0 0 0 0 0 0 0 0 0 0 . 0 0 0 0 0 0
 73      1   1 0 0 0 0 . . 0 0 0 0 0 0 0 . 0 0 0 0 0 0 0 0 0 0 0 0 0 0 0 .
 74      1   1 1 . 0 . . . 0 . . . . . 0 . . . 0 0 0 . 0 0 0 0 . 0 1 . 0 0
 75      1   1 1 . . . . . . . . 0 . . . . . . . . . . . . . 0 . . . . . .
 76      1   6 0 2 . 0 . 0 0 . 0 0 0 0 0 0 0 0 0 0 0 1 . . 2 . . . 1 0 . 0
 77      2   1 . . 0 . . 0 . . 0 . . . 0 . . 0 . . . . . . 0 . 0 . . . 0 .
 78      4   1 0 1 0 . . 0 0 0 0 . 0 0 0 0 0 0 0 0 0 0 0 0 0 0 0 0 . . . 0 . .
 79      4   1 0 0 0 0 0 0 0 0 0 0 0 0 0 0 0 0 0 0 0 0 0 0 0 0 0 0 0 0 0 0
 80      3   3 . . . . . . . . . . . . 0 . . . 0 . . . . . . . . 0 . . . 0 .
 81      1   4 . . . 1 . . . 0 . . . . 0 . . . . . . . . 0 . . 1 . . . . .
 82      1   1 0 0 . . . . . . . . . . . . . . . . . . 0 . . . . . 0 . . . .
 83      1   2 0 . 0 0 0 0 . 0 . . 0 . 0 0 . . 0 . . 0 . . . 0 . . 0 . . 0 .
 84      4   3 0 0 0 0 0 0 0 0 0 0 0 . 0 0 0 0 0 0 0 0 . 0 0 0 0 0 0 0 0 0
 85      3   1 0 0 0 0 0 0 0 0 0 0 . 0 0 0 . 0 . 0 0 . 0 0 0 . 0 0 0 0 0 0 0
```

Data set II (Continued)

Patient ID	31	Months 40	50	53

```
                         Placebo group
 1     . . . . . . . . . . . . . . . . . . . . . . .
 2     . . . . . . . . . . . . . . . . . . . . . . .
 3     . . . . . . . . . . . . . . . . . . . . . . .
 4     . . . . . . . . . . . . . . . . . . . . . . .
 5     . . . . . . . . . . . . . . . . . . . . . . .
 6     . . . . . . . . . . . . . . . . . . . . . . .
 7     . . . . . . . . . . . . . . . . . . . . . . .
 8     . . . . . . . . . . . . . . . . . . . . . . .
 9     . . . . . . . . . . . . . . . . . . . . . . .
10     . . . . . . . . . . . . . . . . . . . . . . .
11     . . . . . . . . . . . . . . . . . . . . . . .
12     . . . . . . . . . . . . . . . . . . . . . . .
13     . . . . . . . . . . . . . . . . . . . . . . .
14     . . . . . . . . . . . . . . . . . . . . . . .
15     . . . . . . . . . . . . . . . . . . . . . . .
16     . . . . . . . . . . . . . . . . . . . . . . .
17     . . . . . . . . . . . . . . . . . . . . . . .
18     . . . . . . . . . . . . . . . . . . . . . . .
19     . . . . . . . . . . . . . . . . . . . . . . .
20     . . . . . . . . . . . . . . . . . . . . . . .
21     . . . . . . . . . . . . . . . . . . . . . . .
22     . . . . . . . . . . . . . . . . . . . . . . .
23     . . . . . . . . . . . . . . . . . . . . . . .
24     . . . . . . . . . . . . . . . . . . . . . . .
25     . . . . . . . . . . . . . . . . . . . . . . .
26     0 . . . . . . . . . . . . . . . . . . . . . .
27     . 0 . . . . . . . . . . . . . . . . . . . . .
28     0 . 0 0 . . . . . . . . . . . . . . . . . . .
29     . . . . . 0 . . . . . . . . . . . . . . . . .
30     . . . . . 0 . . . . . . . . . . . . . . . . .
31     0 . . . . . 0 . . . . . . . . . . . . . . . .
32     0 . . . . 0 . . . 0 . . . . . . . . . . . . .
33     . 0 . 1 . . 0 . . 3 . . . . . . . . . . . . .
34     . . . . 0 0 . . . . 0 . . . . . . . . . . . .
35     . . . 0 . . 0 . . . . . 0 . . . . . . . . . .
36     . 0 . . 0 . . . . . . . 0 . . . . . . . . . .
37     . . 0 . . 0 . . 0 . 0 . . 0 . . . . . . . . .
38     . 0 . . 0 . . . 0 . . 0 . . 0 . . . . . . . .
39     0 . . 0 . . 0 . 0 . . . . . 0 . . 0 . . . . .
40     . . . . 0 . . . . 0 . . . 0 . . . 0 . . . . .
41     . . . . 1 . . . . . . . 0 . . . 0 . . 0 . . .
42     . . 0 . 0 . 0 . . . 0 . . 0 . . 0 . . . . . 0
```

Data set II (Continued)

```
Patient                 Months
  ID    31              40              50     53
  43    0 . . . 0 . . . . 0 . . . 3 . . . . 2 . 1
  44    . . . . 0 . . . . 0 . 0 . . . 0 . . . . .
  45    . . . 4 . . 0 . 1 . . 1 . . 0 . . 1 . . 1 .
  46    . . 0 . . 0 . . . 9 . . 0 0 0 . . 0 . . . 0
  47    . . 1 . . . 0 . . . 0 . . . 0 . . . 1 . . 0 .
                      Thiotepa group
  48    . . . . . . . . . . . . . . . . . . . . . . .
  49    . . . . . . . . . . . . . . . . . . . . . . .
  50    . . . . . . . . . . . . . . . . . . . . . . .
  51    . . . . . . . . . . . . . . . . . . . . . . .
  52    . . . . . . . . . . . . . . . . . . . . . . .
  53    . . . . . . . . . . . . . . . . . . . . . . .
  54    . . . . . . . . . . . . . . . . . . . . . . .
  55    . . . . . . . . . . . . . . . . . . . . . . .
  56    . . . . . . . . . . . . . . . . . . . . . . .
  57    . . . . . . . . . . . . . . . . . . . . . . .
  58    . . . . . . . . . . . . . . . . . . . . . . .
  59    . . . . . . . . . . . . . . . . . . . . . . .
  60    . . . . . . . . . . . . . . . . . . . . . . .
  61    . . . . . . . . . . . . . . . . . . . . . . .
  62    . . . . . . . . . . . . . . . . . . . . . . .
  63    . . . . . . . . . . . . . . . . . . . . . . .
  64    . . . . . . . . . . . . . . . . . . . . . . .
  65    . . . . . . . . . . . . . . . . . . . . . . .
  66    . . . . . . . . . . . . . . . . . . . . . . .
  67    . 0 . . 3 0 . . . . . . . . . . . . . . . . .
  68    . . . . . . . . 0 . . . . . . . . . . . . . .
  69    . . 8 . 0 9 8 . 0 . . . . . . . . . . . . . .
  70    . 3 . 0 . . . . . 0 . . . . . . . . . . . . .
  71    . . . . . . . . . 2 . . . . . . . . . . . . .
  72    0 0 0 0 . 0 0 . . . 0 . . . . . . . . . . . .
  73    0 0 0 0 0 . . . . . 0 . . . . . . . . . . . .
  74    . 0 0 . . 0 0 . . . . . 0 . . . . . . . . . .
  75    . . . . . . . . . . . . . 0 . . . . . . . . .
  76    . . . . . . . 8 . . 0 . . 0 . . . . . . . . .
  77    . . 0 . . . . . 0 . . . . . 0 . . . . . . . .
  78    . . . 0 . . . . . 0 . . . . 0 . . . . . . . .
  79    . 0 0 0 0 0 . . . . . . . . . 0 . . . . . . .
  80    . . . . . . . . . . 0 . . . . . 0 . . . . . .
  81    0 . 0 . . 0 . . . . . 0 . . . 1 . . 0 . . . .
  82    . 0 . . . . . . 0 . . . . . 0 . . 0 . . 0 . . .
  83    . 0 . . . . . 2 . . 0 . . . 0 . . 0 . . 0 . .
  84    0 0 0 0 . 0 . . 0 . . 0 . . 0 . . 0 . . . . .
  85    0 0 0 0 0 . . . . . 0 . . . . . . . . . . . .
```

9 Some Sets of Data

Table 9.3. Data set III—Observed information for the skin cancer trial: observation times in days (t) and # of new skin cancers (N)

			Observation number											
ID	Covariates		1	2	3	4	5	6	7	8	9	10	11	12
						DFMO group								
1	(2, 56, M)	t	180	350	538	742	924	1,100	1,287	1,498	1,680	1,778		
		N_1	0	0	0	0	0	0	1	0	0	2		
		N_2	0	0	0	0	0	0	0	0	0	0		
2	(9, 76, M)	t	180	370	412	543	606	747	873	1,337				
		N_1	0	0	0	0	0	0	0	0				
		N_2	1	4	0	6	0	0	0	0				
3	(7, 76, F)	t	264	362	633	721	994	1,357	1,440	1,788				
		N_1	0	0	0	0	0	0	0	0				
		N_2	0	0	1	0	1	1	1	0				
4	(1, 49, F)	t	99	131	188	342	523	722	910	1,085	1,275	1,457	1,793	
		N_1	0	0	0	0	0	0	0	0	0	0	0	
		N_2	0	0	0	0	0	0	0	0	0	0	0	
5	(5, 64, F)	t	154	352	532	632	820	1,213	1,409	1,453	1,621	1,795		
		N_1	0	0	0	0	1	0	0	1	0	0		
		N_2	0	0	0	1	0	0	0	0	1	0		
6	(1, 82, M)	t	44	179	371	511	840							
		N_1	0	0	0	0	0							
		N_2	0	0	0	0	0							
7	(3, 53, M)	t	179	364	378	544	728	908	1,118	1,309	1,489	1,670	1,770	
		N_1	0	0	0	0	0	0	1	0	0	0	0	
		N_2	0	0	0	0	0	0	0	0	0	0	0	
8	(3, 50, M)	t	151	350	515	718	900	1,068	1,257	1,460	1,656	1,797		
		N_1	0	0	0	0	2	0	0	0	0	0		
		N_2	0	0	0	0	1	0	0	0	0	0		
9	(2, 80, F)	t	182	229	264	462	550	1,280	1,698					
		N_1	0	0	0	0	0	0	0					
		N_2	0	0	0	0	0	0	0					
10	(4, 60, F)	t	176	233	393	575	759	939	1,120	1,304	1,367	1,493	1,688	1,759
		N_1	0	0	0	0	0	0	0	2	0	0	0	0
		N_2	0	0	0	0	0	0	0	0	0	0	0	0
11	(2, 59, F)	t	168	373	538	723	910	1,108	1,288	1,499	1,682	1,778		
		N_1	0	0	0	0	0	0	0	0	0	0		
		N_2	0	0	0	0	0	0	0	0	0	0		
12	(1, 56, F)	t	173	229	355	523	728	916	1,120	1,296	1,370	1,405	1,832	
		N_1	0	0	0	0	0	0	0	0	0	0	0	
		N_2	0	0	0	0	0	0	0	0	0	0	0	
13	(3, 75, M)	t	745	937	1,107	1,288	1,658	1,847						
		N_1	0	1	0	0	0	0						
		N_2	1	0	1	0	4	3						
14	(13, 51, M)	t	25	181	284	662	840	1,050	1,391	1,573				
		N_1	1	0	0	2	1	0	1	0				
		N_2	0	0	0	0	0	0	0	0				
15	(2, 57, M)	t	152	256	328	517	711	894	1,070	1,250	1,293	1,432	1,622	1,777
		N_1	1	0	0	0	0	0	0	0	0	0	0	0
		N_2	0	0	0	0	1	0	0	0	0	0	0	0

Data set III (Continued)

ID	Covariates		1	2	3	4	5	6	7	8	9	10	11	12
							Observation number							
16	(1, 56, M)	t	180	344	543	732	921	1,183	1,306	1,517	1,789			
		N_1	0	0	0	0	0	0	0	0	0			
		N_2	0	0	0	0	0	0	0	0	0			
17	(4, 52, M)	t	167	349	756	1,660								
		N_1	0	0	0	0								
		N_2	0	0	0	1								
18	(3, 72, F)	t	155	295	343	364	377	523	712	896	1,065	1,247	1,358	1,441
		N_1	0	0	0	0	0	0	0	0	0	0	0	0
		N_2	0	0	0	0	0	0	0	0	0	0	0	0
19	(2, 68, F)	t	186	413	442	781	965	1,189	1,412					
		N_1	0	1	0	0	0	0	1					
		N_2	0	0	0	1	0	0	1					
20	(1, 69, F)	t	209	288	389	425	454	579	643	840				
		N_1	0	0	0	0	0	0	0	0				
		N_2	0	0	0	0	0	0	0	0				
21	(3, 76, M)	t	187	369	541	573	751	901	937					
		N_1	0	0	0	0	0	0	1					
		N_2	0	0	0	0	0	0	0					
22	(5, 61, F)	t	155	190	344	526	568	599	722	925	1,100	1,109	1,379	1,554
		N_1	0	0	0	0	0	0	0	1	0	0	0	1
		N_2	0	0	0	0	0	0	0	0	0	0	0	0
23	(14, 70, F)	t	187	376	511	684	699	720	869	939	992	1,174	1,288	1,344
		N_1	0	0	0	0	0	0	0	0	2	0	0	0
		N_2	2	0	0	1	1	1	0	3	2	4	1	0
24	(4, 70, F)	t	73	182	416	612	806	868	1,052	1,201	1,239	1,253	1,421	1,596
		N_1	0	0	0	2	0	1	0	0	0	0	2	1
		N_2	0	0	0	0	0	0	0	0	0	0	0	0
25	(3, 73, M)	t	184	364	554	735	918	1,142	1,176	1,415	1,599	1,779		
		N_1	0	0	0	0	1	0	1	0	0	0		
		N_2	0	0	0	0	0	0	0	0	0	0		
26	(7, 67, M)	t	167	204	246	363	951	1,455	1,826					
		N_1	0	0	0	0	0	0	1					
		N_2	0	0	0	0	0	0	0					
27	(1, 50, F)	t	182	362	545	910	1,645							
		N_1	0	0	0	0	0							
		N_2	0	0	0	0	0							
28	(5, 77, F)	t	11	149	507	604	766	952	1,325	1,689				
		N_1	0	0	0	1	0	0	0	0				
		N_2	0	0	0	0	0	0	0	0				
29	(1, 49, M)	t	73	358	972									
		N_1	0	0	0									
		N_2	0	0	0									
30	(6, 72, F)	t	126	188	271	289	471	652	870	1,237	1,602	1,723		
		N_1	0	0	0	0	0	0	0	0	0	0		
		N_2	0	0	0	0	1	0	0	0	0	0		

9 Some Sets of Data

Data set III (Continued)

ID	Covariates		\multicolumn{12}{c}{Observation number}											
			1	2	3	4	5	6	7	8	9	10	11	12
31	(6, 65, M)	t	171	318	559	775	784	997	1,413	1,461	1,690	1,708		
		N_1	0	0	0	2	0	0	1	0	0	0		
		N_2	0	0	0	0	0	0	0	1	0	0		
32	(1, 69, M)	t	148	330	512	524	577	694	823					
		N_1	0	0	0	0	0	0	0					
		N_2	0	0	0	0	0	0	0					
33	(1, 76, F)	t	182	369	553	770	846	993	1,008	1,082				
		N_1	0	0	0	0	0	0	0	0				
		N_2	0	0	0	0	0	0	0	0				
34	(2, 75, F)	t	179	354	568	799	839	981	1,188	1,420	1,602	1,783		
		N_1	0	0	0	0	0	0	0	0	0	0		
		N_2	0	0	0	0	1	0	0	0	0	0		
35	(1, 56, M)	t	182	357	546	728	903	1,092	1,129	1,227	1,274	1,800		
		N_1	0	0	0	0	0	0	0	0	0	0		
		N_2	0	0	0	0	0	0	0	0	0	0		
36	(4, 66, F)	t	126	176	290	338	547	729	909	1,091	1,282	1,463	1,651	1,798
		N_1	0	0	0	0	0	0	0	0	0	0	0	0
		N_2	0	0	0	0	0	0	0	0	0	1	0	0
37	(7, 61, M)	t	181	364	547	730	821	925	944	1,211	1,770			
		N_1	1	0	1	0	0	1	0	1	1			
		N_2	0	0	0	0	0	0	0	0	0			
38	(2, 69, F)	t	54	76	168	532	690	1,047	1,726					
		N_1	0	0	0	1	1	0	0					
		N_2	0	0	0	0	0	0	0					
39	(2, 51, F)	t	193	425	640	838	1,033	1,223	1,452	1,641	1,795			
		N_1	0	0	0	0	1	0	0	0	0			
		N_2	0	0	0	0	0	0	0	0	0			
40	(2, 52, M)	t	177	365	587	804	986	1,170	1,350	1,532	1,700			
		N_1	0	0	0	0	0	0	0	0	0			
		N_2	0	0	0	0	0	0	0	0	0			
41	(1, 58, M)	t	199	379	540	729	899	1,081	1,262	1,444	1,682	1,794		
		N_1	0	0	0	0	0	0	0	0	0	0		
		N_2	0	0	0	0	0	0	0	0	0	0		
42	(2, 41, F)	t	65	177	366	520	554	707	903	1,098	1,318	1,498	1,709	1,827
		N_1	0	0	0	0	1	0	0	0	0	0	0	0
		N_2	0	0	0	0	1	0	0	0	0	0	0	0
43	(1, 40, F)	t	83	189	371	581	763	969	1,168	1,358	1,547	1,722		
		N_1	0	0	0	0	0	0	0	0	0	0		
		N_2	0	0	0	0	0	0	0	0	0	0		
44	(1, 54, M)	t	181	363	428	552	1,141	1,741						
		N_1	0	0	0	0	0	0						
		N_2	0	0	0	0	0	0						
45	(1, 59, M)	t	81	175	260	557	922	1,230	1,483	1,791				
		N_1	0	0	0	0	0	1	0	0				
		N_2	0	0	0	0	0	0	0	0				

Data set III (Continued)

ID	Covariates		1	2	3	4	5	6	7	8	9	10	11	12
							Observation number							
46	(2, 44, M)	t	184	365	554	800	1,023	1,205	1,304	1,492	1,695	1,786		
		N_1	0	2	3	0	1	2	1	0	0	1		
		N_2	0	0	0	0	0	0	0	0	0	0		
47	(1, 50, F)	t	186	364	546	963	1,155	1,358	1,547	1,722				
		N_1	0	0	0	0	0	0	0	0				
		N_2	0	0	0	0	0	0	0	0				
48	(1, 47, M)	t	180	584	963	1,328	1,693							
		N_1	0	0	0	0	0							
		N_2	0	0	0	0	0							
49	(1, 70, M)	t	186	355	383	479	1,125	1,775						
		N_1	0	0	0	0	1	1						
		N_2	0	0	0	0	0	0						
50	(2, 52, M)	t	152	334	1,368	1,608								
		N_1	0	0	0	0								
		N_2	0	0	0	0								
51	(1, 56, M)	t	189	371	588	765	792	968	1,148	1,330	1,506	1,694	1,780	
		N_1	0	0	0	0	0	0	0	0	0	0	0	
		N_2	0	0	0	0	0	0	0	0	0	0	0	
52	(1, 71, M)	t	176	357	394	432	607	686	1,283	1,373	1,741			
		N_1	0	0	0	0	0	0	0	0	0			
		N_2	0	0	0	0	0	0	0	1	0			
53	(2, 50, F)	t	167	350	379	533	714	895	1,260	1,632	1,715			
		N_1	0	1	0	0	1	0	0	2	0			
		N_2	0	0	0	1	0	0	0	0	0			
54	(5, 78, M)	t	69	104	112	238	567	894						
		N_1	0	1	0	0	1	1						
		N_2	0	0	0	0	0	0						
55	(11, 63, M)	t	158	347	397	529	657	700	840	963	979	1,707		
		N_1	0	0	0	1	0	0	0	0	0	0		
		N_2	0	0	0	1	0	0	0	0	0	0		
56	(1, 77, M)	t	90	190	428	538	720	764	926	1,108	1,114	1,311	1,520	1,723
		N_1	0	0	0	0	0	0	0	0	0	1	0	0
		N_2	0	0	0	0	0	0	0	0	0	0	0	0
57	(6, 59, M)	t	172	361	405	475	476	607	698	775	873	963	1,070	1,160
		N_1	1	0	0	1	0	0	0	0	0	0	0	0
		N_2	0	0	0	0	0	0	0	0	0	0	0	0
58	(10, 75, M)	t	174	339	363	587	817	1,049	1,231	1,417	1,599	1,796		
		N_1	0	0	0	1	1	0	0	0	0	0		
		N_2	0	0	0	1	1	0	1	1	0	0		
59	(11, 67, M)	t	191	372	386	573	762	924	1,106	1,261	1,442	1,652	1,793	
		N_1	1	1	0	1	0	0	0	0	0	0	0	
		N_2	0	0	0	0	0	0	0	0	1	0	0	
60	(1, 55, M)	t	140	322	504	686	868	1,115	1,310	1,493	1,674	1,786		
		N_1	0	0	0	0	0	0	0	0	0	0		
		N_2	0	0	0	0	0	0	0	0	0	0		

9 Some Sets of Data

Data set III (Continued)

ID	Covariates		1	2	3	4	5	6	7	8	9	10	11	12
61	(2, 69, M)	t	161	229	263	334	358	518	700	748	873	1,070	1,281	1,516
		N_1	0	0	0	0	0	0	0	0	0	0	0	0
		N_2	0	0	0	0	0	0	0	0	0	0	0	0
62	(1, 69, M)	t	199	381	595	623	778	967	1,200	1,374	1,556	1,737		
		N_1	0	0	0	0	0	0	0	0	0	0		
		N_2	0	0	0	0	0	0	0	0	0	0		
63	(3, 56, M)	t	196	375	567	749	931	1,127	1,351	1,519	1,708			
		N_1	0	0	0	0	0	0	0	1	0			
		N_2	1	0	0	0	0	0	0	0	0			
64	(2, 46, F)	t	20	30	176	548	1,674							
		N_1	0	0	0	0	0							
		N_2	0	0	0	0	0							
65	(1, 71, F)	t	274	530	698	897	1,139							
		N_1	0	0	0	0	0							
		N_2	0	0	0	0	0							
66	(3, 42, M)	t	20	146	158	326	507	692	866	1,053	1,235	1,417	1,600	1,781
		N_1	0	1	0	0	0	0	0	0	0	0	0	0
		N_2	0	0	0	0	0	0	0	0	0	0	0	0
67	(1, 55, F)	t	221											
		N_1	0											
		N_2	0											
68	(2, 45, M)	t	191	357	799									
		N_1	0	0	0									
		N_2	0	0	0									
69	(3, 44, F)	t	189	371	562	685	745	911	1,093	1,339	1,520	1,707	1,787	
		N_1	0	0	0	0	0	0	1	0	0	0	0	
		N_2	0	0	0	0	0	0	0	0	0	0	0	
70	(1, 75, M)	t	182	365	570	750	947	1,130	1,317	1,499	1,681	1,788		
		N_1	0	0	0	0	0	0	1	0	0	0		
		N_2	0	0	0	0	0	0	0	0	0	0		
71	(2, 70, M)	t	161	336	539	718	910	1,084	1,201	1,470	1,665			
		N_1	0	0	0	0	0	0	0	0	0			
		N_2	0	0	0	0	0	0	0	0	0			
72	(2, 63, M)	t	168	259	349	546	624	671	727	891	1,072	1,291	1,476	1,659
		N_1	0	0	0	0	0	0	0	0	0	1	0	0
		N_2	0	0	1	1	0	0	0	0	0	0	0	0
73	(2, 70, M)	t	179	383	580	767	949	971						
		N_1	0	0	0	0	0	0						
		N_2	0	0	1	0	0	0						
74	(9, 64, M)	t	177	188	202	379	743	1,113	1,666					
		N_1	1	0	0	0	0	1	0					
		N_2	0	0	0	0	0	1	1					
75	(3, 78, M)	t	96	198	439	637	1,037	1,405						
		N_1	0	0	0	0	0	0						
		N_2	0	0	0	0	0	0						

Data set III (Continued)

							Observation number						
ID	Covariates		1	2	3	4	5	6	7	8	9	10	11	12
76	(2, 49, M)	t	184	364	402	567	770	786	952	1,141	1,323	1,505	1,688	
		N_1	0	0	0	0	0	0	0	0	0	0	0	
		N_2	0	0	0	0	0	0	0	0	0	0	0	
77	(2, 72, M)	t	191	371	406	569	751	931	1,114	1,294	1,477	1,658	1,793	
		N_1	0	0	0	0	0	0	0	0	0	0	0	
		N_2	0	0	0	0	0	0	0	0	0	0	0	
78	(1, 67, M)	t	181	364	554	719	901	1,083	1,279	1,450	1,632	1,791		
		N_1	0	0	0	0	0	0	0	0	0	0		
		N_2	0	0	0	0	0	1	1	0	0	0		
79	(3, 61, M)	t	182	365	573	754	936	1,121	1,204	1,308	1,540	1,741		
		N_1	0	0	0	0	0	0	0	0	1	0		
		N_2	0	0	0	0	0	0	0	0	0	0		
80	(5, 63, F)	t	181	292	658	1,190	1,642							
		N_1	0	1	0	0	2							
		N_2	0	0	0	0	0							
81	(2, 44, M)	t	213	360	584	767	949	1,102	1,279	1,470	1,659			
		N_1	0	0	0	0	0	0	0	0	0	0		
		N_2	0	0	0	0	0	0	0	0	0	0		
82	(2, 67, M)	t	34	62	94	336	700	1,710						
		N_1	0	0	0	0	0	0						
		N_2	0	0	0	0	0	0						
83	(5, 63, M)	t	182	364	406	545	721	895	1,252	1,469	1,611	1,674	1,820	
		N_1	0	0	0	0	0	0	0	0	1	0		
		N_2	0	0	1	0	1	0	0	0	0	2		
84	(2, 71, F)	t	182	376	573	754	936	1,038	1,091	1,323	1,503	1,685		
		N_1	0	0	0	0	0	0	0	0	0			
		N_2	1	0	0	0	0	0	0	0	0			
85	(1, 63, M)	t	181	330	356	523	707	894	1,078	1,258	1,469	1,667	1,797	
		N_1	0	0	0	0	0	0	0	0	0	0	0	
		N_2	0	1	0	0	0	0	0	0	0	0	0	
86	(2, 76, F)	t	161	176	210	238	595	959						
		N_1	0	0	0	0	0	0						
		N_2	0	0	0	0	0	0						
87	(1, 49, F)	t	186	368	551	665	956	1,134	1,314	1,490	1,670			
		N_1	0	0	0	0	0	0	0	0	0			
		N_2	0	0	0	0	0	0	0	0	0			
88	(1, 52, M)	t	189	371	549	735	918	1,099	1,247	1,479	1,617			
		N_1	0	0	0	0	0	0	0	0	0			
		N_2	0	0	0	0	0	0	0	0	0			
89	(15, 67, F)	t	175	357	539	742	924	1,142	1,323	1,505	1,695			
		N_1	1	0	1	0	0	1	0	0				
		N_2	0	0	0	0	0	0	0	0				
90	(1, 66, M)	t	176	400	430	456	591	592	1,326	1,578				
		N_1	0	0	0	0	0	0	0					
		N_2	0	0	0	0	0	0	0					

9 Some Sets of Data

Data set III (Continued)

ID	Covariates		1	2	3	4	5	6	7	8	9	10	11	12
								Observation number						
91	(1, 51, F)	t	86	91	112	163	394	582	763	953	1,137	1,330	1,513	1,695
		N_1	1	1	0	0	2	0	0	0	0	0	0	0
		N_2	0	0	0	0	2	0	0	0	0	0	0	0
92	(3, 55, F)	t	175	392	581	770	959	1,141	1,330	1,512	1,694			
		N_1	0	0	0	0	0	0	1	0	0			
		N_2	0	0	0	0	0	0	0	0	0			
93	(2, 53, F)	t	135	316	506	680	717	871	884	1,079	1,276	1,424	1,598	
		N_1	0	0	0	0	0	0	0	0	0	0	2	
		N_2	0	0	0	0	0	0	0	0	0	0	0	
94	(1, 59, F)	t	175	386	583	763	959	1,141	1,323	1,512	1,694			
		N_1	0	0	0	0	0	0	0	0	0			
		N_2	0	0	0	0	0	0	0	0	0			
95	(2, 76, F)	t	62	160	334	517	692	817	874	1,042	1,407			
		N_1	0	0	1	0	1	0	0	0	0			
		N_2	0	0	0	0	0	0	0	0	0			
96	(6, 78, M)	t	140	344	539	762	972	1,282	1,483					
		N_1	0	0	0	0	0	0	0					
		N_2	0	0	0	0	0	2	1					
97	(2, 59, M)	t	210	385	575	756	939	1,125	1,309	1,532				
		N_1	0	0	0	0	1	0	0	0				
		N_2	0	0	0	0	1	0	0	0				
98	(4, 62, M)	t	239	428	593	776	978	1,160	1,344	1,526	1,721			
		N_1	1	0	0	0	0	0	0	0	0			
		N_2	0	0	0	0	0	0	0	0	0			
99	(1, 53, F)	t	27	188	379	559	743	945	1,127					
		N_1	0	0	0	0	0	0	0					
		N_2	0	0	0	0	0	0	0					
100	(12, 74, M)	t	183	249	338	521	688	875	1,086	1,281	1,463	1,666		
		N_1	0	0	0	0	0	0	0	0	0	0		
		N_2	0	0	0	0	0	0	0	1	0	0		
101	(1, 69, M)	t	120	303	340	716	744	877	1,051	1,296	1,492	1,681		
		N_1	0	0	0	0	0	0	0	1	0	1		
		N_2	0	0	0	0	0	0	0	0	0	0		
102	(3, 67, M)	t	56	201	218	391	701							
		N_1	0	0	0	0	0							
		N_2	0	0	0	0	0							
103	(27, 73, F)	t	168	350	582	596	764	940	1,106	1,322	1,496	1,658		
		N_1	0	0	0	0	0	1	0	1	1	0		
		N_2	0	0	1	0	0	0	0	0	0	0		
104	(6, 53, M)	t	147	329	490	672	854							
		N_1	0	0	0	1	0							
		N_2	0	0	0	0	0							
105	(6, 73, F)	t	121	309	485	749	1,126	1,181	1,547					
		N_1	0	0	0	0	0	0	0					
		N_2	0	0	0	0	1	0	0					

Data set III (Continued)

ID	Covariates		Observation number											
			1	2	3	4	5	6	7	8	9	10	11	12
106 (2, 77, M)		t	172	398	516	699	1,064	1,290	1,395					
		N_1	0	1	0	0	0	1	0					
		N_2	0	0	0	0	0	1	0					
107 (4, 79, M)		t	188	377	553	594	733	861	936	1,077	1,336			
		N_1	0	0	0	0	0	0	0	0	0			
		N_2	0	0	0	0	0	0	0	0	1			
108 (1, 45, M)		t	62	188	365	573	762	941						
		N_1	0	0	0	0	0	0						
		N_2	0	0	0	0	0	0						
109 (7, 71, M)		t	159	359	546	730	912	1,092	1,274	1,498				
		N_1	0	1	0	1	0	0	1	0				
		N_2	0	0	0	0	0	0	0	0				
110 (2, 66, M)		t	181	363	533	712	894	1,077	1,261	1,441	1,630			
		N_1	0	0	0	0	0	1	0	0	0			
		N_2	0	0	0	0	0	0	0	0	0			
111 (1, 70, M)		t	180	371	552	733	914	1,098	1,279	1,463				
		N_1	0	0	0	0	1	0	0	0				
		N_2	0	0	0	0	0	0	0	0				
112 (1, 64, F)		t	168	355	538	721	896	1,083	1,260	1,441	1,623			
		N_1	0	0	0	0	0	0	0	0	0			
		N_2	0	0	0	0	0	0	0	0	0			
113 (2, 56, M)		t	175	364	733	971								
		N_1	0	0	0	0								
		N_2	0	0	0	0								
114 (1, 66, F)		t	181	229	356	420	504	1,433						
		N_1	0	0	0	0	0	0						
		N_2	0	0	0	0	0	0						
115 (3, 73, F)		t	177	358	552	749	937	1,115	1,295	1,458				
		N_1	0	0	0	0	0	0	0	0				
		N_2	0	0	0	0	0	0	0	0				
116 (1, 58, M)		t	154	247	335	517	699	884	1,073	1,302	1,437			
		N_1	0	0	0	0	0	0	0	0	0			
		N_2	0	0	0	0	0	0	0	0	0			
117 (3, 53, M)		t	79	108	118	252	301	489	785					
		N_1	0	0	0	0	0	0	0					
		N_2	0	0	0	0	0	0	0					
118 (1, 66, M)		t	180	363	544	762	971	1,169	1,351	1,538				
		N_1	0	1	0	0	1	0	0	0				
		N_2	0	0	0	0	0	0	0	0				
119 (2, 46, M)		t	175	358	650	679	791							
		N_1	0	1	3	1	3							
		N_2	0	0	0	0	0							
120 (2, 54, M)		t	174	296	316	357	680	752	1,081	1,276				
		N_1	0	0	0	0	0	0	0	0				
		N_2	0	0	0	0	0	0	0	0				

9 Some Sets of Data

Data set III (Continued)

ID	Covariates		Observation number											
			1	2	3	4	5	6	7	8	9	10	11	12
121	(4, 44, M)	t	168	350	534	721	896							
		N_1	0	0	0	0	0							
		N_2	0	0	0	0	0							
122	(2, 50, F)	t	152	335	515	713	903	1,085	1,251	1,434				
		N_1	0	0	1	0	0	0	0	0				
		N_2	0	0	0	0	0	0	0	0				
123	(3, 49, M)	t	202	391	581	763	958	1,139	1,321	1,506				
		N_1	1	0	1	0	0	0	0	0				
		N_2	0	1	0	0	0	0	1	0				
124	(4, 59, M)	t	188	314	616	812	866	1,364	1,545					
		N_1	0	0	1	1	1	0	0					
		N_2	0	0	0	0	0	0	0					
125	(8, 62, F)	t	108	290	458	638	837	987	1,228	1,465				
		N_1	0	0	0	0	0	0	0	0				
		N_2	0	0	0	0	0	0	0	0				
126	(1, 73, F)	t	141	351	419									
		N_1	0	0	0									
		N_2	0	0	0									
127	(1, 68, F)	t	180	390	424	600	964	1,224	1,418					
		N_1	0	0	0	0	0	0	0					
		N_2	0	0	0	0	0	0	0					
128	(2, 47, F)	t	175	365	559	756	939	1,121	1,303	1,477				
		N_1	0	0	1	0	0	0	0	0				
		N_2	0	0	1	0	0	0	0	0				
129	(3, 50, F)	t	222	383	572	742	855	943	1,126	1,307	1,477			
		N_1	0	0	0	2	0	0	0	1	0			
		N_2	0	0	0	0	0	0	0	0	0			
130	(2, 56, F)	t	180	197	363	370	559	725	755	943	1,148	1,349	1,495	
		N_1	0	0	0	0	0	0	0	0	0	0	0	
		N_2	0	0	0	0	0	0	0	0	0	0	0	
131	(1, 66, F)	t	166	358	516	698	896	1,091	1,273	1,471				
		N_1	0	0	0	0	0	0	0	0				
		N_2	0	0	0	0	0	0	0	0				
132	(1, 44, M)	t	182	409										
		N_1	0	0										
		N_2	0	0										
133	(1, 51, M)	t	159	516	698	880	1,062	1,244	1,426					
		N_1	0	0	0	0	0	0	0					
		N_2	0	0	0	0	0	0	0					
134	(4, 37, F)	t	359	604	623	996	1,018	1,226						
		N_1	1	1	2	1	0	1						
		N_2	1	0	0	0	0	0						
135	(2, 55, F)	t	173	350	578	760	944	1,085	1,355					
		N_1	0	0	0	1	0	0	0					
		N_2	0	0	0	0	0	0	0					

Data set III (Continued)

ID	Covariates		1	2	3	4	5	6	7	8	9	10	11	12
136	(6, 67, M)	t	195	378	562	626	748	1,163	1,294					
		N_1	0	0	0	0	0	0	0					
		N_2	0	1	2	0	0	1	1					
137	(35, 67, M)	t	189	349	425	574	867							
		N_1	2	1	1	0	0							
		N_2	0	0	0	0	0							
138	(1, 63, M)	t	167	350	553	560	742	971	1,168	1,337				
		N_1	0	0	1	0	0	0	0	0				
		N_2	0	0	0	0	0	0	0	0				
139	(2, 71, M)	t	178	332	517	719	899	1,088	1,270					
		N_1	0	0	0	0	0	0	0					
		N_2	0	0	0	0	1	0	0					
140	(7, 48, M)	t	178	379	440	540	722	764	885	1,084	1,253	1,431		
		N_1	0	0	0	0	1	1	0	0	0	0		
		N_2	0	0	0	0	0	0	0	0	0	0		
141	(4, 44, F)	t	158	356	530	570	740	900	1,063	1,242				
		N_1	0	0	2	0	0	0	0	1				
		N_2	0	0	0	0	0	0	0	0				
142	(34, 73, M)	t	103	162	163	253	343	525	705	833	1,083	1,212		
		N_1	0	0	1	1	2	0	0	0	0	0		
		N_2	0	0	0	0	0	0	0	2	0	0		
143	(7, 73, F)	t	110	117	124	135	183	190	219	254	386	589	617	798
		N_1	0	0	0	0	0	0	0	0	0	0	0	2
		N_2	0	0	0	0	0	0	0	0	0	0	0	0

Placebo group

ID	Covariates		1	2	3	4	5	6	7	8	9	10	11	12
144	(2, 61, M)	t	125	179	363	531	735	915	1,103	1,296	1,476	1,663	1,784	
		N_1	0	1	0	0	0	0	1	0	0	0	0	
		N_2	0	0	0	0	0	0	0	0	0	0	0	
145	(11, 65, M)	t	182	364	546	728	912	955	1,138	1,323	1,519	1,743		
		N_1	1	1	0	4	0	2	1	0	1	0		
		N_2	0	0	0	0	0	0	0	0	0	0		
146	(3, 62, F)	t	210	216	337	713	1,031							
		N_1	0	0	0	0	0							
		N_2	0	0	0	0	0							
147	(7, 56, M)	t	190	383	490	566	756	972	1,002	1,240	1,412	1,601	1,631	1,792
		N_1	0	0	0	0	1	1	0	0	0	0	1	1
		N_2	0	0	0	0	0	0	0	0	0	0	0	1
148	(1, 40, M)	t	190	372	567	763	945	1,127	1,309	1,541	1,723			
		N_1	0	0	0	0	0	0	0	0	0			
		N_2	0	0	0	0	0	0	0	0	0			
149	(1, 67, M)	t	186	362	564	755	925	1,120	1,301	1,483	1,665	1,791		
		N_1	0	0	0	0	0	0	0	0	0	0		
		N_2	0	0	0	0	0	0	0	0	0	0		
150	(6, 75, M)	t	204	302	499	707	911	1,102	1,256	1,470	1,702	1,793		
		N_1	0	0	0	0	0	0	0	0	0	0		
		N_2	0	0	0	0	0	0	0	0	0	1		

9 Some Sets of Data

Data set III (Continued)

ID	Covariates		\multicolumn{12}{c}{Observation number}

ID	Covariates		1	2	3	4	5	6	7	8	9	10	11	12
151	(2, 57, F)	t	176	364	545	743	925	1,106	1,288	1,470	1,651	1,794		
		N_1	0	0	0	0	0	0	0	0	0	0		
		N_2	0	0	0	0	0	0	0	0	0	0		
152	(16, 78, M)	t	183	366	569	757	940	1,011	1,024					
		N_1	1	0	0	0	1	0	0					
		N_2	0	0	0	0	0	0	0					
153	(2, 51, M)	t	21	188	370	552	734	918	1,457	1,709				
		N_1	0	0	0	0	0	0	1	0				
		N_2	0	0	0	0	0	0	0	0				
154	(1, 66, M)	t	182	362	533	695	901	1,268	1,343	1,531	1,713			
		N_1	0	0	0	0	0	0	0	0	0			
		N_2	0	0	0	0	0	0	1	1	0			
155	(3, 74, M)	t	179	392	586	614	642	837	893	1,372	1,798			
		N_1	0	0	1	0	0	0	0	0	0			
		N_2	0	0	0	0	0	0	0	0	0			
156	(26, 63, M)	t	177	282	357	393	610	792	996	1,183	1,394	1,575	1,772	
		N_1	1	0	0	1	0	0	0	0	0	2	0	
		N_2	0	0	0	0	0	0	0	0	0	0	0	
157	(1, 51, F)	t	135	323	504	686	903	1,099	1,309	1,484	1,669	1,799		
		N_1	0	0	0	0	0	0	0	0	0	0		
		N_2	0	0	0	0	0	0	0	0	0	0		
158	(1, 50, M)	t	62	188	191	197	230	238	268	387	517	545	692	818
		N_1	0	2	0	0	1	0	0	0	3	0	0	0
		N_2	0	2	0	0	0	0	0	1	0	0	0	1
159	(1, 75, F)	t	180											
		N_1	0											
		N_2	0											
160	(6, 52, M)	t	126	313	501	693	868	1,049	1,230	1,421	1,610	1,747	1,777	
		N_1	1	1	1	0	2	0	1	1	0	0	1	
		N_2	0	0	0	1	0	0	0	0	0	0	0	
161	(2, 76, F)	t	193	375	559	621	741	936	1,119	1,153	1,187	1,250	1,302	1,370
		N_1	0	0	0	0	0	0	0	0	0	0	0	0
		N_2	0	0	0	0	0	0	0	0	0	0	0	0
162	(17, 73, M)	t	182	357	549	589	661	745	939	1,088	1,129	1,282	1,336	1,449
		N_1	0	0	0	0	0	0	0	0	1	1	0	1
		N_2	0	1	0	1	0	0	1	1	0	0	0	1
163	(12, 71, F)	t	188	357	538	733	916	1,098	1,281	1,484	1,671	1,783		
		N_1	0	0	1	1	0	1	1	0	0	0		
		N_2	0	0	0	0	0	0	0	0	0	0		
164	(3, 42, F)	t	127	314	502	698	796	866	1,048	1,204	1,390	1,579	1,747	
		N_1	0	0	0	1	0	0	0	0	0	0	0	
		N_2	0	1	0	0	0	0	0	0	0	0	0	
165	(34, 47, F)	t	189	302	414	525	718	903	1,098	1,191	1,299	1,461	1,657	1,799
		N_1	0	0	0	0	2	0	2	0	0	3	0	0
		N_2	1	0	0	0	0	1	0	3	0	0	0	0

Data set III (Continued)

ID	Covariates		1	2	3	4	5	6	7	8	9	10	11	12
166	(3, 78, M)	t	180	374	430	441	559	600	644	700	740	776	884	1,075
		N_1	0	0	0	0	0	0	0	0	0	0	0	0
		N_2	0	1	0	0	0	0	0	0	0	0	0	0
167	(9, 49, F)	t	185	367	549	731	947	1,156	1,284	1,415	1,599	1,781		
		N_1	2	2	3	2	0	2	1	2	0	2		
		N_2	0	0	0	0	0	0	0	0	0	0		
168	(7, 61, M)	t	113	177	324	371	772							
		N_1	0	0	0	0	0							
		N_2	1	0	0	0	0							
169	(1, 60, M)	t	181	323	532	705	876	1,051	1,231	1,412	1,595	1,776		
		N_1	0	0	0	0	0	0	0	1	0	1		
		N_2	0	0	0	0	0	0	0	0	0	0		
170	(2, 62, F)	t	180	362	559	748	910	1,090	1,335	1,519	1,762			
		N_1	0	0	0	0	0	0	0	0	0			
		N_2	0	0	0	0	0	0	0	0	0			
171	(6, 75, F)	t	197	379	581	633	763	945	1,129	1,309	1,480	1,669	1,799	
		N_1	0	0	0	0	0	0	0	0	0	1	1	
		N_2	0	0	0	0	0	0	0	0	0	0	0	
172	(3, 48, M)	t	196	337	519	701	889	1,065	1,247	1,435	1,618	1,799		
		N_1	0	0	2	0	0	0	0	0	1	0		
		N_2	0	0	0	0	0	0	0	0	1	0		
173	(1, 72, F)	t	104	189	287	477	653	835	1,008	1,197	1,358	1,583	1,766	
		N_1	0	0	0	0	0	0	0	0	0	0	0	
		N_2	0	0	0	2	0	0	0	0	0	0	0	
174	(8, 56, F)	t	194	302	393	567	757	820	960	1,146	1,316	1,497	1,674	1,797
		N_1	0	0	0	0	1	0	0	0	0	0	0	0
		N_2	0	0	0	0	0	0	0	0	0	0	1	0
175	(8, 64, F)	t	175	221	364	553	735	840	917	1,099	1,281	1,470	1,652	1,778
		N_1	0	0	0	2	0	0	0	0	3	0	0	0
		N_2	0	0	0	0	0	0	0	0	1	0	0	0
176	(7, 56, M)	t	172	344	522	732	900	1,091	1,259	1,440	1,616	1,791		
		N_1	1	0	0	0	0	0	0	1	0	0		
		N_2	0	0	0	0	0	0	0	1	0			
177	(1, 58, F)	t	153	336	517	699	882	1,071	1,252	1,434	1,616	1,793		
		N_1	0	0	0	0	0	0	0	0	0	0		
		N_2	0	0	0	0	0	0	0	0	0	0		
178	(1, 50, M)	t	180	344	505	686	855	1,055	1,281	1,503	1,706			
		N_1	0	0	0	0	0	0	0	0	0			
		N_2	0	0	0	0	0	0	0	0	0			
179	(1, 64, F)	t	188	368	545	733	826	978	1,180	1,285	1,469	1,650	1,785	
		N_1	0	0	0	0	0	0	0	0	0	0	0	
		N_2	0	0	0	0	0	0	0	0	0	0		
180	(2, 56, F)	t	154	197	334	516	698	883	1,065	1,246	1,427	1,608		
		N_1	0	0	0	0	0	1	0	0	0	0		
		N_2	0	0	0	0	0	0	0	0	0	0		

9 Some Sets of Data   243

Data set III (Continued)

ID	Covariates		Observation number											
			1	2	3	4	5	6	7	8	9	10	11	12
181	(1, 46, F)	t	162	308	490	675	724	857	1,052	1,232	1,417	1,631	1,787	
		N_1	0	0	0	0	0	0	0	0	0	0	0	
		N_2	0	0	0	0	0	0	0	0	0	0	0	
182	(4, 42, F)	t	71	162	343	547	730	923	1,105	1,301	1,483	1,675	1,808	
		N_1	1	0	0	0	0	0	0	0	0	0	0	
		N_2	0	0	0	0	0	0	0	0	0	0	0	
183	(8, 63, M)	t	147	246	261	352	569	674	855	1,045	1,234	1,282	1,415	1,494
		N_1	1	0	0	0	1	0	0	0	1	0	0	0
		N_2	0	0	0	0	0	0	1	0	0	1	1	0
184	(6, 64, M)	t	113	200	382	564	746	932	1,114	1,299	1,469	1,665		
		N_1	0	0	0	0	0	0	0	0	0	0		
		N_2	0	0	0	0	0	0	0	0	0	0		
185	(1, 51, M)	t	173	354	389	431	465	558	658	770	922			
		N_1	0	0	0	0	0	0	0	0	0			
		N_2	0	0	0	0	0	0	0	0	0			
186	(9, 67, F)	t	199	381	595	623	778	967	1,200	1,247	1,374	1,737		
		N_1	0	0	0	1	0	0	0	0	1	0		
		N_2	0	0	0	0	0	0	0	0	0	0		
187	(3, 77, M)	t	191	387	583	784	986	1,169	1,350	1,532	1,792			
		N_1	0	0	0	0	0	0	0	0	0			
		N_2	0	0	0	0	0	0	0	0	0			
188	(9, 61, F)	t	111	305	462	486	671	851	1,063	1,301	1,488	1,677	1,795	
		N_1	0	0	0	0	0	2	0	0	2	1	1	
		N_2	0	0	0	0	0	0	0	0	0	0	0	
189	(2, 44, F)	t	38	176	225	339	394	541	750	1,044	1,204	1,386	1,568	1,879
		N_1	0	0	0	0	0	0	0	0	0	0	0	0
		N_2	0	0	0	0	0	0	0	0	0	0	0	0
190	(21, 64, M)	t	119	295	476	660	686	826	1,017	1,204	1,386	1,575	1,771	
		N_1	0	0	0	0	0	0	0	0	0	0	0	
		N_2	1	0	1	0	0	0	0	1	0	1	1	
191	(1, 67, M)	t	182	364	567	744	890	1,098	1,282	1,485	1,637	1,850		
		N_1	0	0	0	0	0	0	1	0	0	0		
		N_2	0	0	0	0	0	0	0	1	0	1		
192	(1, 45, M)	t	175	357	572	755	935	1,141	1,327	1,510	1,701			
		N_1	0	0	0	0	0	0	0	0	0			
		N_2	0	0	0	0	1	0	0	0	0			
193	(15, 70, F)	t	157	337	533	642	745	934	1,122	1,309	1,492	1,674	1,779	
		N_1	1	0	0	0	1	0	1	2	2	1	0	
		N_2	0	1	0	0	0	0	0	0	0	0	0	
194	(1, 69, M)	t	149	329	518	703	893	1,068	1,253	1,449	1,633	1,660	1,793	
		N_1	0	0	0	0	0	0	0	0	0	0	0	
		N_2	0	0	0	0	0	0	0	0	0	1	0	
195	(4, 69, M)	t	174	356	552	726	929	1,127	1,302	1,505	1,674			
		N_1	0	0	0	0	0	1	0	0	0			
		N_2	0	0	0	0	0	0	0	0	0			

Data set III (Continued)

ID	Covariates		Observation number											
			1	2	3	4	5	6	7	8	9	10	11	12
196	(4, 65, M)	t	43	88	170	239	358	394	533	714	876	1,054	1,078	1,269
		N_1	0	0	0	0	1	0	1	0	0	0	0	0
		N_2	0	0	0	0	0	0	0	0	0	0	0	0
197	(1, 47, F)	t	168	350	548	737	911	1,093	1,275	1,457	1,638	1,779		
		N_1	0	0	0	0	0	0	0	0	0	0		
		N_2	0	0	0	0	0	0	0	0	0	0		
198	(3, 62, M)	t	154	322	525	707	860	1,058	1,253	1,443	1,686			
		N_1	0	0	0	0	0	0	0	0	0			
		N_2	0	0	0	0	0	1	0	1	1			
199	(1, 39, M)	t	165	347	539	719	902	1,111	1,294	1,483	1,666	1,791		
		N_1	0	0	0	0	0	0	1	0	0	0		
		N_2	0	0	0	0	0	0	0	0	0	0		
200	(21, 55, M)	t	193	378	566	784	959	1,148	1,319	1,510	1,699	1,789		
		N_1	1	1	0	1	2	0	0	2	0	0		
		N_2	0	0	0	0	0	0	0	0	1	0		
201	(2, 55, M)	t	44	177	359	554	721	958	1,122	1,283	1,465	1,645	1,792	
		N_1	0	0	0	1	0	0	2	0	0	1	0	
		N_2	0	0	0	0	0	1	0	0	0	0	0	
202	(2, 76, F)	t	140	321	351	517	707	882	979	1,014	1,084	1,611		
		N_1	0	0	0	0	0	0	0	0	0	0		
		N_2	0	0	0	0	0	0	0	0	2	0		
203	(6, 63, F)	t	160	342	532									
		N_1	1	1	1									
		N_2	0	0	0									
204	(1, 54, F)	t	176	329	528	696	920	1,095	1,277	1,464	1,646	1,781		
		N_1	0	0	0	0	0	0	0	0	0	0		
		N_2	0	0	0	0	0	0	0	0	0	0		
205	(2, 76, M)	t	167	386	531	714	883	1,078	1,259	1,437	1,617	1,812		
		N_1	0	0	0	0	0	0	0	0	0	0		
		N_2	0	0	0	0	0	0	0	0	0	0		
206	(3, 73, F)	t	180	364	551	736	757	826	924	1,111	1,293	1,394	1,736	
		N_1	0	0	0	0	0	0	0	0	0	1	0	
		N_2	0	0	0	0	0	0	0	0	0	0	1	
207	(2, 60, F)	t	145	175	356	537	747	938	1,112	1,303	1,483	1,671		
		N_1	0	0	0	0	0	0	0	0	0	0		
		N_2	0	0	0	0	0	0	0	0	0	0		
208	(2, 49, M)	t	208	385	574	754	944	1,125	1,309	1,489	1,672			
		N_1	0	0	0	0	0	0	0	0	0			
		N_2	0	0	0	0	0	0	0	0	0			
209	(2, 63, F)	t	138	526										
		N_1	0	0										
		N_2	0	0										
210	(1, 63, F)	t	175	357	538	709	890	1,077	1,259	1,448	1,623	1,787		
		N_1	0	0	0	0	0	0	0	0	0	0		
		N_2	0	0	0	0	0	0	0	0	0	0		

9 Some Sets of Data

Data set III (Continued)

ID	Covariates		1	2	3	4	5	6	7	8	9	10	11	12
211	(2, 78, M)	t	147	328	524	707	887	1,069	1,252	1,434	1,616			
		N_1	0	0	0	0	0	0	1	0	0			
		N_2	1	0	0	0	0	0	0	0	0			
212	(2, 40, M)	t	179	389	657	844	1,026	1,217	1,399	1,586	1,768			
		N_1	0	0	0	0	0	0	0	0	0			
		N_2	0	0	0	0	0	0	0	0	0			
213	(3, 57, M)	t	104	286	468	655	832	1,014	1,203	1,399	1,488	1,555		
		N_1	0	0	0	0	0	0	0	0	0	0		
		N_2	0	0	0	0	0	0	0	0	0	0		
214	(1, 43, M)	t	152	334										
		N_1	0	0										
		N_2	0	0										
215	(7, 68, F)	t	55	68	173	424	446	705	783	1,529				
		N_1	0	0	0	0	0	1	0	0				
		N_2	0	0	0	0	0	0	0	0				
216	(2, 76, F)	t	145	327	552	590	618	698	1,091	1,280	1,476	1,715		
		N_1	0	0	0	0	0	0	0	0	0	0		
		N_2	0	0	0	0	0	0	0	0	1	0		
217	(2, 62, M)	t	180	377	569	616	706	756	936	1,135	1,328	1,511	1,708	
		N_1	0	1	1	0	0	0	0	0	0	1	0	
		N_2	0	0	0	0	0	0	0	0	0	0	0	
218	(3, 52, F)	t	188	404	574	784	973	1,168	1,355	1,540	1,720			
		N_1	0	0	0	0	1	1	0	1	1			
		N_2	0	0	0	0	0	0	0	0	0			
219	(2, 59, M)	t	175	407	589	778	960	1,066	1,149	1,338	1,527	1,736		
		N_1	2	0	0	0	0	1	0	0	0	1		
		N_2	0	1	0	0	0	0	0	0	0	0		
220	(1, 52, F)	t	175	329	511	708	890	1,072	1,268	1,443	1,646			
		N_1	0	0	0	0	0	0	0	0	0			
		N_2	0	0	0	0	0	0	0	0	0			
221	(1, 78, M)	t	314	563	650	752	754	1,185	1,704					
		N_1	0	0	0	0	0	0	2					
		N_2	0	0	0	0	0	0	0					
222	(1, 59, F)	t	308	663										
		N_1	0	0										
		N_2	0	0										
223	(17, 74, M)	t	168	399	582	672	743	882	919	1,185	1,345	1,526		
		N_1	3	1	0	1	2	0	1	2	0	0		
		N_2	0	0	0	1	0	0	0	0	0	1		
224	(1, 55, M)	t	140	336	518	707	946	1,128	1,310	1,518	1,672			
		N_1	0	0	0	0	0	0	0	0	0			
		N_2	0	0	0	0	0	0	0	0	0			
225	(12, 63, M)	t	42	124	208	420	502	637	819	1,006	1,070	1,188	1,370	1,558
		N_1	1	0	1	0	0	0	1	0	1	0	0	1
		N_2	0	0	0	1	0	0	0	0	0	0	0	0

Data set III (Continued)

ID	Covariates		Observation number											
			1	2	3	4	5	6	7	8	9	10	11	12
226	(1, 49, F)	t	182	364	546	735	917	1,099	1,279	1,463	1,650			
		N_1	0	0	0	0	0	0	0	0	0			
		N_2	0	0	0	0	0	0	0	0	0			
227	(2, 75, M)	t	172	355	545	699	741	811	923	1,399				
		N_1	0	0	1	0	1	0	0	0				
		N_2	0	0	0	0	0	1	0	0				
228	(10, 51, M)	t	183	372	539	728	749	910	1,087	1,281	1,464	1,652		
		N_1	0	0	0	0	0	0	0	0	0			
		N_2	0	0	0	0	0	0	0	0	0			
229	(5, 69, M)	t	78	152	519	1,380	1,581							
		N_1	0	0	0	1	0							
		N_2	0	0	0	0	0							
230	(2, 79, M)	t	154	336	511	698	957	1,393						
		N_1	0	0	0	0	0	0						
		N_2	0	0	0	1	0	0						
231	(2, 58, M)	t	175	359	386	548	729	945	1,128	1,379	1,548			
		N_1	0	0	0	0	0	0	0	0	0			
		N_2	0	0	0	0	0	0	0	0	0			
232	(1, 73, M)	t	107	182	358	540	640	679	723	904	1,093	1,270	1,451	1,654
		N_1	1	0	0	0	0	0	0	0	1	0	0	0
		N_2	0	0	0	0	0	0	0	0	0	0	0	0
233	(1, 60, M)	t	182	364	567	734	918	1,088	1,282	1,468	1,651			
		N_1	0	0	0	0	0	0	0	0	0			
		N_2	0	0	0	0	0	0	0	0	0			
234	(2, 68, M)	t	21	28	73	164	352	541	553	722	904	1,185	1,360	1,533
		N_1	0	1	0	0	0	0	0	0	0	0	0	0
		N_2	0	0	0	0	0	0	0	0	0	0	0	0
235	(2, 53, M)	t	65	245	427	610	829	1,032	1,197	1,401	1,589			
		N_1	0	0	0	0	0	0	0	0	1			
		N_2	0	0	0	0	0	0	0	0	0			
236	(6, 55, M)	t	174	364	547	727	924	1,135	1,315	1,499				
		N_1	1	1	0	0	1	0	0	1				
		N_2	0	0	0	0	0	0	0	0				
237	(7, 73, F)	t	82	89	112	187	370	517	734	1,139	1,504	1,545		
		N_1	0	0	0	0	1	0	0	0	0	0		
		N_2	1	0	0	0	0	1	0	0	0	0		
238	(2, 63, M)	t	118	313	490	769	979	1,167	1,376					
		N_1	0	0	0	0	1	0	0					
		N_2	0	0	0	0	0	0	0					
239	(4, 67, M)	t	64	254	329	583	737	918	923	1,100	1,282			
		N_1	0	0	1	0	0	0	0	0	0			
		N_2	1	1	0	0	0	0	0	0	1			
240	(3, 74, M)	t	185	368	571	754	886	1,055	1,244	1,426	1,615			
		N_1	0	1	0	1	1	2	0	0	0			
		N_2	0	0	0	1	0	0	0	1	0			

9 Some Sets of Data

Data set III (Continued)

ID	Covariates		\multicolumn{12}{c}{Observation number}										
			1	2	3	4	5	6	7	8	9	10	11	12
241	(1, 58, F)	t	93	175	379	406	548	798	974	1,131	1,309			
		N_1	0	0	0	0	0	0	0	0	0			
		N_2	0	0	0	0	0	0	0	0	0			
242	(9, 79, F)	t	82	145	365	511	700	1,069	1,310					
		N_1	0	0	0	1	0	0	0					
		N_2	0	0	0	0	0	1	1					
243	(5, 54, M)	t	203											
		N_1	0											
		N_2	0											
244	(22, 54, M)	t	61	69	279	326	572	818	1,140	1,329	1,510			
		N_1	2	0	1	0	0	1	0	1	0			
		N_2	0	0	2	0	2	0	1	2	1			
245	(6, 57, M)	t	150	297	329	472	668	852	1,032	1,217	1,399	1,588		
		N_1	0	0	0	0	0	0	0	0	0	0		
		N_2	0	0	0	0	0	0	0	0	0	0		
246	(2, 59, F)	t	162	393	400	590	760	772	792	794	856	927	1,312	
		N_1	0	0	0	0	0	0	0	1	0	0	0	
		N_2	0	0	0	0	0	0	0	0	0	0	0	
247	(12, 76, F)	t	179	361	544	726	908	1,097	1,273	1,454				
		N_1	0	0	0	0	3	0	0	0				
		N_2	0	0	0	0	0	0	0	0				
248	(1, 66, M)	t	141	331	519	750	987	1,154	1,359	1,575				
		N_1	0	1	0	0	0	0	0	0				
		N_2	0	0	0	0	0	0	0	0				
249	(4, 69, F)	t	225	575	734	980	1,239							
		N_1	0	0	0	0	0							
		N_2	0	0	0	1	0							
250	(2, 46, F)	t	32	144	360	520	564	702	882	1,085	1,148	1,382		
		N_1	0	1	0	0	0	0	0	1	0	0		
		N_2	0	0	0	0	0	0	0	0	0	0		
251	(2, 60, M)	t	205	384	582	610	790	833	972	1,102	1,154	1,336	1,518	
		N_1	0	0	1	0	0	1	0	0	0	1	0	
		N_2	0	0	0	0	0	1	0	0	0	0	0	
252	(6, 68, M)	t	194	377	552	733	957	1,141	1,323	1,511				
		N_1	0	0	0	0	0	0	0	0				
		N_2	0	0	1	0	0	0	0	0				
253	(10, 66, F)	t	209	384	573	776	973	1,154	1,337	1,546				
		N_1	0	0	4	0	0	1	2	0				
		N_2	1	0	0	0	0	0	0	0				
254	(5, 71, F)	t	134	315	509	693	873	1,064	1,245	1,427				
		N_1	0	0	0	0	0	0	0	0				
		N_2	0	0	0	0	0	0	0	0				
255	(1, 48, F)	t	196	370	565	747	936	1,126	1,308	1,503				
		N_1	0	0	0	0	0	0	0	0				
		N_2	0	0	0	0	0	0	0	0				

Data set III (Continued)

ID	Covariates		1	2	3	4	5	6	7	8	9	10	11	12
								Observation number						
256	(2, 52, M)	t	187	378	600	782	971	1,151	1,335	1,522				
		N_1	0	0	0	0	0	0	0	0				
		N_2	0	0	0	0	0	0	0	0				
257	(1, 39, M)	t	190	380	580	813	1,063	1,266	1,420					
		N_1	0	0	0	0	0	0	0					
		N_2	0	1	0	0	0	0	0					
258	(6, 54, F)	t	127	334	509	743	894	1,051	1,219	1,414				
		N_1	2	0	0	0	1	0	0	0				
		N_2	0	0	0	0	0	0	0	0				
259	(8, 75, M)	t	182	362	583	679	817	1,163						
		N_1	0	0	2	0	1	1						
		N_2	0	0	0	1	0	0						
260	(3, 77, F)	t	133	322	323	503	693	861	938					
		N_1	0	0	0	0	0	0	0					
		N_2	0	0	0	0	0	0	0					
261	(1, 40, M)	t	182	353										
		N_1	0	0										
		N_2	0	0										
262	(9, 64, M)	t	239	380	386	430	483	604	793	1,038	1,219	1,442		
		N_1	0	0	0	0	0	0	0	0	0	0		
		N_2	0	1	0	0	1	0	0	0	0	0		
263	(10, 58, M)	t	181	194	370	549	728	859	888	1,041	1,187	1,369		
		N_1	0	1	0	0	0	0	0	0	0	0		
		N_2	0	0	0	0	0	0	0	0	0	0		
264	(11, 65, M)	t	70	196	379	567	573	663	825	846	1,034	1,293		
		N_1	1	0	0	2	0	0	0	0	0	1		
		N_2	0	0	0	0	0	0	0	0	0	0		
265	(2, 46, F)	t	182	357	519	700	892	1,137	1,312	1,459				
		N_1	0	0	0	0	0	0	0	0				
		N_2	0	0	0	0	0	0	0	0				
266	(1, 57, F)	t	47	170	215	335	537	769	889	1,023	1,225	1,386		
		N_1	0	0	0	0	0	0	0	0	0	0		
		N_2	0	0	0	0	0	0	0	0	0	0		
267	(8, 66, M)	t	168	202	332	421	477	686	833	1,050	1,101	1,273	1,427	
		N_1	0	1	0	2	1	0	1	0	0	0	1	
		N_2	0	0	0	0	0	0	1	1	0	0	0	
268	(2, 49, M)	t	191	384	405	566	957	1,097						
		N_1	0	0	0	0	0	1						
		N_2	0	0	0	0	0	0						
269	(2, 67, M)	t	201	383	579	762	962	1,137	1,321					
		N_1	0	0	0	0	0	0	0					
		N_2	0	0	0	0	0	0	0					
270	(1, 71, M)	t	175	334	516	712	901	1,090	1,252	1,433				
		N_1	0	0	0	0	0	0	0	0				
		N_2	0	0	0	0	0	0	0	0				

9 Some Sets of Data

Data set III (Continued)

ID	Covariates		1	2	3	4	5	6	7	8	9	10	11	12
							Observation number							
271	(2, 67, F)	t	226	405	587	772	946	1,129	1,309					
		N_1	0	0	0	0	0	0	0					
		N_2	0	0	0	0	0	0	0					
272	(1, 51, M)	t	176	364	472	659	855	1,037	1,213	1,379				
		N_1	0	0	0	0	0	0	0	0				
		N_2	0	0	0	0	0	0	0	0				
273	(2, 47, M)	t	183	309	497	596	776	968	1,161	1,308				
		N_1	0	0	1	0	0	0	0	0				
		N_2	0	0	0	0	0	0	0	0				
274	(9, 34, M)	t	195	378	566	692	1,061							
		N_1	0	1	4	3	1							
		N_2	0	0	0	0	0							
275	(7, 42, F)	t	152	341	515	698	866	1,081	1,265	1,440				
		N_1	0	0	0	0	0	1	0	0				
		N_2	0	0	0	0	0	0	0	0				
276	(5, 67, M)	t	181	203										
		N_1	1	0										
		N_2	0	0										
277	(17, 51, M)	t	138	154	315									
		N_1	0	0	0									
		N_2	0	3	0									
278	(2, 48, F)	t	145	332	403	509	669	885	1,075	1,292	1,440			
		N_1	0	0	0	0	0	0	0	0	0			
		N_2	0	0	0	0	0	0	0	0	0			
279	(1, 52, F)	t	185	369	381	551	731	913	1,095	1,284				
		N_1	0	0	1	0	0	0	1	0				
		N_2	0	0	0	0	0	0	0	0				
280	(3, 66, M)	t	138	321	334	502	630	790	973	1,111	1,258	1,420		
		N_1	0	0	0	0	0	0	0	0	0	0		
		N_2	0	0	0	0	0	0	0	0	0	0		
281	(4, 68, M)	t	175	349	510	691	873	1,055	1,237	1,419				
		N_1	0	0	0	0	0	0	0	1				
		N_2	0	0	0	0	0	0	0	0				
282	(1, 77, F)	t	115	242	354									
		N_1	1	0	0									
		N_2	0	0	0									
283	(1, 42, F)	t	179	368	544	731	906	1,096	1,280					
		N_1	0	0	0	0	0	0	0					
		N_2	0	0	0	0	0	0	0					
284	(2, 54, M)	t	125	146	153	308	568	869						
		N_1	0	0	0	0	0	0						
		N_2	0	0	0	0	0	0						
285	(1, 52, F)	t	124	300	469	882	1,064	1,246	1,433					
		N_1	0	0	0	0	0	0	0					
		N_2	0	0	0	0	0	0	0					

Data set III (Continued)

ID	Covariates		Observation number											
			1	2	3	4	5	6	7	8	9	10	11	12
286	(2, 52, F)	t	128	314	499	679	860	1,042	1,224	1,420				
		N_1	1	0	0	0	0	0	0	0				
		N_2	0	0	0	0	0	0	0	0				
287	(1, 41, M)	t	182	420	600	805	986	1,260						
		N_1	0	0	0	0	0	0						
		N_2	0	0	0	0	0	0						
288	(10, 63, M)	t	161	301	487	637	802	945	1,063					
		N_1	0	0	0	0	0	0	1					
		N_2	0	0	0	0	0	0						
289	(4, 50, M)	t	178	360	670	949	1,210							
		N_1	0	0	1	0	0							
		N_2	0	0	0	0	0							
290	(28, 75, M)	t	12	206	238	318	381	592	753	958	1,046	1,102	1,326	1,403
		N_1	1	1	0	0	0	0	2	1	1	0	0	0
		N_2	0	2	0	0	1	1	1	3	2	2	3	0

9 Some Sets of Data   251

Data set III (Continued)

ID	Covariates		Observation number				
			13	14	15	16	17
			DFMO group				
18	(3, 72, F)	t	1,622	1,793			
		N_1	0	0			
		N_2	0	0			
22	(5, 61, F)	t	1,765				
		N_1	0				
		N_2	0				
23	(14, 70, F)	t	1,560	1,729			
		N_1	0	0			
		N_2	1	0			
24	(4, 70, F)	t	1,778				
		N_1	3				
		N_2	0				
57	(6, 59, M)	t	1,257	1,517	1,622		
		N_1	0	0	0		
		N_2	0	0	0		
61	(2, 69, M)	t	1,713				
		N_1	0				
		N_2	0				
72	(2, 63, M)	t	1,765				
		N_1	0				
		N_2	0				
143	(7, 73, F)	t	896	1,002	1,107	1,694	
		N_1	0	0	0	2	
		N_2	1	0	0	0	
			Placebo group				
158	(1, 50, M)	t	1,014	1,352	1,766		
		N_1	0	0	1		
		N_2	0	0	1		
162	(17, 73, M)	t	1,631	1,791			
		N_1	0	1			
		N_2	1	0			
166	(3, 78, M)	t	1,440	1,742			
		N_1	0	0			
		N_2	1	0			
183	(8, 63, M)	t	1,647	1,794			
		N_1	0	1			
		N_2	0	1			
196	(4, 65, M)	t	1,458	1,640	1,823		
		N_1	0	0	0		
		N_2	1	0	0		
290	(28, 75, M)	t	1,419	1,466	1,508	1,704	174
		N_1	0	0	0	0	0
		N_2	3	1	2	1	1

References

Aalen, O. O. (1975). *Statistical inference for a family of counting processes.* Ph.D. Thesis, University of California, Berkeley.

Aalen, O. O. (1978). Nonparametric inference for a family of counting processes. *The Annals of Statistics*, **6**, 701–726.

Akaike, H. (1973). Maximum likelihood identification of Gaussian autoregressive moving average models. *Biometrika*, **60**, 255–265.

Albert, P. S. (1991). A two-stage Markov mixture model for a time series of epileptic seizure counts. *Biometrics*, **47**, 1371–1381.

Allison, P. D. (1984). *Event history analysis: regression for longitudinal event data.* Sage Publications, Inc.

Andersen, P. K. and Borgan, O. (1985). Counting process models for life history data: a review. *Scand. J. Stat.* **12**, 97–158.

Andersen, P. K., Borgan, O., Gill, R. D. and Keiding, N. (1993). *Statistical models based on counting processes.* Springer-Verlag, New York.

Andersen, P. K. and Gill, R. D. (1982). Cox's regression model for counting processes: A large sample study. *The Annals of Statistics*, **10**, 1100–1120.

Andersen, P. K. and Klein, J. P. (2004). Multi-state models for event history analysis. *Statistical Methods in Medical Research*, **11**, 91–115.

Andersen, P. K. and Klein, J. P. (2007). Regression analysis for multistate models based on a pseudo-value approach, with applications to bone marrow transplantation studies. *Scandinavian Journal of Statistics*, **34**, 3–16.

Andrews, D. F. and Herzberg, A. M. (1985). *Data: A collection of problems from many fields for the student and research worker.* Springer-Verlag, New York.

Bacchetti, P., Boylan, R. D., Terrault, N. A., Monto, A. and Berenguer, M. (2010). Non-Markov multistate modeling using time-varying covariates, with application to progression of liver fibrosis due to Hepatitis C following liver transplant. *The International Journal of Biostatistics*, **6**, Article 7.

Balakrishnan, N. and Zhao, X. (2009). New multi-sample nonparametric tests for panel count data. *The Annals of Statistics*, **37**, 1112–1149.

Balakrishnan, N. and Zhao, X. (2010a). A nonparametric test for the equality of counting processes with panel count data. *Computational Statistics and Data Analysis*, **54**, 135–142.

Balakrishnan, N. and Zhao, X. (2010b). A class of multi-sample nonparametric tests for panel count data. *Ann. Inst. Stat. Math.*

Barlow, R., Bartholomew, D., Bremner, J. and Brunk, H. (1972). *Statistical inference under order restrictions*. New York: John Wiley.

Bartholomew, D. J. (1983). Some recent developments in social statistics. *International Statistical Review*, **51**, 1–9.

Bean, S. J. and Tsokos, C. P. (1980). Developments in non-parametric density estimation. *Int. Statist. Rev.*, **48**, 267–287.

Beebe, K. R., Pell, R. J. and Seasholtz, M. B. (1998). *Chemometrics: A practical guide*. John Wiley & Sons, Inc.

Breiman, L. (1996). Heuristics of instability and stabilization in model selection. *The Annals of Statistics*, **24**, 2350–2383.

Breslow, N. E. (1984). Extra-Poisson variation in log-linear models. *Applied Statistics*, **33**, 38–44.

Breslow, N. E. (1990). Tests of hypotheses in overdispersed Poisson regression and other quasi-likelihood models. *Journal of the American Statistical Association*, **85**, 565–571.

Buzkova, P. (2010). Panel count data regression with informative observation times. *The International Journal of Biostatistics*, **6**, article 30.

Byar, D. P. (1980). The veterans administration study of chemoprophylaxis for recurrent stage I bladder tumors: comparison of placebo, pyridoxine, and topical thiotepa. In *Bladder Tumors and Other Topics in Urological Oncology*, eds. Pavone-Macaluso, M., Smith, P. H. and Edsmyn, F., New York: Plenum, 363–370.

Byar, D. P., Blackard, C. and The Veterans Administration Cooperative Urological Research Group (1977). Comparisons of placebo, pyridoxine, and topical thiotepa in preventing recurrence of stage I bladder cancer. *Urology*, **10**, 556–561.

Cai, J. and Schaubel, D. E. (2004). Analysis of recurrent event data. *Handbook of Statistics*, **23**, 603–623.

Cai, Z. and Sun, Y. (2003). Local linear estimation for time-dependent coefficients in Cox's regression models. *Scandinavian Journal of Statistics*, **30**, 93–111.

Cameron, A. C. and Trivedi, P. K. (1998). *Regression analysis of count data*. Econometric Society Monograph, No.30, Cambridge University Press.

Carroll, R. J., Ruppert, D. and Stefanski, L. A. (1995). *Measurement error in nonlinear models*. Chapman & Hall, London.

Chen, B., Yi, G. Y. and Cook, R. J. (2010). Analysis of interval-censored disease progression data via multi-state models under a nonignorable inspection process. *Statistics in Medicine*, **29**, 1175–1189.

References

Chen, B. E., Cook, R. J., Lawless, J. F. and Zhan, M. (2005). Statistical methods for multivariate interval-censored recurrent events. *Statistics in Medicine*, **24**, 671–691.

Chen, B. E. and Cook, R. J. (2003). Regression modeling with recurrent events and time-dependent interval-censored marker data. *Lifetime Data Analysis*, **9**, 275–291.

Chen, H. Y. and Little, R. J. A. (1999). Proportional hazards regression with missing covariates. *Journal of the American Statistical Association*, **94**, 896–908.

Chen, J. and Li, P. (2009). Hypothesis test for normal mixture models: the EM approach. *The Annal of Statistics*, **37**, 2523–2542.

Chen, J. and Tan, X. (2009). Inference for multivariate normal mixtures. *Journal of Multivariate Analysis*, **100**, 1367–1383.

Cheng, G., Zhang, Y. and Lu, L. (2011). Efficient algorithms for computing the non and semi-parametric maximum likelihood estimates with panel count data. *Journal of Nonparametric Statistics*, **23**, 567–579.

Cheng, S. C. and Wei, L. J. (2000). Inferences for a semiparametric model with panel data. *Biometrika*, **87**, 89–97.

Cleveland, W. S. (1979). Robust locally weighted regression and smoothing scatterplots. *Journal of the American Statistical Association*, **74**, 829–836.

Cook, R. J. and Lawless, J. F. (1996). Interim monitoring of longitudinal comparative studies with recurrent event responses. *Biometrics*, **52**, 1311–1323.

Cook, R. J. and Lawless, J. F. (2007). *The statistical analysis of recurrent events*. Springer-Verlag, New York.

Cox, D. R. (1972). Regression models and life-tables. *Journal of the Royal Statistical Society, Series B*, **34**, 187–220.

Cox, D. R. and Miller, H. D. (1965). *The theory of stochastic processes*. London: Chapman and Hall.

Darlington, G. A. and Dixon, S. N. (2013). Event-weighted proportional hazards modelling for recurrent gap time data. *Statstics in Medcine*, **32**, 124–130.

Davis, C. S. and Wei, L. J. (1988). Nonparametric methods for analyzing incomplete nondecreasing repeated measurements. *Biometrics*, **44**, 1005–1018.

Dean, C. B. (1991). Estimating equations for mixed Poisson models. *Estimating Functions*, Ed. Godambe, V. P., Clarendon Press, Oxford, 3546.

DeGruttola, V. and Tu, X. M. (1994). Modeling progression of CD4-Lymphocyte count and its relationship to survival time. *Biometrics*, **50**, 1003–1014.

Dempster, A. P., Laird, N. M. and Rubin, D. B. (1977). Maximum likelihood from incomplete data via the EM algorithm. *Journal of the Royal Statistical Society, Series B*, **39**, 1–38.

Diamond, I. D. and McDonald, J. W. (1991). The analysis of current status data. In *Demographic Applications of Event History Analysis*, eds. Trussel J, Hankinson R, Tilton, J, Oxford University Press, Oxford, U.K.

Dicker, L., Huang, B. and Lin, X. (2012). Variable selection and estimation with the seamless-L_0 penalty. *Statistica Sinica*, to appear.

Diggle, P. J., Liang, K. Y. and Zeger, S. L. (1994). *The analysis of longitudinal data*. Oxford University Press, New York

Elashoff, R. M., Li, G. and Li, N. (2008). A joint model for longitudinal measurements and survival data in the presence of multiple failure types. *Biometrics*, **64**, 762–771.

Fan, J. and Li, R. (2001). Variable selection via nonconcave penalized likelihood and its oracle properties. *Journal of the American Statistical Association*, **96**, 1348–1360.

Fan, J. and Li, R. (2004). New estimation and model selection procedures for semiparametric modeling in longitudinal data analysis. *Journal of the American Statistical Association*, **99**, 710–723.

Fan, J. and Lv, J. (2010). A selective overview of variable selection in high dimensional feature space. *Statistica Sinica*, **20**, 101–148.

Fan, J. and Peng, H. (2004). Nonconcave penalized likelihood with a diverging number of parameters. *The Annals of Statistics*, **32**, 928–961.

Ferguson, T. S. (1973). A Bayesian analysis of some non-parametric problems. *The Annals of Statistics*, **1**, 209–230.

Ferguson, T. S. (1974). Prior distributions on spaces of probability measures. *The Annals of Statistics*, **2**, 615–629.

Fleming, T. R. and Harrington, D. P. (1991). *Counting process and survival analysis*. John Wiley: New York.

Freireich, E. O. et al. (1963). The effect of 6-mercaptopmine on the duration of steroid induced remission in acute leukemia. *Blood*, **21**, 699–716.

French, J. L. and Ibrahim, J. G. (2002). Bayesian methods for three-state model for rodent carcinogenicity studies. *Biometrics*, **58**, 906–916.

Gail, M. H., Santner, T. J. and Brown, C. C. (1980). An analysis of comparative carcinogenesis experiments based on multiple times to tumor. *Biometrics*, **36**, 255–266.

Gaver, D. P. and O'Muircheartaigh, I. G. (1987). Robust empirical Bayes analyses of event rates. *Technometrics*, **29**, 1–15.

Gehan, E. A. (1965). A generalized Wilcoxon test for comparing arbitrarily singly-censored samples. *Biometrika*, **52**, 203–223.

Gentlemen, R. C., Lawless, J. F. and Lindsey, J. C. (1994). Multi-state Markov models for analysing incomplete diseases history data with illustrations for HIV disease. *Statistics in Medicine*, **13**, 805–821.

Ghosh, D. and Lin, D. Y. (2000). Nonparametric analysis of recurrent events and death. *Biometrics*, **56**, 554–562.

Ghosh, D. and Lin, D. Y. (2002). Marginal regression models for recurrent and terminal events. *Statistica Sinica*, **12**, 663–688.

References

Ghosh, D. and Lin, D. Y. (2003). Semiparametric analysis of recurrent events in the presence of dependent censoring. *Biometrics*, **59**, 877–885.

Gibbons, J. D. and Chakraborti, S. (2011). *Nonparametric statistical inference*, 5th ed., Chapman & Hall.

Gladman, D. D., Farewell, V. T. and Nadeau, C. (1995). Clinical indicators of progression in psoriatic arthritis (PsA): multivariate relative risk model. *Journal of Rheumatology*, **22**, 675–679.

Gómez, G., Calle, M. L. and Oller, R. (2004).] Frequentist and Bayesian approaches for interval-censored data. *Statistics Papers*, **2**, 139–173.

Gómez, G., Espinal and Lagakos, S. W. (2003).] Inference for a linear regression model with an interval-censored covariate. *Statistics in Medicine*, **22**, 409–425.

Groeneboom, P. and Wellner, J. A. (2001). Computing Chernoff's distribution. *Journal of Computational & Graphical Statistics*, **10**, 388–400.

Hart, J. D. (1986). Kernel regression estimation using repeated measurements data. *Journal of the American Statistical Association*, **81**, 1080–1088.

He, X. (2007). Semiparametric analysis of panel count data. *Ph.D. Dissertation*, University of Missouri, Columbia.

He, X., Tong, X. and Sun, J. (2009). Semiparametric analysis of panel count data with correlated observation and follow-up times. *Lifetime Data Analysis*, **15**, 177–196.

He, X., Tong, X., Sun, J. and Cook, R. J. (2008). Regression analysis of multivariate panel count data. *Biostatistics*, **9**, 234–248.

Hinde, J. (1982). Compound Poisson regression models. In *GLIM 82: Proceedings of the International Conference in Generalized Linear Models*, R. Gilchrist, (ed.), Berlin: Springer-Verlag, 109–121.

Hougaard, P. (2000). *Analysis of multivariate survival data*. Statistics for Biology and Health. Springer-Verlag, New York.

Hsieh, H. J., Chen, T. H-H. and Chang, S. H. (2002). Assessing chronic disease progression using non-homogeneous exponential regression Markov models: An illustration using a selective breast cancer screening in Taiwan. *Statistics in Medicine*, **21**, 3369–3382.

Hu, X. J. and Lagakos, S. W. (2007). Nonparametric estimation of the mean function of a stochastic process with missing observations. *Lifetime Data Analysis*, **13**, 51–73.

Hu, X. J., Lagakos, S. W. and Lockhart, R. A. (2009a). Marginal analysis of panel counts through estimating functions. *Biometrika*, **96**, 445–456.

Hu, X. J., Lagakos, S. W. and Lockhart, R. A. (2009b). Generalized least squares estimation of the mean function of a counting process based on panel counts. *Statistica Sinica*, **19**, 561–580.

Hu, X. J. and Lawless, J. F. (1996). Estimation of rate and mean function from truncated recurrent event data. *Journal of the American Statistical Association*, **91**, 300–310.

Hu, X. J., Sun, J. and Wei, L. J. (2003). Regression parameter estimation from panel counts. *Scand. Journal of Statistics*, **30**, 25–43.

Huang, C. Y. and Wang, M. C. (2004). Joint modeling and estimation for recurrent event processes and failure time data. *Journal of the American Statistical Association*, **99**, 1153–1165.

Huang, C. Y., Wang, M. C. and Zhang, Y. (2006). Analyzing panel count data with informative observation times. *Biometrika*, **93**, 763–775.

Huang, X. and Liu, L. (2007). A joint frailty model for survival and gap times between recurrent events. *Biometrics*, **63**, 389–397.

Ibrahim, J. G., Chen, M.-H. and Sinha, D. (2001). *Bayesian survival analysis*. Springer-Verlag: New York.

Ii, Y., Kikuchi, R., and Matsuoka, K. (1987). Two-dimensional (time and multiplicity) statistical analysis of multiple tumors. *Mathematical Bioscience*, **84**, 1–21.

Ishwaran, H. and James, L. F. (2004). Computational methods for multiplicative intensity models using weighted gamma processes: proportional hazards, marked point processes, and panel count data. *Journal of the American Statistical Association*, **99**, 175–190.

Jamshidian, M. (2004). On algorithms for restricted maximum likelihood estimation. *Computational Statistics and data Analysis*, **45**, 137–157.

James, L. F. (2003). Bayesian calculus for gamma processes with applications to semiparametric intensity models. *Sankhya A*, **65**, 196–223.

Jin, Z., Liu, M., Albert, S. and Ying, Z. (2006). Analysis of longitudinal health-related quality of life data with terminal events. *Lifetime Data Analysis*, **12**, 169–190.

Johnson, R. A. and Wichern, D. W. (2002). *Applied multivariate statistical analysis*. Fifth edition, Prentice Hall, Inc.

Joly, P. and Commenges, D. (1999). A penalized likelihood approach for a progressive three-state model with censored and truncated data: Application to AIDS. *Biometrics*, **55**, 887–890.

Joly, P., Commenges, D., Helmer, C. and Letenneur, L. (2002). A penalized likelihood approach for an illness-death model with interval-censored data: Application to age-specific incidence of dementia. *Biostatistics*, **3**, 433–443.

Joly, P., Durand, C., Helmer, C. and Commenges, D. (2009). Estimating life expectancy of demented and institutionalized subjects from interval-censored observations of a multi-state model. *Statistical Modelling*, **9**, 345–360.

Kalbfleisch, J. D. and Lawless, J. F. (1985). The analysis of panel data under a Markov assumption. *Journal of the American Statistical Association*, **80**, 863–871.

Kalbfleisch, J. D., Lawless, J. F. and Robinson, J. A. (1991). Methods for the analysis and prediction of warranty claims. *Technometrics*, **33**, 273–285.

Kalbfleisch, J. D. and Prentice, R. L. (2002). *The statistical analysis of failure time data*. Second edition, John Wiley: New York.

Kay, R. (1986). A Markov model for analyzing cancer markers and diseases states in survival studies. *Biometrics*, **42**, 855–865.

References

Kim, Y-J. (2006). Analysis of panel count data with dependent observation times. *Communications in Statistics - Simulation and Computation*, **35**, 983–990.

Kim, Y-J. (2007). Analysis of panel count data with measurement errors in the covariates. *Journal of Statistical Computation and Simulation*, **77**, 109–117.

Klein, J. P. and Moeschberger, M. L. (2003). *Survival analysis*, Springer-Verlag: New York.

Lagakos, S. W. and Louis, T. (1988). Use of tumour lethality to interpret tumorigenicity experiments lacking cause-of-death data. *Applied Statistics*, **37**, 169–179.

Langohr, K., Gómez, G. and Muga, R. (2004). A parametric survival model with an interval-censored covariate. *Statistics in Medicine*, **23**, 3159–3175.

Lawless, J. F. (1987a). Regression methods for Poisson process data. *Journal of the American Statistical Association*, **82**, 808–815.

Lawless, J. F. (1987b). Negative binomial and mixed Poisson regression. *Canadian Journal of Statistics*, **15**, 209–225.

Lawless, J. F. and Nadeau, J. C. (1995). Some simple robust methods for the analysis of recurrent events. *Technometrics*, **37**, 158–168.

Lawless, J. F. and Zhan, M. (1998). Analysis of interval-grouped recurrent-event data using piecewise constant rate functions. *Canadian Journal of Statistics*, **26**, 549–565.

Lee, L-Y. (2008). Nonparametric and semiparametric models for multivariate panel count data. *Ph.D. Dissertation*, University of Wisconsin-Madison.

Lee, M-L. T. (2004). *Analysis of microarray gene expression data*. Kluwwe Academis Publishers.

Li, N. (2011). Semiparametric transformation models for panel count data. *Ph.D. Dissertation*, University of Missouri, Columbia.

Li, N., Park, D-H., Sun, J. and Kim, K. (2011). Semiparametric transformation models for multivariate panel count data with dependent observation process. *The Canadian Journal of Statistics*, 39, 458–474.

Li, N., Sun, L. and Sun, J. (2010). Semiparametric transformation models for panel count data with dependent observation processes. *Statistics in Biosciences*, **2**, 191–210.

Li, N., Zhao, H. and Sun, J. (2013). Semiparametric transformation models for panel count data with correlated observation and follow-up times. *Statistics in Medicine*, in press.

Li, Y., Suchy, A. and Sun, J. (2010). Nonparametric treatment comparison for current status data. *Journal of Biometrics & Biostatistics*, 1, 102.

Liang, K. Y. and Zeger, S. L. (1986). Longitudinal data analysis using generalized linear models. *Biometrika*, **73**, 13–22.

Liang, Y., Lu, W.B. and Ying, Z. (2009). Joint modeling and analysis of longitudinal data with informative observation times. *Biometrics*, **65**, 377–384.

Lin, D. Y., Wei, L. J., Yang, I. and Ying, Z. (2000). Semiparametric regression for the mean and rate functions of recurrent events. *Journal of Royal Statistical Society Ser B*, **62**, 711–730.

Lin, D. Y., Wei, L. J. and Ying, Z. (1993). Checking the Cox model with cumulative sums of martingale-based residuals. *Biometrika*, **80**, 557–572.

Lin, D. Y., Wei, L. J. and Ying, Z. (2001). Semiparametric transformation models for point processes. *Journal of the American Statistical Association*, **96**, 620–628.

Lin, D. Y. and Ying, Z. (2001). Nonparametric tests for the gap time distributions of serial events based on censored data. *Biometrics*, **57**, 369–375.

Lin, H., Scharfstein, D. O. and Rosenheck, D. O. (2004). Analysis of longitudinal data with irregular outcome-dependent follow-up. *Journal of Royal Statistical Society, Series B*, **66**, 791–813.

Lindsey, J. C. and Ryan, L. M. (1993). A three-state multiplicative model for rodent tumorigenicity experiments. *Applied Statistics*, **42**, 283–300.

Little, R. J. A. and Rubin, D. B. (1987). *Statistical analysis with missing data*, John Wiley: New York.

Liu, L., Huang, X. and O'Quigley, J. (2008). Analysis of longitudinal data in the presence of informative observational times and a dependent terminal event, with application to medical cost data. *Biometrics*, **64**, 950–958.

Liu, L., Wolfe, R. A. and Huang, X. (2004). Shared frailty models for recurrent events and a terminal event. *Biometrics*, **60**, 747–756.

Liu, M. and Ying, Z. (2007). Joint analysis of longitudinal data with informative right censoring. *Biometrics*, **63**, 363–371.

Louis, T. (1982). Finding the observed information matrix when using the EM algorithm. *Journal of the Royal Statistical Society, Series B*, **44**, 226–233.

Lu, M., Zhang, Y. and Huang, J. (2007). Estimation of the mean function with panel count data using monotone polynomial splines. *Biometrika*, **94**, 705–718.

Lu, M., Zhang, Y. and Huang, J. (2009). Semiparametric estimation methods for panel count data using monotone B-splines. *Journal of the American Statistical Association*, **104**, 1060–1070.

Luo, X. H. and Huang, C. Y. (2010). A comparison of various rate functions of a recurrent event process in the presence of a terminal event. *Statistical Methods in Medical Research*, **19**, 167–182.

Mallows, C. L. (1973). Some comments on Cp. *Technometrics*, **15**, 661–675.

McCulluagh, P. and Nelder, J. A. (1989). *Generalized linear models*. Chapman and Hall, London.

Mclachlan, G. and Peel, D. (2000). *Finite mixture models*. Wiley: New York.

Nelson, W. B. (2003). *Recurrent events data analysis for product repairs, disease recurrences, and other applications*. ASA-SIAM Series on Statistics and Applied Probability, **10**.

Nielsen, J. D. and Dean, C. B. (2008). Clustered mixed nonhomogeneous Poisson process spline models for the analysis of recurrent event panel data. *Biometrics*, **64**, 751–761.

Park, D-H. (2005). Semiparametric and nnonparametric methods for the analysis of longitudinal data. *Ph.D. Dissertation*, University of Missouri, Columbia.

Park, D-H., Sun, J. and Zhao, X. (2007). A class of two-sample nonparametric tests for panel count data. *Communication in Statistics: Theory Methods*, **36**, 1611–1625.

Pepe, M. S. and Cai, J. (1993). Some graphical displays and marginal regression analyses for recurrent failure times and time dependent covariates. *Journal of the American Statistical Association*, **88**, 811–820.

Pepe, M. S. and Fleming, T. R. (1989). Weighted Kaplan-Meier statistics: a class of distance tests for censored survival data. *Biometrics*, **45**, 497–507.

Prentice, R. L. (1982). Covariate measurement errors and parameter estimation in a failure time regression model. *Biometrika*, **69**, 331–342.

Robertson, T., Wright, F. T. and Dykstra, R. (1988). *Order restricted statistical inference*. John Wiley & Sons, New York.

Robison, L., Mertens, A., Boice, J., et al. (2002). Study design and cohort characteristics of the childhood cancer survivor study: A multi-institutional collaborative project. *Medical and Pediatric Oncology*, **38**, 229–239.

Rosen, O., Jiang, W. and Tanner, M. A. (2000). Mixtures of marginal models. *Biometrika*, **87**, 391–404.

Rosenberg, P. S. (1995). Hazard function estimation using B-splines. *Biometrics*, **51**, 874–887.

Roy, J. and Lin, X. (2002). Analysis of multivariate longitudinal outcomes with nonignorable dropouts and missing covariates: Changes in methadone treatment practices. *Journal of the American Statistical Association*, **97**, 40–52.

Schaubel, D. E. and Cai, J. (2004). Regression methods for gap time hazard functions of sequentially ordered multivariate failure time data. *Biometrika*, **91**, 291–303.

Scheike, T. H. and Martinussen, T. (2004). On estimation and tests of time-varying effects in the proportional hazards model. *Scandinavian Journal of Statistics*, **31**, 51–62.

Schoenfeld, D. (1982). Partial residuals for the proportional hazards regression model. *Biometrika*, **69**, 239–241.

Schumaker, L. (1981). *Spline functions: Basic theory*. New York: Wiley.

Schwartz, G. (1978). Estimating the dimension of a model. *The Annals of Statistics*, **6**, 461–464.

Severini, T. A. and Wong, W. H. (1992). Profile likelihood and conditionally parametric models. *The Annals of Statistics*, **20**, 1768–1802.

Singer, B. and Spilerman, S. (1976a). The representation of social processes by Markov models. *American Journal of Sociology*, **82**, 1–54.

Singer, B. and Spilerman, S. (1976b). Some methodological issues in the analysis of longitudinal surveys. *Annals Economic and Sociological Measurement*, **5**, 447–474.

Song, X., Davidian, M. and Tsiatis, A.A. (2002). A semiparametric likelihood approach to joint modeling of longitudinal and time-to-event data. *Biometrics*, **58**, 742–753.

Song, X., Mu, X. and Sun, L. (2012). Regression analysis of longitudinal data with time-dependent covariates and informative observation times. *Scandinavian Journal of Statistics*, to appear.

Song, X. and Wang, C. Y. (2008). Semiparametric approaches for joint modeling of longitudinal and survival data with time-varying coefficients. *Biometrics*, **64**, 557–566.

Staniswalls, J. G., Thall, P. F. and Salch, J. (1997). Semiparametric regression analysis for recurrent event interval counts. *Biometrics*, **53**, 1334–1353.

Sun, J. (1999). A Nonparametric test for current status data with unequal censoring. *J. R. Statist. Soc. B*, **61**, 243–250.

Sun, J. (2006). *The statistical analysis of interval-censored failure time data*. Springer: New York.

Sun, J. (2009). Panel count data. *Handbook of Statistical Methods in Life and Health Sciences*, Editor: Balakrishnan, N., John Wiley & Sons. Ltd.

Sun, J. and Fang, H. B. (2003). A nonparametric test for panel count data. *Biometrika*, **90**, 199–208.

Sun, J. and Kalbfleisch, J. D. (1993). The analysis of current status data on point processes. *Journal of the American Statistical Association*, **88**, 1449–1454.

Sun, J. and Kalbfleisch, J. D. (1995). Estimation of the mean function of point processes based on panel count data. *Statistica Sinica*, **5**, 279–290.

Sun, J. and Matthews, D. E. (1997). A random-effect regression model for medical follow-up studies. *Canadian Journal of Statistics*, **25**, 101–111.

Sun, J., Park, D-H., Sun, L. and Zhao, X (2005). Semiparametric regression analysis of longitudinal data with informative observation times. *Journal of the American Statistical Association*, **100**, 882–889.

Sun, J and Rai, S. N. (2001). Nonparametric tests for the comparison of point processes based on incomplete data. *Scand Journal Statistics*, **28**, 725–732.

Sun, J., Sun, L. and Liu, D. (2007a). Regression analysis of longitudinal data in the presence of informative observation and censoring times. *Journal of the American Statistical Association*, **102**, 1397–1406.

Sun, J., Tong, X. and He, X. (2007b). Regression analysis of panel count data with dependent observation times. *Biometrics*, **63**, 1053–1059.

Sun, J. and Wei, L. J. (2000). Regression analysis of panel count data with covariate-dependent observation and censoring times. *Journal of the Royal Statistical Society, Series B*, **62**, 293–302.

Sun, L., Guo, S. and Chen, M. (2009a). Marginal regression model with time-varying coefficients for panel data. *Communications in Statistics, Theory and Methods*, **38**, 1241–1261.

Sun, L., Park, D. and Sun, J. (2006). The additive hazards model for recurrent gap times. *Statistica Sinica*, **16**, 919–932.

References

Sun, L., Song, X., Zhou, J. and Liu, L. (2012). Joint analysis of longitudinal data with informative observation times and a dependent terminal event. *Journal of the American Statistical Association*, **107**, 688–700.

Sun, L. and Tong, X. (2009). Analyzing longitudinal data with informative observation times under biased sampling. *Statistics and Probability Letter*, **79**, 1162–1168.

Sun, L., Zhu, L. and Sun, J. (2009b). Regression analysis of multivariate recurrent event data with time-varying covariate effects. *Journal Multivariate Analysis*, **100**, 2214–2223.

Sun, Y. (2010). Estimation of semiparametric regression model with longitudinal data. *Lifetime Data Analysis*, **16**, 271–298.

Sun, Y. and Wu, H. (2005). Semiparametric time-varying coefficients regression model for longitudinal data. *Scandinavian Journal of Statistics*, **32**, 21–47.

Susko, E., Kalbfleisch, J. D. and Chen, J. (1998). Constrained nonparametric maximum-likelihood estimation for mixture models. *Canadan Journal of Statistics*, **26**, 601–617.

Thall, P. F. (1988). Mixed Poisson likelihood regression models for longitudinal interval count data. *Biometrics*, **44**, 197–209.

Thall, P. F. and Lachin, J. M. (1988). Analysis of recurrent events: nonparametric methods for random-interval count data. *Journal of the American Statistical Association*, **83**, 339–347.

Tibshirani, R. J. (1996). Regression shrinkage and selection via the lasso. *Journal of the Royal Statistical Society, Series B*, **58**, 267–288.

Tibshirani, R. J. (1997). The lasso method for variable selection in the Cox model. *Statstics in Medicine*, **16**, 385–395.

Tibishirani, R. and Hastie, T. (1987). Local likelihood estimation. *Journal of the American Statistical Association*, **82**, 559–567.

Titman, A. C. (2011). Flexible nonhomogeneous Markov models for panel observed data. *Biometrics*, **67**, 780–787.

Tong, X., He, X., Sun, L. and Sun, J. (2009). Variable selection for panel count data via nonconcave penalized estimating function. *Scandinavian Journal of Statistics*, **36**, 620–635.

Tsiatis, A. A. and Davidian, M. (2004). An overview of joint modeling of longitudinal and time-to-event data. *Statistica Sinica*, **14**, 793–818.

Tsiatis, A. A., DeGruttola, V. and Wulfsohn, M. S. (1995). Modeling the relationship of survival to longitudinal data measured with error. Applications to survival and CD4 counts in patients with AIDS. *Journal of the American Statistical Association*, **90**, 27–37.

Tuma, N. B. and Robins, P. K. (1980). A dynamic model of employment behavior: An application to the Seattle and Denver income maintenance experiments. *Econometrica*, **48**, 1031-1-52.

Vermunt, J. K. (1997). *Log-linear models for event histories*. Sage Publications Inc: Newbury Park, CA.

Wand, M. P. and Jones, M. C. (1995). *Kernel smoothing.* Chapman & Hall, London.

Wang, M. C. and Chen, Y. Q. (2000). Nonparametric and semiparametric trend analysis of stratified recurrence time data. *Biometrics*, **56**, 789–794.

Wang, M. C., Qin, J. and Chiang, C. T. (2001). Analyzing recurrent event data with informative censoring. *Journal of the American Statistical Association*, **96**, 1057–1065.

Wang, P., Puterman, M. L., Cockburn, I. and Le, N. (1996). Mixed Poisson regression models with covariate dependent rates. *Biometrics*, **52**, 381–400.

Wasserman, S. (1980). Analyzing social networks as stochastic processes. *Journal of the American Statistical Association*, **75**, 280–294.

Wedel, M., Desarbo, W. S., Bult, J. R. and Ramaswamy, V. (1993). A latent class Poisson regression model for heterogeneous count data. *Journal of Applied Econometrics*, 8, 397–411.

Wei, L. J., Lin, D. Y. and Weissfeld, L. (1989). Regression analysis of multivariate incomplete failure time data by modeling marginal distributions. *Journal of the American Statistical Association*, **84**, 1065–1073.

Wellner, J. A. and Zhang, Y. (2000). Two estimators of the mean of a counting process with panel count data. *The Annal of Statistics*, **28**, 779–814.

Wellner, J. A. and Zhang, Y. (2007). Two likelihood-based semiparametric estimation methods for panel count data with covariates. *The Annals of Statistics*, **35**, 2106–2142.

Wellner, J. A., Zhang, Y. and Liu, H. (2004). A semiparametric regression model for panel count data: when do pseudo-likelihood estimators become badly inefficient? *Proceedings of the Second Seattle Symposium in Biostatistics*, Springer, New York, 143–174.

White, H. (1982). Maximum likelihood estimation of misspecified models. *Econometrica*, **50**, 1–25.

Wulfsohn, M. S. and Tsiatis, A. A. (1997). A joint model for survival and longitudinal data measured with error. *Biometrics*, **53**, 330–339.

Yamaguchi, K. (1991). *Event history analysis.* Sage Publications, Inc.

Yan, J. and Huang, J. (2012). Model selection for Cox models with time-varying coefficients. *Biometrics*, **68**, 419–428.

Ye, Y., Kalbfleisch, J. D. and Schaubel, D. E. (2007). Semiparametric analysis of correlated recurrent and terminal events. *Biometrics*, **63**, 78–87.

Yi, G. Y. and Lawless, J. F. (2012). Likelihood-based and marginal inference methods for recurrent event data with covariate measurement error. *Canadian Journal of Statistics*, **40**, 530–549.

Zeng, D. and Cai, J. (2010). A semiparametric additive rate model for recurrent events with an informative terminal event. *Biometrika*, **97**, 699–712.

Zhang, C. (2010). Nearly unbiased variable selection under minimax concave penalty. *The Annals of Statistics*, **38**, 894–942.

Zhang, H., Sun, J. and Wang, D. (2013a). Variable selection and estimation for multivariate panel count data via the seamless-L_0 penalty. *The Canadian Journal of Statistics*, in press.

Zhang, H. Zhao, H., Sun, J., Wang, D. and Kim, K. M. (2013b). Regression analysis of multivariate panel count data with an informative observation process. *Journal of Multivariate Analysis*, **119**, 71–80.

Zhang, Y. (2002). A semiparametric pseudolikelihood estimation method for panel count data. *Biometrika*, **89**, 39–48.

Zhang, Y. (2006). Nonparametric K-sample test with panel count data. *Biometrika*, **93**, 777–790.

Zhang, Y. and Jamshidian, M. (2003). The gamma-frailty Poisson model for the nonparametric estimation of panel count data. *Biometrics*, **59**, 1099–1106.

Zhang, Y. and Jamshidian, M. (2004). On algorithms for NPMLE of the failure function with censored data. *Journal of Computational and Graphical Statistics*, **13**, 123–140.

Zhang, Z., Sun, L., Zhao, X. and Sun, J. (2005). Regression analysis of interval censored failure time data with linear transformation models. *The Canadian Journal of Statistics*, **33**, 61–70.

Zhao, H., Li, Y. and Sun, J. (2013a). Analyzing panel count data with dependent observation process and a terminal event. *The Canadian Journal of Statistics*, **41**, 174–191.

Zhao, H., Li, Y. and Sun, J. (2013b). Semiparametric analysis of multivariate panel count data with dependent observation process and terminal event. *Journal of Nonparametric Statistics*, **25**, 379–394.

Zhao, H., Virkler, K. and Sun, J. (2013c). Nonparametric comparison for multivariate panel count data. *Communications in Statistics - Theory and Methods*, to appear.

Zhao, Q. and Sun, J. (2006). Semiparametric and nonparametric analysis of recurrent events with observation gaps. *Computational Statistics and Data Analysis*, **51**, 1924–1933.

Zhao, X. and Sun, J. (2011). Nonparametric comparison for panel count data with unequal observation processes. *Biometrics*, **67**, 770–779.

Zhao, X., Balakrishnan, N. and Sun, J. (2011a). Nonparametric inference based on panel count data (with discussion). *Test*, 20, 1–71.

Zhao, X. and Tong, X. (2011). Semiparametric regression analysis of panel count data with informative observation times. *Computational Statistics and Data Analysis*, **55**, 291–300.

Zhao, X., Tong, X. and Sun, J. (2013). Robust estimation for panel count data with informative observation times. *Computational Statistics and Data Analysis*, **57**, 33–40.

Zhao, X., Tong, X. and Sun, L. (2012). Joint analysis of longitudinal data with dependent observation times. *Statistics Sinica*, **22**, 317–336.

Zhao, X., Zhou, J. and Sun, L. (2011b). Semiparametric transformation models with time-varying coefficients for recurrent and terminal events. *Biometrics*, **67**, 404–414.

Zhao, X. and Zhou, X. (2012). Modeling gap times between recurrent events by marginal rate function. *Computational Statistics and Data Analysis*, **56**, 370–383.

Zhou, H. and Pepe, M. S. (1995). Auxilliary covariate data in failure time regression analysis. *Biometrika*, **82**, 139–149.

Zhu, L., Sun, J., Srivastava, D. K., Tong, X., Leisenring, W., Zhang, H., and Robison, L. L. (2011a). Semiparametric transformation models for joint analysis of multivariate recurrent and terminal events. *Statistics in Medicine*, **30**, 3010–3023.

Zhu, L., Sun, J., Tong, X. and Pounds, S. (2011b). Regression analysis of longitudinal data with informative observation times and application to medical cost data. *Statistics in Medicine*, **30**, 1429–1440.

Zhu, L., Sun, J., Tong, X. and Srivastava, D. K. (2010). Regression analysis of multivariate recurrent event data with a dependent terminal event. *Lifetime Data Analysis*, **16**, 478–490.

Zhu, L., Tong, X., Zhao, H., Sun, J., Srivastava, D., Leisenring, W. and Robison, L. (2013). Statistical analysis of mixed recurrent event data with application to cancer survivor study. *Statistics in Medicine*, to appaer.

Zou, H. (2006). The adaptive lasso and its oracle properties. *Journal of the American Statistical Association*, **101**, 1418–1429.

Index

Aalen, O.O., 10, 11, 211
Akaike, H., 191
Albert, P.S., 33
Allison, P.D., 1
Andersen, P.K., 2, 3, 10, 12, 15–17, 52, 69, 91, 111, 119, 205, 206
Andrews, D.F., 8
Asymptotic properties, 57, 96, 97, 103, 108
    asymptotic distribution, 26, 28, 101, 107, 112, 131, 147, 149, 164, 165, 173, 180, 181
    asymptotic normality, 30, 32, 38, 40, 160, 202, 209, 219
    consistency, 26, 30, 32, 38, 40, 101, 103, 107, 131, 146, 147, 164, 173, 180, 202
        L_2-consistency, 94

Bacchetti, P., 211
Balakrishnan, N., 76, 78–80, 89
Barlow, R.E., 53, 94
Bartholomew, D.J., 190
Bean, S.J., 65
Beebe, K.R., 189
Bootstrap procedure, 97, 128
Borgan, O., 10
Box-Cox transformation, 110, 137, 144
Breiman, L., 191
Breslow estimator, 105, 146
Breslow, N.E., 23, 44
Brownian motion, 57
Byar, D.P., 8

Cai, J., 2, 143, 163, 221
Cai, Z., 221
Cameron, A.C., 23, 27, 44
Carroll, R.J., 212, 217
Chakraborti, S., 134

Chen, B., 205, 206
Chen, B.E., 169, 186, 222
Chen, H.Y., 222
Chen, J., 217
Chen, Y.Q., 2, 221
Cheng, G., 119
Cheng, S.C., 119, 202
Cleveland, W.S., 69
Commenges, D., 205, 212
Cook, R.J., 2, 5, 13, 16, 69, 75, 90, 91, 111, 113, 115, 119, 143, 144, 181, 222
Counting process, 2, 3, 8, 10–12, 15–17, 19, 56, 92, 104, 122, 162, 175
    Cox intensity model, 12
    intensity process, 3, 12, 15, 17, 19, 20, 71, 90, 91
    mean function estimation, 57
    multiplicative intensity model, 11
Cox, D.R., 10, 99, 207, 210
Cross-sectional studies, 53
Current status data, 2, 32, 54, 73, 75, 95, 99

Darlington, G.A., 221
Davidian, M., 153, 187
Davis, C.S., 74
Dean, C.B., 23, 119, 212, 218–220
DeGruttola, V., 153
Dempster, A.P., 36
Diamond, I.D., 2
Dicker, L., 192, 195
Diggle, P.J., 91, 119
Dirichlet process, 213, 214
Dixon, S.N., 221

Elashoff, R.M., 153
EM algorithm, 36–38, 51, 64, 121, 125, 126, 129

Estimating equation approach, 44, 91, 92,
    97–109, 119, 120, 143, 156, 171
  generalized estimating equation, 35, 39,
    91, 119

Failure time data, 2, 3, 18, 22, 75, 90, 92,
    114, 122, 155, 157, 170, 211, 212, 214,
    216, 221
  accelerated failure time model, 152
  additive hazards model, 152
  censoring, 2, 143
  hazard function, 90, 98, 123, 145, 211
  interval-censored, 19
  leukemia data, 3
  linear transformation model, 152
  log-rank test, 72
  multivariate, 221
  proportional hazards model, 92, 98, 124,
    145, 198, 211
  right-censored, 4, 19, 72, 99
  survival function, 90, 157
  truncation, 2
Fan, J., 191, 194
Fang, H., 72, 73, 89
Fenchel duality theorem, 49
Ferguson, T.S., 214
Fleming, T.R., 105, 157
Follow-up process, 121, 123, 128, 220
  dependent terminal event, 143, 151, 187,
    205
  terminal event, 122, 142–145, 151–153
Frailty model, 122, 143
Freireich, E.O., 3, 4
French, J.L., 205

Gómez, G., 212, 222
Gail, M.H., 4
Gamma distribution, 25, 31, 35, 97
Gamma function, 25
Gamma process, 213
Gaussian process, 116, 132, 152, 174
Gaver, D.P., 5, 6
Gehan, E.A., 3, 4
Generalized isotonic regression estimator,
    57, 58, 60, 62, 70
Gentleman, R.C., 210
Ghosh, D., 143–145, 152
Gibbons, J.D., 134
Gill, R.D., 10, 12
Gladman, D.D., 166, 206
Goodness-of-fit test, 92, 109, 115–116, 120,
    130, 131, 135, 139, 141, 152, 153, 171,
    173, 176
Groeneboom, P., 57

Harrington, D.P., 105
Hart, J.D., 62
Hastie, T., 69
He, X., 8, 119, 124, 128, 153, 164, 165, 186
Herzberg, A.M., 8
Hinde, J., 44
Hougaard, P., 155
Hsieh, H.J., 205, 212
Hu, X.J., 8, 44, 57, 58, 60, 70, 105, 107
Huang, C.Y., 8, 124, 128, 143–145, 152,
    187
Huang, J., 221
Huang, X., 221

Ibrahim, J.G., 205, 212
Ii, Y., 32
Illness-death model, *see* Multi-state model
Inverse probability weighting technique,
    143, 146
Ishwaran, H., 213, 214, 221
Isotonic regression, 52, 61
  max-min formula, 53, 94
  pool-adjacent-violators algorithm, 53, 94
  up-and-down algorithm, 53, 94
Isotonic regression estimator, 48, 51, 52,
    55–58, 63, 69, 71, 72, 74, 76–78, 80,
    84, 86, 88, 89, 94, 95, 133, 157–160,
    222
Iterative convex minorant algorithm, 50,
    60

James, L.F., 213, 214, 221
Jamshidian, M., 51, 69, 96
Jin, Z., 153, 187
Johnson, R.A., 189
Joint model approach, 153, 155
Joly, P., 205, 212
Jones, M.C., 16, 62, 65

Kalbfleisch, J.D., 1, 2, 4, 5, 19, 32, 52, 53,
    69, 72, 73, 75, 89, 90, 99, 101, 152,
    157, 190, 205, 206, 208, 211
Kay, R., 211
Kernel estimation, 62, 64, 65, 67
  bandwidth, 16, 64, 65, 216
  Gaussian kernel, 65, 67
  kernel estimator, 16, 64, 88
  kernel function, 16, 64, 65, 213, 216
Kim, Y.-J., 152, 212, 216
Klein, J.P., 1, 2, 205, 206
Kolomogorov-Smirnov test, 134

Lachin, J.M., 6, 33, 57, 63, 69, 75, 89
Lagakos, S.W., 70, 205
Langohr, K., 222

Index

Lawless, J.F., 2, 5, 13, 16, 19, 23, 31, 33, 34, 36, 38, 40, 42–44, 51, 69, 75, 90, 91, 101, 102, 104, 111, 113, 115, 119, 143, 144, 181, 190, 205, 206, 208, 211, 214, 221
Least squares, 58, 59, 70
Lee, L-Y., 186
Lee, M.T., 189
Li, N., 9, 75, 112, 139, 153, 180, 181, 186
Li, P., 217
Li, R., 191, 194
Li, Y., 89
Liang, K.Y., 40
Liang, Y., 153
Likelihood function, 20, 24, 25, 28, 30–32, 35, 37, 38, 49, 51, 63, 68, 94, 95, 125, 129, 207, 209, 210, 212, 213, 218
  conditional likelihood, 30
  Fisher information matrix, 32, 38
  local likelihood, 69
  maximum likelihood estimator, 24, 25, 28, 30, 36, 38, 158, 208, 210
  maximum partial likelihood estimator, 146
  partial likelihood, 10, 101
  penalized likelihood, 68, 69, 189
  profile likelihood, 44, 211
  pseudo-likelihood, 51, 93–96, 117, 215, 216
  pseudo-maximum likelihood estimator, 27
Lin, D.Y., 1, 2, 12, 69, 109, 110, 114–116, 137, 143–146, 152, 212, 214, 221
Lin, H., 153
Lin, X., 153
Lindsey, J.C., 205
Little, R.J.A., 222
Liu, L., 143, 153, 187, 221
Liu, M., 153
Longitudinal data, 3, 91, 114, 119, 122, 153, 187, 214, 220, 221
Longitudinal process, 137
Louis, T., 38, 129, 205
Lu, M., 34, 70, 95, 96, 119
Luo, X.H., 144, 145, 152
Lv, J., 191

Mallows, C.L., 191
Marginal model approach, 143, 153, 155, 156, 185
Martingale, 11, 15
  covariance process, 12
  Gaussian martingale, 17
  variance process, 12

269

Martinussen, T., 221
Matthews, D.E., 119, 221
McCulluagh, P., 39
McDonald, J.W., 2
Mclachlan, G., 212
Mean function, see Recurrent event process
Miller, H.D., 10, 207, 210
Model misspecification, 129, 142
Moeschberger, M.L., 1, 2
Multi-state model, 189, 190, 205–212
  illness-death model, 205, 206, 212
  irreversible, 212
  Markov chain, 13, 205, 207, 211
  progressive, 212
  transition intensity matrix, 13, 22, 205, 207, 208, 210
  transition probability matrix, 13, 22, 205, 207, 210
Multiplicative intensity model, 16

Nadeau, J.C., 2, 13, 69, 101, 102, 104
Negative binomial distribution, 25, 51, 97
Negative binomial process, 31, 51
Nelder, J.A., 39
Nelson, J.D., 119
Nelson, W.B., 1
Nelson-Aalen estimator, 15, 16, 52, 53, 63
Newton-Raphson algorithm, 36, 64, 94, 173, 209
Nielsen, J.D., 119, 212, 218–220
Nonparametric estimation, 15–16, 21, 47, 48, 69
Nonparametric maximum likelihood estimator, 16, 48–53, 55, 56, 69, 71, 76–79, 81, 84, 88–90, 95
Nonparametric maximum pseudo-likelihood estimator, see Isotonic regression estimator

O'Muircheartaigh, I.G., 5, 6
Observation process, 2, 3, 20, 45, 71, 72, 78, 81, 84, 87, 89, 91, 97, 103, 106, 108, 110, 121–123, 128, 129, 133–136, 139, 142, 144, 145, 153, 156, 160, 170, 171, 175, 176, 183, 185–187, 198, 200, 220
  dependent, 20, 121, 122, 128, 136, 152, 170, 178
  empirical, 74, 85, 157, 160
  independent, 21, 24, 48, 70, 121, 137, 153, 156, 161, 162, 176, 205, 207, 212, 215, 221
  informative, 20, 21, 44, 121, 137, 178, 212
  unequal, 84

Panel count data
  arthritis data
    analysis of, 166–169
  bladder tumor data, 7–8, 136, 143, 223, 227
    analysis of, 86, 133–135, 139–141, 149–151
  gallstone data, 6–7
    analysis of, 54–56, 61–62, 67, 82, 116–118
  Gallstone study, 223, 224
  reliability data, 5–6
    analysis of, 54, 65–66
  skin cancer data, 9, 171, 178, 223, 231
    analysis of, 158–159, 175–176, 183–185, 195–197
Park, D-H., 74, 89, 221
Peel, D., 212
Peng, H., 191
Pepe, M.S., 2, 157, 212, 214
Piecewise procedure, 23, 43
  piecewise constant function, 34, 43, 63, 119, 211
Poisson distribution, 5, 14, 24, 25, 28, 218
  mixed, 25
Poisson model, 23, 119, 120
  latent class, 28
  mixed, 28, 39
Poisson process, 14, 20, 30, 33, 39, 44, 51, 56, 58, 68, 73, 83, 91, 95, 97, 117, 119, 120, 129, 134, 142, 169, 185, 220
  mixed, 23, 29, 30, 32, 39, 44, 91, 97, 169
  non-homogeneous, 16, 23, 29, 30, 35, 48–51, 92–95, 97, 110, 117, 123, 128, 136, 179, 186, 187, 215–217, 220
Prentice, R.L., 1, 2, 4, 19, 72, 75, 90, 99, 101, 152, 157, 212, 214
Proportional mean model, *see* Recurrent event process
Proportional rate model, *see* Recurrent event process

Rai, S.N., 89, 90, 221
Rate function, *see* Recurrent event process
Recurrent event data, 2, 3, 12, 19, 20, 75, 90, 91, 104, 107, 110, 111, 124, 142–144, 152, 163, 181, 187, 190, 199, 200, 214, 221, 222
  analysis of, 14–18
  mammary tumor data, 4
Recurrent event process, 19–21, 23, 24, 39, 44, 45, 48, 62, 71, 72, 77, 78, 81, 86, 87, 89, 91, 97, 103, 109, 117, 119, 121–123, 128, 129, 135, 136, 142, 144, 151, 153, 155, 156, 160, 161, 169–171, 176, 178, 185, 187, 189, 190, 205, 212, 213, 215, 217, 220, 222
  additive mean model, 144
  conditional mean model, 178, 187
  gap time, 221
  marginal mean model, 161
  mean function, 12, 16, 17, 19–21, 39, 43, 47, 48, 51, 58, 63–65, 68, 69, 71–74, 76–78, 80, 83, 84, 86, 87, 89, 91, 92, 95, 97, 98, 109, 119, 123, 130, 133, 137, 144, 151, 155–157, 159–162, 165, 168, 171, 185, 200, 213, 220
    conditional, 178, 185
    marginal, 171, 185
  proportional mean model, 13, 24, 91, 92, 108, 109, 117–119, 122, 123, 144, 155, 161, 163, 197, 200, 204, 215, 221
  proportional rate model, 13, 35, 104, 106, 110, 119, 130, 136, 145, 178, 179, 211
  rate function, 12, 17, 21, 29–32, 34, 35, 41, 43, 44, 48, 62, 65, 68, 69, 71, 91, 155, 217, 221
    conditional, 185
    marginal, 185
  semiparametric transformation model, 92, 109–116, 118, 122, 136–139, 153, 161, 178, 204
Reliability study, 1, 5, 53
Residual process, 115, 132, 139, 152, 173
Robertson, T., 53, 94
Robins, P.K., 211
Robison, L., 199
Robust estimation, 129–136, 142
Rosen algorithm, 96
Rosen, O., 212, 217
Rosenberg, P.S., 69
Roy, J., 153
Rubin, D.B., 222
Ryan, L.M., 205

Schaubel, D.E., 163, 221
Scheike, T.H., 221
Schoenfeld, D., 152
Schumaker, L., 95
Schwartz, G., 191
Semiparametric transformation model, *see* Recurrent event process
Sensitivity analysis, 129
Severini, T.A., 44
Singer, B., 190
Smoothing estimation, 44, 64–65, 119
  B-spline, 69, 95, 96, 119, 211, 217

Index

M-spline, 69
penalized spline, 119
scatterplot smoothing, 69
Song, X., 153, 221
Spilerman, S., 190
Spline function, *see* Smoothing estimation
Staniswalls, J.G., 44, 119, 221
Sun, J., 2, 5, 6, 8, 19, 32, 52, 53, 69, 72, 73, 84, 85, 88–90, 100–102, 115, 119, 128, 137, 152, 153, 221
Sun, L., 153, 221
Sun, Y., 119, 221
Susko, E., 217

Tan, X., 217
Terminal event, *see* Follow-up process
Thall, P.F., 6, 19, 30, 32, 33, 51, 57, 63, 69, 75, 89
Three-state model, *see* Illness-death model
Tibshirani, R.J., 69, 191
Time-to-event data, *see* Failure time data
Titman, A.C., 211
Tong, X., 153, 197
Trivedi, P.K., 23, 27, 44
Tsiatis, A.A., 153, 187, 214
Tsokos, C.P., 65
Tu, X.M., 153
Tuma, N.B., 211
Tumorigenicity experiment, 1, 2, 32, 205

Vermunt, J.K., 1, 27, 119

Wand, M.P., 16, 62, 65
Wang, C.Y., 221
Wang, M.C., 1, 2, 124, 143, 187, 221
Wang, P., 212
Wasserman, S., 190

Wedel, M., 28
Wei, L.J., 8, 19, 74, 100–102, 119, 170, 202
Wellner, J.A., 8, 48, 50, 51, 53, 56, 69, 95, 119
White, H., 26, 40, 219
Wichern, D.W., 189
Wilcoxon-like rank test, 75
Wong, W.H., 44
Wu, H., 221
Wulfsohn, M.S., 214

Yamaguchi, K., 1
Yan, J., 221
Ye, Y., 143, 187
Yi, G.Y., 214
Ying, Z., 153, 212, 214, 221

Zeger, S.L., 40
Zeng, D., 143
Zhan, M., 19, 34, 36, 38, 40, 42, 43, 119, 221
Zhang, C., 192
Zhang, H,, 198
Zhang, H., 173, 174, 186, 193, 194, 197
Zhang, Y., 8, 48, 50, 51, 53, 56, 69, 80, 88, 89, 94–96
Zhang, Z., 114
Zhao, H., 147, 149, 153, 157, 158, 160, 186, 187
Zhao, Q., 221
Zhao, X., 2, 76, 78–80, 84, 85, 88, 89, 131, 132, 143, 153, 221
Zhou, H., 212, 214
Zhou, X., 221
Zhu, L., 153, 190, 199, 202
Zou, H., 191

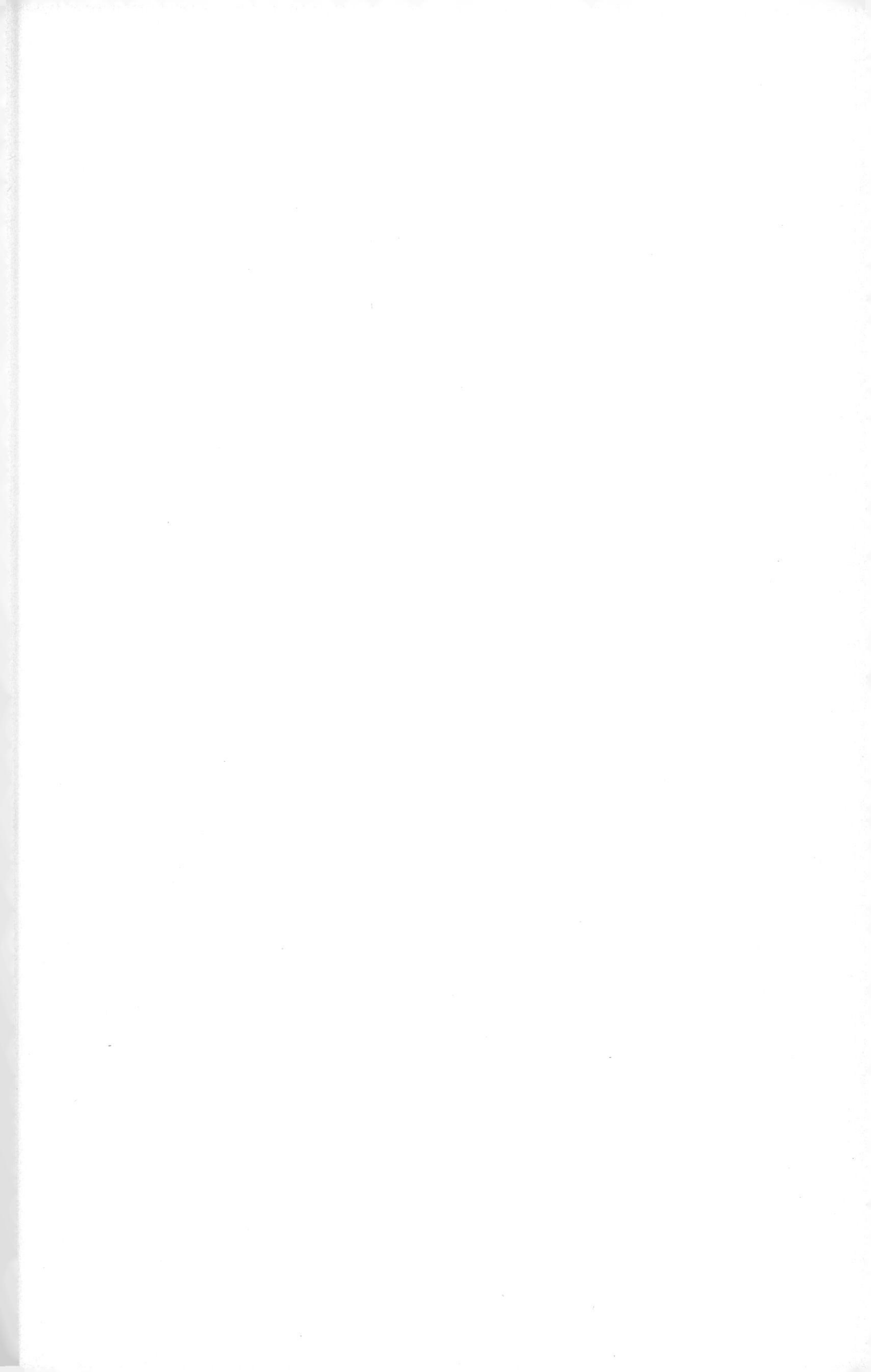

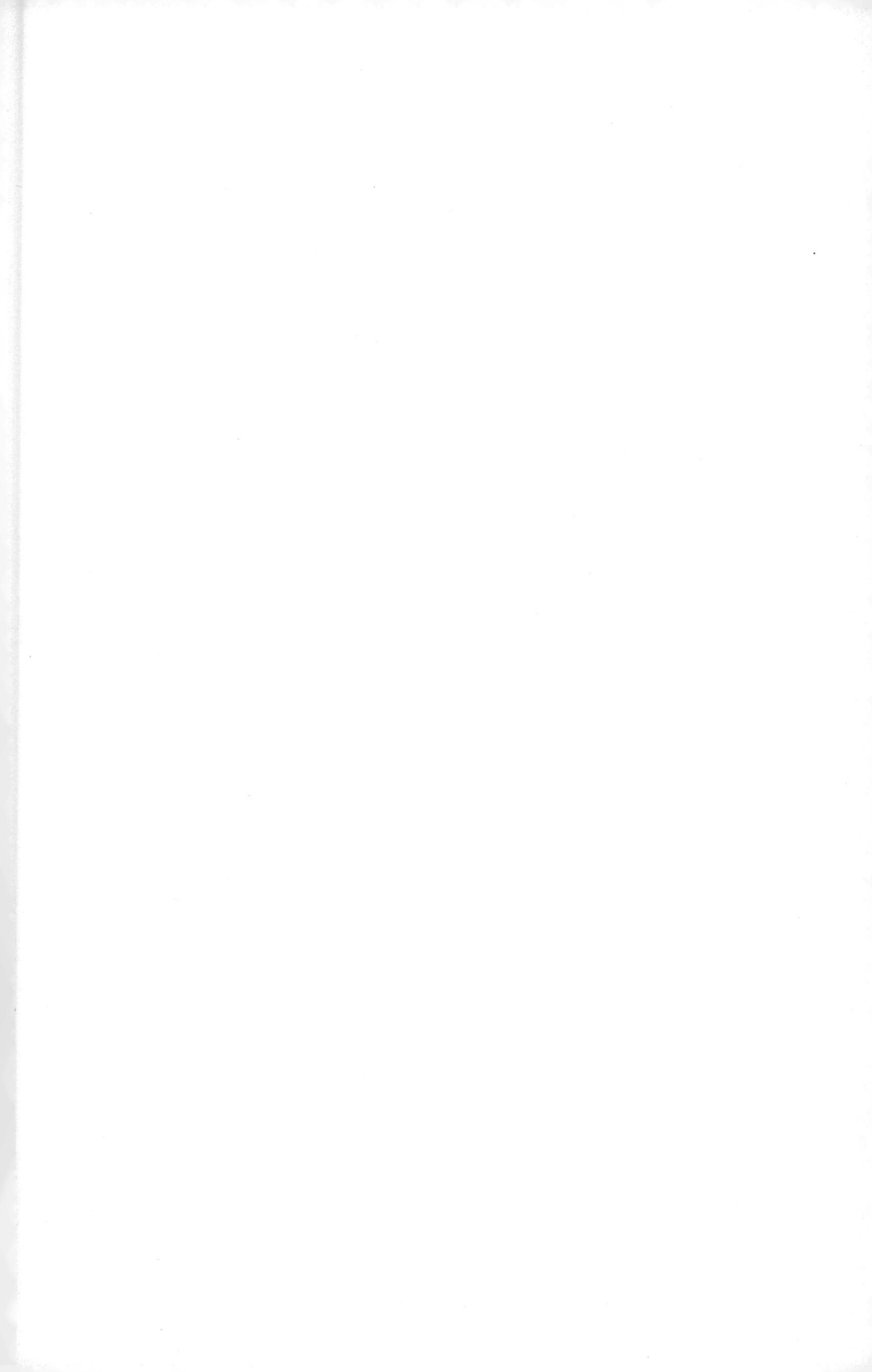

Printed by Printforce, the Netherlands